Award-winning writer, t___ of numerous bestsellers, Lesli___ the press as 'the guru of health and fitness a___ most original voice in health'. A shining example of energy and commitment, she is highly respected for her thorough reporting. Leslie was born in California, and is the daughter of jazz musician Stan Kenton. After leaving Stanford University she journeyed to Europe in her early twenties, settling first in Paris then in Britain where she has since remained. She has raised four children on her own by working as a television broadcaster, novelist, writer and teacher on health and for fourteen years she was editor at *Harpers & Queen*.

Leslie's writing on mainstream health is internationally known and has appeared in *Vogue*, the *Sunday Times*, *Cosmopolitan* and the *Daily Mail*. She is the author of many other health books including: *The New Raw Energy* and *Raw Energy Recipes* – co-authored with her daughter Susannah – *The New Ultrahealth*, *The New Joy of Beauty*, *The New Ageless Ageing*, *Cellulite Revolution*, *10 Day Clean-Up Plan*, *Endless Energy*, *Nature's Child*, *Lean Revolution* and the *10 Day De-Stress Plan*. She turned to fiction with *Ludwig* – her first novel. Former consultant to a medical corporation in the USA and to the Open University's Centre of Continuing Education, Leslie's writing has won several awards including the PPA 'Technical Writer of the Year'. Her work was honoured by her being asked to deliver the McCarrison Lecture at the Royal Society of Medicine. In recent years she has become increasingly concerned not only with the process of enhancing individual health but also with re-establishing bonds with the earth as a part of helping to heal the planet.

PASSAGE TO POWER

Natural Menopause Revolution

Leslie Kenton

Vermilion
LONDON

For the hundreds of thousands of women who courageously seek ways and means of living their full potential for health, creativity and freedom, each in her own way. This book is dedicated to you.

14

Text copyright © Leslie Kenton 1996

The right of Leslie Kenton to be identified as the author of this book has been asserted by her in accordance with the Copyright, Designs and Patents Act, 1988

First published in the United Kingdom in 1995 by Ebury Press
First paperback edition published in the United Kingdom in 1996 by Vermilion

This paperback edition published in the United Kingdom in 1998 by Vermilion
an imprint of Ebury Press
Random House,
20 Vauxhall Bridge Road,
London SW1V 2SA

www.eburypublishing.co.uk

Addresses for companies within
he Random House Group Limited can be found at:
www.randomhouse.co.uk/offices.htm

The Random House Group Limited Reg. No. 954009

A CIP catalogue record for this book
is available from the British Library

ISBN 9780091815943

The Random House Group Limited supports The Forest Stewardship Council (FSC®), the leading international forest certification organisation. Our books carrying the FSC label are printed on FSC® certified paper. FSC is the only forest certification scheme endorsed by the leading environmental organisations, including Greenpeace. Our paper procurement policy can be found at www.randomhouse.co.uk/environment

Printed and bound in Great Britain by Clays Ltd, St Ives PLC

Acknowledgements

There are so very many people who have either helped me learn what I needed to know in order to write this book or painstakingly read the manuscript and given me their comments and suggestions that it would be impossible to list them all. There are a few, however, who must be thanked by name: Dr John Lee, Dr Robert Jacobs, the late Dr Dagmar Leichti von Brasch, Dr Michael Harner, Dr Barry Durrant-Peatfield, Doctor Shamim Daya, Dr John Howard, Dr Ellen Grant, Dr Peter Mansfield, Dr Gordon Latto, Willa Shaffer, Celia Wright, Sandra Ingerman, Sandra Coney, Barbara Sommers and Rhodri Thomas. I am also enormously grateful to my assistant Yvette Brown – The Fox – for her tenacity in seeing me through the task of researching and writing and to Sarah Wallace who has with such care and skill edited the book.

Leslie Kenton
Pembrokeshire 1995

Contents

The Science of Myth

Rites and Rituals

Author's Note

The content of this book is intended for informational purposes only. I am only a reporter. None of the suggestions or information is meant in any way to be prescriptive. Any attempt to treat a medical condition should always come under the direction of a competent physician – preferably one knowledgeable about nutrition and natural methods of healing. Neither the publishers nor the author can accept responsibility for injuries or illness arising out of a failure by a reader to take medical advice.

I want to make it clear that I have no commercial interest in any product, treatment or organization mentioned in this book. However, I have long sought to learn more about whatever can help us to live at a high level of energy, intelligence and creativity, for it is my belief that the more each one of us is able to re-establish harmony within ourselves and with our environment, the better equipped we shall be to wrestle with the challenges now facing our planet.

THE MYTHS OF SCIENCE

Chapter One
Bloodless Revolution

Power, energy and freedom. These are meant to be the rewards of menopause. This is a book about how as women we can bring them into being. It is *not* about how to cope with the 'horrors of the change'. *Passage to Power* explores the transformation in a woman's life that takes place between the ages of 35 and 60 as a journey towards individual freedom. Along the way the book takes a cold, hard look at HRT, exposes the common misconception that menopause is an 'oestrogen deficiency disease', and scrutinizes the rampant misinformation surrounding the use of prescription hormones – sadly even among many otherwise competent doctors who use them too often because they simply don't know what else to do. It also gathers together diverse information about simple yet effective actions an informed woman can take to improve her physical health and appearance as well as to maximize her energy and to enhance the quality of her life, whatever her age. And it probes the spiritual nature of the menopause passage which must be experienced through myth and ritual, archetypes and dreams.

For ten years people have been saying to me 'write a book on menopause'. I have always refused. 'I can't until I've experienced it,' I used to say. When, finally, menopause arrived I was unprepared for it. Despite my knowledge about health I did not know what to expect. Neither had I any idea of the freedom that is available to us on the other side of the menopause passage. The freedom of which I speak is not the 'freedom' that advertisers would have us believe comes with owning a pair of Levi 501's or popping in a tampon so that we can swim during a period. It is a freedom of body and soul which enables each woman to experience unfettered her full potential for aliveness. Only by doing this can we call forth our greatest gifts both for our own personal fulfilment and to share with our culture and the planet.

Freedom to Be

Despite demands for equal rights at work and our desire to take control of our lives, such freedom too often still eludes us. On a physical level, the proliferation of poisonous chemicals in our environment and the widespread use of chemically grown convenience foods depleted of essential minerals and trace elements have dangerously eroded our freedom to be healthy; so much so that we now experience a Pandora's box of ailments – from infertility and PMS to cancers of the womb and breasts – with a frequency and intensity unprecedented in history.

Meanwhile, driven by a desire to exploit the largest commercial market in the world, drug manufacturers spend a fortune each year in an attempt to convince governments, doctors and the public that using their products is the only choice available to women for contraception and to treat the problems which arise as menopause approaches. Faced with the prospect of a menopause portrayed increasingly as dangerous to body and psyche – an event which, it is intimated, can turn an attractive woman into an old hag – women can become frightened into complying, sometimes to their long-term detriment. Rather like the temple guardians (statues of threatening animals placed at the door of sacred buildings to dissuade the faint-hearted from entering), our fears of menopause need to be seen for the paper dragons they are. Only then will we be able to pass through the doorway which menopause opens to us and return with the boons of meaning, purpose and freedom that have been hidden for too long.

On a psychospiritual level, too, we are still seeking to define ourselves as women – not as beings *equal* or *superior* to men or as *counterparts* to men – but rather as creatures in our own right, capable of making autonomous decisions and of tapping our resources for creativity and joy. The knowledge and power which enables a woman to play an active role in supporting her own hormonal changes can restore a woman's faith in the miraculous ability of her body to rebalance and heal itself. Menopause can reconnect a woman to her core values, helping her rediscover her connections with the earth. A woman who *knows* such connectedness seldom needs to rely on high-tech medical intervention or prescription. Such are the goals of natural menopause.

To experience menopause as a passage to power a woman needs two kinds of knowledge. First she needs scientific information to help discern fact from fiction as well as self-help techniques and natural products to support the transformation taking place in her body and her life. Secondly, she needs knowledge of the soul – access to myths, symbols and rituals which help her reconnect with the deepest levels of intuition and instinct. As I began to explore the rich interactions between mind and body via hormones, I realized that the two are inextricably woven together.

The Myths of Science

In our society the basic approach to health has tended to separate body, mind and spirit, and opt for symptomatic treatment of ailments with little concern for the underlying effects on the person being treated. As a result we now live in a world where it is easy for a woman's biochemistry to become distorted by declining physical activity, the proliferation of highly processed convenience foods, and the rise of a whole new – as yet largely unrecognized – phenomenon known as *oestrogen dominance*. Now, instead of the oestrogens playing their essential roles within the rich symphony of steroid hormones in a woman's body, they have begun to overshadow the other players, some would say creating biochemical dissonance and undermining our mental and physical health.

Oestrogen dominance has developed for many reasons, including the widespread use of oestrogen-based oral contraceptives and the exponential spread of chemicals in our environment which are *oestrogen mimics*. Their presence in such force undermines the natural oestrogen/progesterone balance and synergy in a woman's body – sometimes with devastating consequences. Every woman needs to be aware of the potential dangers of the 'sea of oestrogens' in which we now live. She also needs to know what steps she can take both personally and politically to help counter it. Sadly, most still remain largely ignorant of its existence. As a result we continue to place responsibility for our lives in the hands of others – doctors, drug companies, government agencies – who we are told will fix things for us. Too often, instead of making use of these agencies to serve our needs, we allow them to become our masters. It is a tendency which needs to be overcome.

This has already started to happen. There is mounting dissatisfaction among women who continue to be told that drug-based HRT is the only answer to mid-life depression, hot flushes, loss of sexual appetite and early ageing, probably because such advice goes strangely against our deepest intuition. For many who have followed it, the use of hormonal drugs has ultimately created more problems that it has solved.

There is also a growing sense among women that osteoporosis – female plague of the late twentieth century – *is* stoppable and that we as women need only to understand what is causing this galloping consumption of our bones and take effective action to stop it. How we do this is another question this book addresses.

At the same time more and more women in mid-life instinctively feel it should not be necessary to fill their bodies with drugs to keep them from falling apart nor should they have to plaster their faces with pricey cosmetics to keep their skin from looking like an alligator's rear end. Although scientific information and simple do-it-yourself techniques for natural menopause are readily available, seldom are they drawn together for easy access and use. Neither are they promoted simply because most are not commercial – there is little money to be made from them.

Among so many women there exists a deep dissatisfaction with the negative image of the postmenopausal woman and the loss of respect for the female that western society promulgates. Finally, there is a mounting insistence by women worldwide that we will not only find a way to dream our dreams but, as our childbearing years come to an end, turn our dreams into reality.

The Science of Myth

The loss of respect for the female in our world is paralleled in a lack of respect for the earth. We keep looking for solutions to the ecological crisis on the planet, in the same way that we keep reading books about redefining what it means to be female, yet neither brings us much closer to being able to regenerate the earth or ourselves. Perhaps we have been looking in the wrong place. Perhaps we need for a time to abandon the language of science and turn to myth. Mythological symbols and rituals are readily available on which women can draw. They explore the nature of what it is to be female and the meaning implicit in our life changes, yet we have mostly forgotten them. Symbols and myth no longer play an important part in the linear, left-brain education we receive. Together, as women, we now need to move beyond science and explore the archetypal processes involved in the transformations that take place as we move out of our childbearing years and towards the years of the crone.

Crone is a much maligned word. It tends to be used to describe the postmenopausal woman only in her negative aspect – the crone as hag, an ugly old woman. When we fall prey to the false notion that hormone drugs hold all the answers to a menopausal woman's worries, then the medical-industrial complex continues to feed our fear of the crone as a negative archetype and blinds us to her wisdom and her beauty. An important part of every woman's menopausal journey is meeting the crone face to face in *all* her mythological aspects – from dark witch to gloriously ripe wise woman. When you befriend the crone she shares her power with you. She can help a woman to forge a new, more authentic life for herself as well as create rich new bonds with other women and with the planet. For crone is a word which carries great beauty and power hidden within its original meaning which can help a woman connect with her own infinite female wisdom. The crone can help us dream our dreams afresh. Embracing her wholeheartedly gives each of us access to new energies and healing abilities which not only benefit ourselves but can also help us to guide others.

Call to Revolution

In recent years we have witnessed a revolution in pregnancy and natural childbirth. Where once women were dazzled by high-tech medical intervention at birth, and all too willingly surrendered their bodies to epidurals, episiotomies and foetal monitoring equipment, in the last 20 years this has changed. We have witnessed a demand for natural childbirth, breast-feeding and good mother–child bonding. And there has developed a growing willingness by hospitals and government agencies to provide the environment for them. It is women themselves, led by a handful of visionary doctors and thinkers, such as Frédéric Leboyer, Michel Odent and Pierre Vellay, who have helped to make the world aware of the importance of natural childbirth and who have encouraged us to insist upon it for the physical and spiritual welfare of ourselves and our children.

Now we are poised at the brink of a new revolution. This time it is a revolution in women's natural health care which focuses on the years just before, during and after menopause. This gentle yet persistent uprising takes its impetus from two sources: first, from an urgent demand among women for profound change; and second, from a group of pioneers who present us with the means for bringing it about. A growing number of scientists and doctors now seriously challenge the wisdom of established medical practice – the doling out of potent drug-based hormones from puberty onwards and the widespread propaganda which accompanies it. Such practices, they insist, are seriously undermining the long-term health and fertility of women as well as poisoning the environment. These scientists and experts are not trying to damn HRT but rather to put it in perspective. They insist that, while it may be useful for short periods in the small number of women who actually *need* extra oestrogen, the use of drug-based hormones for most women is costly in financial and physical terms. At grass-roots level more and more women's voices rise up against the use of oestrogens and progestogen drugs in the 'treatment' of menopause because they have been shown to carry side-effects.

The reason for protest is simple. It is *our* bodies which have to bear the consequences. We sense that whatever menopause may be it most certainly is not a disease in need of urgent treatment. The guidance we need as women to accomplish our ends both spiritually and physically is already available so long as we are willing to look for it and so long as we adamantly refuse to buy into the fear-mongering world that would make of every menopausal woman a 'patient' for the rest of her life. While researching this book I became aware that the whole idea of menopause as a disease to be treated has largely been concocted by multinational pharmaceutical companies in need of a new market for their drugs. Such books as Sandra Coney's *The Menopause Industry* should be read by any woman wanting to understand the ins and outs of the medical-industrial complex and how it functions. Once you have the facts, the question becomes what then *is* menopause all about? How do we – each one of us – make our own passage to power? These are some of the issues that this book attempts to address.

Male and Female – Dry and Moist

The male-orientated western world in which we live is linear and hierarchical. The world of the female is cyclical. The female is moist, the male is dry. The female, like the ancient goddess in whose image she is made, is infinitely generous. Her generosity takes many forms. When Christianity came to Ireland the Irish hung on to their goddess, carving her into the walls of their churches. Sometimes she is depicted sitting on a pig, sometimes she has a huge vagina which she holds open with her hands. In the eighteenth and nineteenth centuries most of these figures were removed. For what most terrifies the male is the absolute licentiousness of female generosity. It is a power which is completely free, which cannot be bought or sold, manipulated or exploited and which is continually fuelled by the seasons, nature, by our friendship with each other and our bonds to the earth. No wonder our materialistic world has devised ingenious ways of trying to contain women's wildness. Control a woman's hormones and you may for a time be able to contain her wildness. Yet locked within the wildness of woman is her only true experience of freedom and meaning as well as her sense of connection to the planet. No woman can live without these things for long. It is my belief that the time has come for the wild female energies to be set free.

The pioneers behind the bloodless revolution have already done much of the groundwork that can help us do this. These men and women come from many disciplines. They are scientists and thinkers, psychologists, doctors, herbalists, healers and shamans. In the next decade a few are likely to be household names but the chances are you will not have heard of most of them. For the pioneers of the bloodless revolution belong to no great corporation. Their work, much of which you will find described in the pages that follow (together with references at the back of the book so it can be examined further), helps point the way to orchestrating positive changes in our lives. The responsibility for making practical use of what they have to offer is our own.

Pioneers for Change

Mythologists Demetra George and Joseph Campbell and storyteller Clarissa Pinkola Estés have uncovered many of the myths and archetypes we can draw on to help us come fully into our spiritual power. New Zealand health educator Sandra Coney, biologist Renata Klein, and her medical scientist colleague Lynette Dumble in Australia, have all painstakingly amassed information about menopause, the menopausal woman and the undermining effect which the medical-industrial complex and its insistence on the widespread use of HRT is having on women. Then there are the *wise women* – such as author Susun Weed and midwife Willa Shaffer – who have spent decades resurrecting long-forgotten female secrets about how to use readily available plants for fertility and the treatment of women troubles – even for natural birth control. Another pioneer in the bloodless revolution is Sandra Ingerman. A practising shaman, Ingerman has devoted her life to teaching a simple technique that can help people retrieve aspects of their own soul from which they have become separated. Soul retrieval, however it comes, is at the crux of a woman's passage to power.

On the science side, biochemist Dr Ray Peat has shared with all willing to listen his research into steroid hormones. It has led to a profound understanding of the mechanisms by which many of women's illnesses – both mental and physical – develop and may be healed *naturally*. In Canada, endocrinologist Dr Jerilynn Prior at the University of British Columbia claims to have uncovered the real reasons behind the plague of osteoporosis and infertility which we in the industrial world are now experiencing. At the University of Cambridge, Professor of Clinical Gerontology Kay-Tee Khaw investigates how lifestyle and diet can influence a woman's experience of menopause, drawing upon new knowledge in biochemistry and nutrition. A handful of courageous British physicians such as Dr Shirley Bond, Dr Shamim Daya, Dr Patrick Kingsley, Dr Barry Durrant-Peatfield and Dr Yehudi Gordon are already helping individual women find their way. Meanwhile, expert in natural hormones and brain chemistry, researcher in twenty-first-century energy medicine, Dr Robert Jacobs heads charitable trusts in Britain and the United States where the lives of seriously ill people are transformed from sickness into health. The charities also focus on helping people who are well to maximize their energies to become super-healthy. Jacobs and his wife, body therapist Beth Jacobs, use leading-edge techniques to regenerate and rejuvenate women, enabling them to experience better health, greater clarity and more control over their destiny. Finally – and in many ways the most important pioneer of all in the bloodless revolution – there is American physician Dr John Lee.

Let There Be Light

Lee is a family doctor who has spent the last fifteen years exploring the actions of a *natural* plant-derived form of progesterone available to women in most countries without prescription. Together with a good diet and lifestyle changes he has found that this natural hormone is capable of eliminating much of the suffering associated with both PMS and menopause. Thousands of women in the western world now use natural progesterone – generally in the form of a non-prescription cream which you rub on the body – and claim they have not only had relief from female symptoms but experience increased vitality, better skin and renewed emotional balance. Many who have been through the transformations which natural progesterone can bring consider them little short of miraculous. Contrary to traditional medical thinking, Dr Lee believes that the use of natural progesterone together with dietary and lifestyle change can not only stop osteoporosis but actually *reverse* it – even in women aged 70 or more. Lee, who discovered this, now spends his life researching, lecturing and giving help to doctors, scientists and women who want to find their way out of the labyrinth of suffering. Yet he adamantly refuses to accept any money for any of what he does. He is determined to maintain his own autonomy and to return the power for wellbeing where he believes it belongs – firmly in the hands of the individual woman.

Without the painstaking devotion of these pioneers for change there would be no bloodless revolution. However, just as so-called common people have created the basis for every popular movement for change in the past, it is only we women that can bring the revolution that has now been seeded into full flower. This is how change has always happened throughout history, whether the revolutionaries have been seeking democratic representation or the end of slavery. Sometimes history books give the impression that successful movements come about solely because of their leaders – that it was Nelson Mandela and Martin Luther King who brought about the civil rights movement. But these men were not the civil rights movement. Their names appear in history books because lots of people whose names you never know or whose names are long forgotten were working for change. So it is with the bloodless revolution. When you have enough women devoting themselves to change then pathfinders like Jerilynn Prior, John Lee, Sandra Coney and Demetra George become well known. But that is only because at grassroots level somebody – in this case we women ourselves – is doing the work.

This process has already begun. Groups of women in Canada, the United States, Britain, Australia, South Africa and New Zealand are already demanding *another way*. They want to know about herbs and homeopathic remedies. They are rediscovering alternatives based on long traditions of use in natural medicine, hard-core scientific findings and current clinical use. They are also exploring how natural hormones like progesterone and leading-edge substances such as melatonin, DMAE and L-pyroglutamic acid can be used to balance brain and mood, to heighten immunity and to slow down ageing. Such women want to *experience* how various natural substances act upon their bodies. They are demanding methods of self-care that take into account how spirit and body interact and support each other, and they are not content with palliative symptomatic treatments which carry the threat of dangerous side-effects. The time has come, they insist, for us to stop thinking of ourselves as victims – victims of cancer, of PMS, menopausal trauma or anything else. When you see yourself in the role of a victim nothing can help you. Only when we let go of the victim role can we begin to take an active part in our own transformation.

Call to Adventure

The radical and fundamental changes which take place in a woman's life around the time of menopause are not signs of decay or pathology but rather a *call to adventure* signalling the beginning of each woman's archetypal *hero's journey* to her core. When a woman makes such a journey she discovers that menopause is not only a time for grieving over past mistakes and irredeemable losses, it is also a time of rejoicing. It is a time to regenerate and rejuvenate our bodies using a combination of ancient principles and leading-edge science. Most of all, menopause is a time of celebration, that our creativity is no longer bound to our obligations as a member of the human race to propagate the species. Often for the first time in a woman's life, her creativity can be set free for use in whatever way the whispers of her soul dictate.

To me there is little more exciting than being present at

the beginning of the bloodless revolution – a quiet moment which promises to bring better health and greater autonomy in its wake. This is where we now stand. This book is designed to serve as a traveller's companion – a guide to both the scientific and the mythological aspects of the menopausal journey. In many ways it is rather like a collection of rudimentary maps to which a woman can turn in the course of planning and carrying out her own hero's journey. The book is divided into three parts: the Myths of Science, the Science of Myth, and a practical section called Rites and Rituals. As a whole the book explores the experience of menopause from its spiritual and psychological roots to its hormonal interactions. It draws together the work of trailblazers from a great variety of fields and presents it in a way that hopefully can help a woman wanting to take control of her own life to do so with relative ease. It addresses the knowledge which the pioneers have unearthed and some of the visions held for women, not only around the time of menopause itself but during the eight to ten years that precede it as well as the many years afterwards. PMS and osteoporosis, like all the other manifestations of hormonal imbalances, are easiest to prevent by taking action long before menopause arrives. However, no matter what your age or condition it is never too late to benefit from the new knowledge.

Each woman is biochemically and spiritually unique. So is the hero's journey which she must undertake if she is to succeed in her quest for wholeness. Although there are useful allies to be found at every step of the way, like birth and death, a woman's menopause passage is one which, by its very nature, she must make alone. After all, when Arthur's knights set out on their search for the Grail each entered the woods alone at the place where it was darkest, never dreaming to walk a path which another had walked before him. To do so would have dishonoured the quest. Such journeys cannot be codified. They are not package holidays where you pay your money and know exactly what to expect. These are journeys of the soul.

Chapter Two
Cry Freedom

Nobody ever prepares you for menopause. Nobody tells you that if you are going to have hot flushes or emotional instability they are likely to be far worse *before* you stop menstruating than afterwards. Nor does anybody explain that waking regularly at two or three in the morning and lying in bed filled with sadness or fear or anger is likely to be not some aberration of nature but a messenger announcing that menopause is near. Because we are told so little, few women in our culture are prepared for the third movement of the hormonal symphony – menopause – nor for the next phase of their life. They seldom expect the intensity of emotion, both pain and pleasure, that can accompany the end of the child-bearing years.

Perils of Pathology

Too many women in the western world first come upon menopause as a result of some pathological event for which they feel forced to seek medical advice: endometriosis, fibroid tumours, depression, loss of libido, vaginal discomfort during intercourse, or the kind of persistent excessive bleeding that can make a woman weak with anaemia and weary of the struggle. Such symptoms sometimes result in the loss of a womb. It can be easier for doctors to take out something they are not sure how to handle than to struggle with their own frustration and sense of inadequacy while in search of another way. If surgery is not seen to be the answer then often a woman is led to believe that Hormone Replacement Therapy (HRT) is. After all, taking oestrogen is supposed to halt osteoporosis. 'Quite frankly, my dear, I think it would be *dangerous* to try to live without it,' one leading gynaecologist intimated to me recently. 'Be sure to take plenty of calcium pills and drink lots of milk.' The so-called experts often add that HRT is important in preventing early ageing. 'You don't want your skin to go all wrinkled and saggy do you? You don't want your vagina to dry up? And you *do* want to remain *feminine* and *desirable*, don't you? Well don't you?'

Just about everybody who is anybody these days will tell you that menopause is an oestrogen deficiency disease and that you need to take more oestrogen as you approach mid-life. What may surprise you is this: not only is most of such commonly given advice on menopause wrong, a great deal of it can be positively dangerous. Nevertheless, such is the introduction to menopause for almost half of the women in the industrialized world today. It ignores the freedom waiting to be claimed now that the childbearing years have ended – freedom to surrender to passionate love-making without fear of pregnancy, or to refuse sex altogether if we choose and to channel our libido in other directions. Menopause also brings freedom from the emotional ups and downs that commonly accompany the moon cycles of menstruating women as well as the freedom to feel radiantly well. For now you no longer need to be bound into whatever your role has been. Anthropologist Margaret Mead always insisted that passing through menopause brought a woman the gift of 'post-menopausal zest'.

Sadly, the menopausal horror stories we hear today have become so far removed from the positive experience reported by women in the past, and still reported by women in other parts of the world, that it is easy to wonder who is lying. Women have begun to ask themselves just what is going on. Is menopause a cosmic joke – an aberration of evolution? Did nature foul up when she made us this way? Are we *meant* to be over the hill at the age of fifty? Is the doctor right? If we don't take HRT are we going to end up as crumpled old bags in ten years? (Or, even worse, dead after having broken both hips falling down the stairs?) If any of this sounds exaggerated then you have not spent as much time as I have talking with menopausal women in Britain, North America, Australia, New Zealand and South Africa. For these are very much the fears and exhortations to which women are now subjected. It is not easy for a woman to know what to make of it all until she has a good understanding of what takes place when menopause –

the second big initiation – arrives and the third stage of her life begins. Each woman needs to become familiar with what lies behind the various pathologies (illnesses and abnormalities) commonly associated with menopause in the western world as well as how relatively easy it can be to counter them if she chooses, often without having to resort to serious medical intervention of any kind.

What is Menopause?

The first challenge menopause presents a woman is the task of identifying exactly what it is. Apart from those cheerful little booklets on the subject from doctors' surgeries which are thinly disguised vehicles for the sale of Hormone Replacement Therapy (HRT), information is often not readily available. Even most well-written articles in women's magazines and in newspapers closely follow the 'catechism'. In recent decades, backed by major pharmaceutical money, an obsession with HRT has developed. As a result, in the past 30 years, very little objective research into other aspects of menopause and the hormonal changes associated with it has even been carried out. Few doctors are as yet aware of what does exist.

When you examine the studies that have been done into menopause you realize that many of the so-called symptoms of menopause have nothing particularly to do with it. They are instead symptoms of ageing or of physiological imbalances that have developed out of lifestyles that do not give real support to the proper functioning of mind and body, or symptoms of frustration at the very deepest levels of the soul when a woman is trying to live everybody else's life rather than her own. Such *false* menopausal symptoms can include aches and pains, fatigue, digestive disturbances and anxiety – all of which develop when a woman's metabolic processes are no longer functioning as they should be. They may be the result of years of eating convenience foods depleted of essential minerals and trace elements yet replete with trans-fatty acids or junk fats (see Order Out of Chaos, p. 161). They can also develop out of having wrestled with the long-term stress of a marriage that isn't working or a career that demands everything of you yet brings you little satisfaction in return. Around the time of mid-life all of these things get thrown together and wrongly labelled 'the symptoms of menopause'. To treat them as such by papering over the cracks with tranquillizers or hormone drugs (other than temporarily if absolutely necessary) can mean interfering with the power that comes with the menopause journey. It is a journey which, when taken with your eyes open, promises to take you to the very source of your strength and creativity and helps you to make positive changes in your life which can bring about not just palliative and temporary relief from symptoms but long-term improved health and the discovery of new spiritual freedom and power.

Will Menopause Please Stand Up

Back in 1973 two epidemiologists at Oxford, John and Sonja McKinlay, set out to survey the research that had been carried out on menopause. They discovered that there had been very little, and that most of what had been done suffered from serious holes in its methodology. Many studies done did not discriminate between women who had undergone a *surgical menopause* resulting from the removal of their womb or ovaries, and women who had experienced a natural menopause. Even much of the research into HRT which examines the use of oestrogen in relation to osteoporosis is seriously flawed. Certain that oestrogen was the prime factor in preventing osteoporosis, for years researchers paid little attention to whether or not women taking part in various studies had been given anything else as well. Yet when you go back and examine many of the studies frequently cited as 'proof' that oestrogen counters osteoporosis, you find that the women studied had also been given a progestogen or progesterone. Still too few stop to ask the question: 'Is it really oestrogen which is the prime factor in preventing osteoporosis, or might it be something else?' Since the McKinlay research, by far the most revealing investigations into the nature of menopause have been carried out not by medical researchers but by anthropologists, psychologists, sociologists and epidemiologists. As a result, despite all the books and articles on the subject and all the leaflets handed out, surprisingly little objective medical information is available about the menopausal woman. The people who know most about natural menopause are the women themselves who have passed through it.

To some women even a hint that menopause may be on its way seems confirmation that they are 'past it', or 'it's all downhill from here'. At some point in mid-life every woman in our society comes to feel the sadness and frustration which arises because our society links physical ageing to a loss of sexual attractiveness and self-esteem. So when menopause arrives it can seem an unwelcome visitor. Women who have long been at home may find that home and family no longer hold the fascination that they once did, nor do they any longer seem good sources from which to draw a sense of personal identity. Women who have long worked in the world, on the other hand, can come to feel that although they may have achieved the success they once longed for, something fundamental is missing. They ask themselves if life is not passing them by.

As marketing folk worth their salt know full well, the easiest way to sell anything to a woman is to convince her that she is inadequate and in desperate need of whatever is on offer. This is exactly what has happened with HRT. A woman nearing the passage of menopause is particularly vulnerable to such suggestions. If she is told that menopause is a deficiency disease or an inevitable source of struggle, pain and grief, undermining her sexual attractiveness and pushing her over the hill, she is likely to face her future burdened with these notions. Once a woman, even unconsciously, swallows the negative stereotypes that our culture has created about the older woman she opens herself up to the idea that she needs 'treatment'. But take heart. There *is* another way.

Early Start

Strictly speaking, just as the word *menarche* means a woman's first menstrual period, menopause means the last period she will ever have. *Meno* comes from the Greek meaning month and *pause* from *pausis* meaning halt. In common usage, however, when most people speak of menopause, they are talking about the whole of the period a woman goes through – often for years before and after her last menstruation – during which the production of the oestrogens and progesterone slow down, her periods may become irregular and she begins to experience other bodily signs of change from sudden fluctuations in temperature to alterations in sleep patterns. This total transition from childbearing to past-childbearing is properly known as the *climacteric*. And because each woman is a biochemical and physiological individual it can last from a few months to as long as fifteen years.

The climacteric is usually divided into three parts: *perimenopause* to indicate the time when hormonal shifts have already begun but a woman is still menstruating; *menopause*, the time at which the last period occurs; and *postmenopause*, which among wise women was traditionally considered to have begun on the fourteenth moon after a woman's last menstruation since by then her reproductive capacity had most definitely finished. The end of a woman's reproductive life seldom coincides with the time of her last period, in fact. It can either precede the moment of menopause or come afterwards. This is the main reason why it is important to continue to use some sort of contraception for the first year to eighteen months after your last period if you don't want another child.

The physiological cause of menopause is simple. It is not a woman's age which brings it about but rather the 'burning out' of her ovaries when the finite number of eggs she has carried since birth are all used up. Since puberty the ovaries have allowed maybe 400 follicles to ripen while thousands more unneeded and unused eggs have at the same time partly ripened then degenerated and been resorbed into her body. So by the time a woman reaches the age of 45, very few follicles are left waiting to be triggered into action. As the number grows smaller and smaller, follicles begin to mature irregularly. Around the same time the secretion of oestrogens by a woman's ovaries decreases as does the production of progesterone. Then somewhere between the ages of 40 and

50 (although it can happen earlier or later), a woman's sexual cycles often become irregular because ovulation no longer takes place during some of her cycles – even though she may appear to be menstruating as usual. Gradually, this *anovulatory* menstruation begins to occur more often. Anovulatory menstruation is a menstrual period in which, although you bleed as expected – often more heavily than expected – no mature follicle is released from your ovary, so you are not capable of becoming pregnant. It is common in women in the years preceding menopause and is the major reason why fertility drops greatly as women get older. When ovulation does not take place, progesterone levels take a nosedive since no corpus luteum (glandular mass in the ovary formed after ovulation) has been formed to produce the hormone. Very few people – doctors and women alike – are as yet aware of the implications of anovulatory menstruation nor that it can exert powerful negative effects on a woman's body and psyche. Neither do they know how widespread it has become in our society, nor how great a role it is playing in the rise of infertility in the industrialized world, not to mention in the increasing number of women developing negative symptoms from PMS to menstrual flooding.

Egg-free Menstruation

Canadian researcher Jerilynn Prior, chief endocrinologist at the University of British Columbia in Vancouver, has done more than any other scientist to bring to light the significance of anovulatory menstruation. Prior and her colleagues made the important discovery that a substantial proportion of menstruating women, long before menopause, are no longer ovulating. Their finding came out of some original work with women athletes whose periods had stopped as a result of heavy training. After studying female athletes in depth, Prior published a paper describing how it is that women in training for marathon running develop osteoporosis. At that time the medical profession widely believed that this occurs because female athletes are simply not making enough oestrogen. (Most of the medical profession still believes this.) Prior meticulously measured oestrogen levels in these women and discovered they were normal. In the process Prior and her researchers measured a lot of other things too – including the level of progesterone in their subjects. She and her team discovered that it is the progesterone not the oestrogen in these young athletes which becomes depleted. In fact their progesterone levels are not just low, they can be lower than that of a man's. For although the women Prior studied were still menstruating, they were not ovulating. Therefore they were not producing progesterone.

So out of Prior's work an important discovery emerged. The osteoporosis which occurs in women runners is due not to lack of oestrogen as was believed but rather to lack of progesterone. Now this was hot stuff. When Prior's paper was published in a respectable scientific journal it should by rights have tossed a bombshell into the medical world, especially since almost every doctor was giving oestrogen for osteoporosis. Yet nobody seemed to take much notice.

Female Epidemic

Prior then became intrigued to see what was happening to the hormones of ordinary women. Her next paper, which appeared two or three years later, reported on a similar study carried out on non-athletic women in which she discovered that the same thing was happening to them. Many women reaching their mid-thirties have their periods as usual, yet become anovulatory and are therefore deficient in progesterone. When it comes to female athletes, the theory has always been that since they train so hard and keep their body fat so low, the body thinks that it is not able to have a baby so does not make the oestrogen needed and periods cease. This was believed by scientists to be some kind of reflex that happened as a result of a lack of cholesterol – the molecule from which the steroids are made, including progesterone and the oestrogens.

But Prior's second group of women were not doing extra exercise and their body fat levels were normal so something else had to be going on. Whatever it was, unbeknown to the medical world, it had grown to epidemic proportions. Prior and her colleagues discovered that anovulation and a short luteal phase cycle now occurs in up to 50 per cent of North American women's menstrual cycles during the final reproductive years. Just what is it that is causing this epidemic of 35-year-old progesterone-depleted women who are *not* ovulating but *are* developing osteoporosis long before menopause?

It has taken the work of environmental scientists of the calibre of Niels Skakkebaek, researcher at the Rigshopital in Copenhagen, and Richard M. Sharpe of the British Medical Council's Centre for Reproductive Biology in Edinburgh to point the way towards an answer. We in the industrialized world, they tell us, now live immersed in a rising sea of petro-chemical derivatives. They are in our air, our foods and our water. These chemicals include pesticides and herbicides as well as various plastics which all have a phenol ring in common as part of their chemical structure. This means they are capable of mimicking the action of oestrogen in an animal's body and which therefore can also burn out a woman's ovaries, using up her follicles long before their time. When this happens anovulatory menstruation occurs so that progesterone production decreases or even stops altogether – with potentially devastating consequences for some women.

Chemical Seas

The oestrogen-mimicking chemicals which have come to pollute our environment do not break down and disappear. Sprayed on our grain and vegetables, including the corn that is fed to the animals whose meat we eat, these petroleum by-products are fat soluble. They have to be. For only if they are fat-based will they dissolve the insect cuticle so that insects feeding on these plants will be killed. However, these chemicals don't just cease to exist once they have done their insect-killing job. They remain in our foodstuffs. The meat we consume from feed-lot fed animals is full of fat in which these chemicals are stored. The fat we see can always be trimmed off but most fat in meat is marbled into the muscle and cannot be removed.

Such highly polluting petroleum derivatives have by now been spread all over the industrialized world. Thousands of miles from where they were used to spray crops, they can be found in quantity in the fat of Arctic seals. Gradually, over the years, we accumulate these toxins in the fat of our own bodies. Research shows they are found in particularly high quantities in women who develop breast cancer. There is an argument raging in medicine at the moment: it centres on the relationship between a high fat intake and the incidence of breast cancer. In the West we now consume almost half of our calories in the form of fat, and breast cancer incidence continues to rise. Scientists have known for some time that the incidence of breast cancer can be directly correlated with the levels of fat a woman has in her diet. Now, however, a growing number of experts aware of the rise in oestrogen-mimicking chemicals are beginning to suspect that it is not so much the *fat* that predisposes a woman to breast cancer but the *toxins* which have accumulated in the fat that then build up in her body.

The leitmotif running through almost all of the 'menopausal horrors' for which women are put on HRT – and filled full of yet *more* oestrogen – is oestrogen dominance, that is high oestrogen or oestrogen-like chemicals in the presence of a relative insufficiency of progesterone in the woman's body. You find the same hormonal pattern in anovulatory cycles, breast cancer, mood swings, night sweats and fibroids as well as many other illnesses associated with menstruation and menopause. The incidence of fibrocystic breast disease, uterine fibroids, endometriosis, PMS, breast cancer and cancer of the womb has in recent years become alarmingly high and continues to mount in industrialized countries. Yet these conditions used to be rare. They are still virtually unknown in non-industrialized areas of the world where women live mostly on a simple diet of compost-grown local foods.

Egg or No Egg?

It can be hard for a woman to know for sure if her cycles are anovulatory or not. Sometimes periods become irregular, heavier or of longer duration. Sometimes she will have PMS or depression. In many women their periods can seem quite normal. The only way to know for sure is to have a laboratory test done for low serum progesterone (that is low levels of progesterone in the blood) between days 18 and 26 of your menstrual cycle. Most laboratories say day 21 is best. A normal serum progesterone level after ovulation is in the range of 7–28 picograms. If a woman does not ovulate that month then the level tends to be around 0.3 picograms. This is a test that your doctor can order (see Appendix to Resources, p. 513).

Where oestrogen dominance does exist the only way to correct it is to re-establish a good balance between oestrogen and progesterone. This, too, can be easier said than done, especially if your doctor, like many, has been steeped in the dogma of HRT. Adding one of the progestogens which are now frequently used together with oestrogen as part of HRT won't do it. What these synthetics do is to help protect against cancer of the womb if you are on extra oestrogen drugs. But, because all the progestogens are end-molecules, your body cannot use them to make the other steroids it needs for hormonal balance, energy, emotional stability and protection from stress. Only natural progesterone can offer these things. And because the progestogens take up progesterone receptor sites, using them in HRT or contraception further reduces the levels of natural progesterone in your body and can therefore interfere with your body's ability to make more.

Low progesterone levels in a woman experiencing anovulatory menstruation increase oestrogen dominance in her body even further as she gets closer and closer to menopause and the complex hormonal feedback mechanisms between the central control station – the hypothalamus – and its first officer, the pituitary, come into play. This can cause disturbances in the feedback mechanisms involving important hormones such as GnRh, LH and FSH. This creates mood swings, hot flushes and depression, not to mention disruptions in the thyroid and in the functions of the many other organs and systems which the hypothalamus oversees – all common experiences of perimenopausal women in the industrialized world. Dr Barry Durrant-Peatfield, one of Britain's pioneers in the menopause revolution, says of oestrogen dominance:

'Water retention and bloating; increasing enlargement of the bust, mastitis and cystic disease of the breast, weight gain, loss of energy and libido, increased risks of breast and endometrial [womb] cancer and the start of osteoporosis . . . progesterone will stop all of these problems.' He continues: 'This situation is really the start of menopause and the use of progesterone is obviously what is required while the use of oestrogen in this situation, as with HRT, may be quite disastrous.'

Eventually menopause arrives. Oestrogen levels finally fall at the time in a woman's life when they are meant to – usually somewhere between the ages of 45 and 52. Periods become erratic or lighter or irregular in the quantity of blood lost. Eventually they stop altogether since there is now not enough oestrogen to stimulate the proliferation of the endometrium. All of this should take place without much difficulty. Thankfully it still does for most women throughout the world. But in western industrialized society more than half of the female population are now thrown into confusion and forced to suffer the negative symptoms of menopause in no uncertain terms – night sweats, hot flushes, emotional ups and downs, even hirsutism (the appearance of hair in quantity on the face and body).

Oestrogen Deficient – No Way

Just about everyone these days still leaps to the conclusion that menopausal women *need* oestrogen. Many women still believe, and so do their doctors for that matter, that when menstruation finally ceases a woman's oestrogen production falls to nothing. They also think that it is oestrogen which keeps skin young looking and sexuality glowing – both of which are patently untrue. A woman's oestrogen production does not cease at menopause. Only oestrogen production in her ovaries stops so that the monthly build up of the womb lining in preparation for pregnancy doesn't happen. This is why menstruation no longer takes place. However, provided a woman's body is in good balance and she is healthy, the oestrogen she makes now in her fat cells, in her liver, and in her adrenals is all she will ever need. What does cease how-ever – or pretty nearly ceases – as soon as menopause arrives, if not earlier, is the production of progesterone. It can fall to near zero. In an oestrogen-dominant woman this produces some of the symptoms commonly associated with menopause, many of which the average doctor is still trying to 'treat' by giving a woman more oestrogen. In a few women low or no progesterone can lead to hirsutism, as well as to male-pattern baldness often associated with old age. This is because their bodies, in the absence of progesterone, turn towards DHEA (dehydroepiandrostenediol) and the male hormones, such as androstenediol and androstenedione, as the only metabolic pathway left open to the production of the oestrogens.

Knock-on Effects

Because progesterone is a precursor to so many other steroid hormones, when the body's production of it ceases or when oestrogen dominance gets out of hand, other hormones are not produced adequately either. Some progesterone-derived hormones (hormones to which progesterone is a precursor) are brain chemicals which influence the way you think and feel. Others are needed by the body to protect against inflam-mation and early ageing or to sustain libido. The absence of sufficient quantities of these steroids can produce aches and pains in the joints and chronic fatigue as well as depression, hot flushes and anxiety. It can also be a prime cause of the emotional upsets which many women experience in mid-life, where a woman is often urged to 'pull herself together' or branded 'emotionally ill'. Such experiences are most assured-ly *not* a natural part of growing older. They are signs that a woman's hormonal balance needs help.

Too often these days the help that is offered comes automatically in the form of drug-based HRT. The new menopause revolutionaries insist this is usually not the best way to go. It can be far more helpful to a woman and far more protective of her long-term health to look first to her lifestyle and help her make adjustments in the way she eats, the kind of nutritional supplements she uses and introduce her to the remarkable healing and balancing properties of natural plant substances. Often this alone will be enough to restore a high level of balance and wellbeing. Then, if hormones are needed, they claim, it is far better to consider making use of the natural hormones – those which are chemically identical to the hormones her own body produces.

The pioneers are also aware, to a degree that few of their less informed colleagues are, that certain of the natural oestrogens such as oestriol are far safer than others, such as oestrone or oestradiol if for a time a woman needs a little extra oestrogen to protect against vaginal thinning or help her through a rough and tumble period of hot flushes (see p. 135). What is so exciting about the new approach is the way in which its advocates take a genuinely holistic view of women. They know about the dangers of oestrogen dominance and they look for ways not only to help a woman counter it but at the same time enhance her mental clarity and emotional balance so that menopause becomes a true passage to power for each woman. We will be examining closely how they do this in later chapters. First let's take a closer look at the sea of environmental oestrogens in which we now live and examine just how widespread are its potential consequences – not only to the lives of women but to men and children as well as animal life on the planet.

Chapter Three

Sleeping with the Enemy

One of the great ironies at the turn of the millennium is that for almost half a century women have been encouraged to use oestrogens. They have been sold both as a means of birth control and for counteracting negative symptoms experienced at menopause. Yet it turns out that excessive oestrogen may well be the greatest enemy any woman in the industrialized world ever faces. It is a silent enemy present day in day out as we eat, as we work, and as we sleep.

Twentieth-century Plague

Of the thousands of oestrogens and oestrogen-like chemicals which appear to be responsible for the mounting incidence of oestrogen dominance in our culture none appear quite as sinister as *xenoestrogens* – sometimes called xenobiotics. The word *xeno* means strange or foreign. Xenoestrogen is the name given to environmental pollutants and chemicals now widespread in our foods, our air and our water that are capable of disrupting biological processes. They mimic the effects of a woman's own natural oestrogens, and interfere with the balance of oestrogens and progesterone in her body. Because xenoestrogens are taken up by oestrogen receptor sites in the body and because the hormones in the body interact with its organs and systems as well as with each other in highly complex and interdependent ways, they can disrupt the workings of the body as a whole. This group of environmental toxins includes hundreds of bedrock chemicals now widespread in our post-industrial society – from the polycarbonated plastics found in our baby bottles and water jugs and polychlorinated biphenyls (PCBs) used in the manufacture of electronics to highly poisonous pesticides such as DDT and its even more toxic cousin DDE. It also includes dieldrin, toxaphene, mirex, heptachlor and kepone as well as hundreds of other herbicides and pesticides, all of which have an ability to mimic natural oestrogen. Even the breakdown products from many common detergents can do this as can the chlorine compounds now used to bleach paper.

All steroid hormones are derived from cholesterol. However, the oestrogen molecule is unique among the steroids by having a phenol in what chemists call its 'A-ring' in the basic cholesterol framework. So whether oestrogens are made in the body or come in the form of chemical sprays all oestrogens are what is chemically called *phenolated*. None of the other steroid molecules such as testosterone, progesterone or corticosterone have a phenolated A-ring in their molecular structure. A phenolated A-ring is also common among petrochemical by-products, such as the organochlorines and pesticides which get into the food chain. They concentrate in the fat of the animals that we eat and eventually in our own fat. Vegetarians are generally better off than meat eaters in terms of the quantity of xenoestrogens they absorb simply because plants tend to have less fat than animals and what there is tends to be confined to the germ of a grain. Meat, however, is 50 per cent fat or even more, so the great mass of the oestrogenic pollutants in our environment finds its way into our bodies most easily by way of animal fats.

The xenoestrogen resemble other oestrogens in some of the effects they exert on the body. Some resemble them molecularly, others can look quite different. All these chemicals and their breakdown products can enter our bodies. Hormones used in birth control and in hormone replacement are other forms of oestrogens foreign to the human system. Most forms of oestrogens, natural or chemical, are capable of bringing about biochemical changes in the body. Sometimes they are able to attach themselves to receptor sites within the body's cells and prevent the natural hormonal response. Other times they may even stimulate a hormone receptor. Unfortunately oestrogen receptor sites are not particularly choosy. Fraudulent oestrogens in pesticides and other chemicals can just as easily hook to them as the real thing.

Locks and Keys

Cell receptor sites normally trigger genetic activity when a hormone or a vitamin is keyed into them, functioning rather like a key which opens a lock. For a long time scientists believed that each lock would only open when presented with the exact molecular key intended for it. They thought that only the perfect key would turn its 'tumblers' to release the gene action as in the oestrogen-modulated biology of breast growth for instance. Recently, however, they have discovered that many foreign chemicals are also capable of opening up oestrogen receptors. These oestrogen mimics can then fool the body into turning off certain biochemical pathways with the sort of consequences that include the development of cancers of the breast and womb, endometriosis, infertility, and cause changes in the reproductive and hormone systems not only of adults but also of unborn children. This happens in several different ways. Some oestrogen mimic molecules fit into the receptor keyholes but won't fully unlock them, so they don't trigger normal activity on a cellular level. Others behave like poorly cut keys – sometimes they will turn the lock and at others they won't. A third group act like skeleton keys and appear to fit perfectly into a receptor and fully unlock its gene action yet can still bring devastating effects in their wake.

Reproductive Devastation

One of the most infamous of these is the drug diethylstibesterol (DES). Between 1948 and 1971 as many as 6 million women in Europe and the United States took this synthetic form of oestrogen which was enthusiastically toted for its ability to prevent miscarriage. Around the same time – according to John A. McLachlan, a tall, slim, handsome man with a fine sense of humour, who organized the recent world conference sponsored by the National Institute of Environmental Health Sciences (NIEHS) in the United States – some 27 thousand kilos of DES were also given to cattle as a 'growth promoter'. Years down the road, the incidence of abnormalities in the offspring of women treated with DES is still being tallied. Female offspring of women who took it have a high level of T-shaped wombs and other structural abnormalities in their organs predisposing them to sterility. Many male offspring show similar structural abnormalities including a high incidence of undescended testicles and deformed urethras as well as a lowered sperm count. Both males and females show a much higher incidence of certain forms of cancer – from the rare Clear-Cell Vaginal Adenocarcinoma in women to testicular and prostate cancer in men. McLachlan, who is also chief of NIEHS's laboratory on reproductive and developmental toxicology, looks upon the effects of DES on the offspring of mothers given the drug as a model for the kinds of effect xenoestrogens may be having today. DES is the only oestrogenic substance so far known to trigger the body's oestrogen receptor activity even more efficiently than the body's natural oestrogens.

At a recent conference in California called 'Environmental Estrogens: Pathway to Extinction', McLachlan pointed out that screening chemicals using traditional toxicology for their hormonal effects is virtually impossible since these may not show up until the next generation is born. We cannot, he points out, judge a chemical's hormonal activity by any specific attribute of its molecular structure. He therefore suggests that we turn to what he calls 'functional toxicology' when chemicals are defined not by their chemical structure but by how they act on an organism. Chemicals could be tested, for instance, for their ability to occupy, activate or turn off cell receptors. This information could be included with chemical information such as molecular weight, melting point and solubility to help us better anticipate chemical dangers where they are present. So far we are a generation away from this being done. Meanwhile we keep taking more and more xenoestrogens into our bodies.

Secrets of Oestrogen

In order to grasp how xenoestrogens affect the body it is important to know how the natural oestrogens work. There are three major kinds of oestrogens made in the human body: oestradiol (the most common and the most potent), oestriol and oestrone (see also p. 108). These oestrogens are produced mainly in the ovaries although small quantities are secreted from the adrenal glands, the placenta during pregnancy and in fat cells. The oestrogen production in a woman's body begins when she is still a foetus, reaches its peak after puberty and then declines at menopause. While you were in the womb oestrogens stimulated the development of your ovaries and uterus and ensured that you developed properly into a female child. Men, too, produce oestrogen but in much smaller quantities than we do. High oestrogen levels in a male foetus prevent the full development of masculine characteristics needed for a boy even if its genes are programmed to produce a male child. When puberty arrives, oestrogens in a girl encourage the development of breasts and the expansion of the uterus. After that they help regulate the menstrual cycle and play other important roles such as helping to maintain bone mass and keeping blood cholesterol levels in check. When excessive quantities of oestrogen, regardless of source, are present in a young woman's body they will burn out her ovaries and undermine fertility. It is this phenomenon which many eco-scientists believe to be largely responsible for the rapidly decreasing fertility in western women.

Each year evidence mounts further that women in industrialized countries are suffering from an overexposure to oestrogen mimics. In 1960 the chances of a woman developing breast cancer were only one in 20. Today one in nine women are statistically destined to get the disease. Only about 30 per cent of women who get breast cancer now are in what are considered high-risk groups – women who have an early menses, don't breastfeed or breastfeed for a limited period, come from a family with a history of breast cancer, or who have their first pregnancy late in life. A number of studies have recently demonstrated that women exposed to polycyclic aromatic hydrocarbons (PAHs) and polychlorinated biphenyls (PCBs) have a significantly higher rate of breast cancer than women not exposed. Devra Lee Davis at the US Department of Health and Human services is one of the scientists who have closely examined the issue of breast cancer.

She points out that many studies have shown elevated breast cancer rates in women who have worked in the chemical industry and who have been exposed to PCBs or PAHs in drinking water, or who have breast tissue which contains high concentrations of DDT.

Good Guy Oestrogens

To make things even more complicated not all oestrogens or oestrogen-like substances exert the *negative* effect on the body that oestrogen drugs and xenoestrogens can. In the same way that medicine now recognizes that there is a good-guy cholesterol and a bad-guy cholesterol in relation to protecting the body from heart disease, so are there 'good' oestrogens and 'bad' oestrogens. According to Herman Aldercreutz, nutritional chemist at the University of Helsinki, and others, a number of weaker natural oestrogen-like ingredients in foods actually help protect us against cancer of the breast and reproductive system by binding with oestrogen receptor sites so that dangerous strong oestrogenic compounds are not so readily taken up. Many of the best protective foods contain oestrogen-like compounds called isoflavoids. They are found in many of the soya-based foods eaten daily in the Orient, such as tofu, tempeh and miso, as well as in rye bread and in the pulses or legumes such as lentils. A number of other edible plants, including pomegranates and French beans, contain phyto-oestrogens of a different kind which also boast protective properties. At the Children's Hospital Medical Centre in Washington DC, when Kenneth Setchell fed rodents on soya protein he discovered that his animals developed far fewer tumours than animals fed on a soy-free diet. This, plus the fact that Japanese women also eat a great variety of land and sea plants which continually help to detoxify the body, may explain why Orientals still have very low rates of breast cancer and few menopause-related problems compared to Europeans and North Americans. However, when Japanese women move to the United States and take up a western diet, they rapidly develop the same diseases we have.

Not Created Equal

Devra Lee Davis at the United States Department of Health and Human Services is one of the researchers delving into the way in which oestrogens are not all created equal. She says that when the body produces oestradiol this oestrogen can be broken down via two different metabolic pathways. One turns into a form of oestrogen called 16-hydroxy oestrone which can damage DNA – the cell's genetic material. It is the kind of bad-guy oestrogen implicated in triggering breast and testicular cancers. The other metabolic pathway breaks down oestradiol to a form of oestrogen called 2-hydroxy oestrone which is not only harmless but is beginning to be hailed by scientists as beneficial and protective against cancer.

In Germany and the UK, doctors working with natural methods for treating hot flushes and vaginal dryness prescribe phyto-oestrogens in tablet or capsule form or as herbal tinctures or extracts and claim to get excellent results from them. When beneficial phyto-oestrogens bind to oestrogen receptor sites they can not only supply an alternative form of natural oestrogen where needed but, by taking up her oestrogen receptor sites, they may protect the woman from the xenoestrogens in her environment which are continually trying to key into them.

Poisoned Consensus

Less than a year ago some 300 scientists from all over the world gathered at a conference in Washington DC, sponsored by the NIEHS. The intention was to share specific information on the effects that environmental chemicals are now exerting on human and animal health. It was only the third such conference ever held. Mary S. Wolff of New York City's Mount Sinai School of Medicine also reported that DDT and DDE are likely to be playing an important role in the huge rise in breast cancer incidence we are witnessing in the western world. Wolff and her colleagues compared levels of DDE in 58 women with breast cancer with those of 170 women who were cancer-free. All the women were carefully screened so that they matched in age, socio-economic status and every known risk factor. They discovered that the risk of breast cancer was four times greater in the women with the highest levels of DDE than in those with the lowest. The general consensus among conservative scientists investigating the link between environmental chemicals and breast cancer is that as much as a third of breast cancer now developing is directly related to the use of xenoestrogen chemicals in our environment but many experts insist this is far too low an estimate. As far as cancer of the womb is concerned, oestrogen dominance in the body is the *only* known cause of this illness. Meanwhile the whole business of exposure to excessive oestrogenic compounds becomes an increasing worry when you consider that oestrogens are also the hormones most commonly prescribed for women not only for birth control but also for HRT. Exposure to xenoestrogens and environmental pollutants over a period of time, say experts, is exacerbated by oestrogens prescribed as drugs to women and may be producing breast cancer by disrupting the normal processes of cell regulation in breast tissue.

Dr Ana Soto, an endocrinologist at Tufts University in the United States, discovered for herself quite by accident just how powerful an effect a xenoestrogen can exert on breast tissue. She and her colleagues had been experimenting with cancer cells taken from the breast, then cultured. They found the cells would only grow if they were fed oestrogens. In fact the technique Soto was using – bathing the cells with specific chemicals and then recording whether or not the cells proliferate – may one day prove to be an excellent test for whether or not a specific chemical exhibits an oestrogenic effect.

One day the tests simply stopped working. The cancer cells continued to grow even when no oestrogens were fed to them. This had been going on for four months when Soto realized that the manufacturers who made the disposable flasks in which she had been culturing her cells had started to use a different plastic – one that, when it becomes warm, releases minute quantities of the oestrogen-like compound nonylphenol. Her tissues samples were being continually contaminated by these leaking oestrogens. Once Soto determined the cause and changed to glass flasks she found that she could carry on with the experiments as usual but the experience stunned her. It has since made her voice extreme concern about the effect that plastics we use day to day may be exerting upon our health.

The Perils of Plastic

Our world is full of plastics – containers which we use every day to store leftovers in the refrigerator or to cook food in the microwave, cups which we drink coffee from, bottles which our mineral water comes in. Most companies who manufacture plastics are not even aware themselves whether or not their products slough off oestrogen-like molecules. The use of a number of PCBs may have been restricted in many industrialized countries but, like DDT and a few pesticides known to be highly toxic, the products of their breakdown persist in the environment for decades. As endocrinologist David Feldman from Stanford University says: 'It is very possible – and it is frightening – that we may be drowning in a sea of oestrogens.' The xenoestrogens which occur in highest concentrations in many of our effluents are the nonylphenols and octylphenols. These are the break-down products of surfactants in our detergents and common household products, and in spermicides.

While examining fish populations, John P. Sumpter of the Department of Biology and Biochemistry at Brunel University in Uxbridge, discovered that powerful oestrogenic chemicals are being discharged from sewage treatment plants into rivers. More than 70 per cent of the waste water he and his colleagues sampled contained between 0.1 and 5 micrograms per litre of dissolved nonylphenol. He, like most scientists investigating the rising oestrogenic sea, voices great concern for the implications of xenoestrogens in our rivers on human health and on the health of fish and other animals. As far back as the late 1960s, discharges of almost 2 million kilograms of DDT into the coastal waters of Southern California brought about the collapse of the brown pelican and doublecrested cormorant populations. Since then, with the introduction of restrictions on DDT, populations have recovered. However, DDT has a very long half-life. Even were it to be banned worldwide, it would continue to poison the earth for many generations to come. But it is still used in many countries today. DDT is part of a group of xenochemicals which travel easily in the environment and which have been shown capable of inducing and promoting mammary cancers in laboratory animals.

DDE-sexed Alligators

Not long ago in Lake Apopka in Florida wildlife biologists discovered that strange things were happening to the alligators living there. Lake Apopka is a large body of water not far from Disney World with a southern channel on which lies a petrochemical factory making pesticides. A toxic spill took place in 1980 but was forgotten and initially unknown to scientists called in five years later to investigate a decline in the numbers of alligators. The population of alligators in 1980 had been 30 per square kilometre. By 1987 it had dropped to a mere 3 per square kilometre. It was discovered that in those eggs that hatched, the male alligators which emerged from the eggs had abnormally small penises. They were 75 per cent shorter than average. Almost certainly, say scientists investigating the phenomenon, this is the result of residual concentrations of DDE from a lakeside spill of the chemical dicofol and DDT which took place many years before. Following up this hypothesis, Louis J. Guillette, wildlife endocrinologist at the University of Florida, experimented with these xenoestrogens. He discovered that painting alligator eggs with the same doses of DDE which are now present in concentrations in the lake (such low doses that they can only be measured in parts per billion) brings about the same reproductive problems in laboratory animals. Only 10 per cent of the treated eggs hatch and most of these animals turn out to be female.

Alligators are not the only beasts being affected by the 'feminization' of the environment. Wildlife biologist Michael

Fry, a bird physiologist from the University of California at Davis, has examined birds in areas where concentrations of PCBs are high and found that female gulls are producing extra egg-laying organs while males have a mixture of female and male reproductive structures. At the University of Texas David Crews works with turtle eggs. He reports that even very low doses of oestrogen-mimicking chemicals applied to the shells of turtle eggs can cause ovary formation in otherwise male turtles. Meanwhile in Europe and North America a group of studies have been carried out to investigate the decline of certain species including gulls, turtles, frogs, deer and alligators. Different animal experts report the same apparent causes – the females of these species have enlarged ovaries. Like consistently anovulatory women, their egg follicles have been burned out and are simply gone.

The old saying 'these days a man is only half his grandfather' may no longer be hyperbole. Speaking at the international conference held last year, Danish endocrinologist Niels Skakkebaek, a researcher at the Rigshopital in Copenhagen, and Richard M. Sharpe of the British Medical Research Council Centre for Reproductive Biology in Edinburgh, presented strong evidence that the increased incidence of male birth defects, testicular cancer and prostate cancer is likely to be the result of exposure to environmental xenoestrogens begun while the male foetus is still in the womb. After carrying out a 21-country study of semen quality which analysed records from 50 years starting in 1938, Skakkebaek and his colleagues reported in 1992 that there has been a 50 per cent drop in sperm counts worldwide. During this same period the incidence of testicular cancer has tripled in many countries while that of prostate cancer has doubled. Meanwhile in Germany, researchers have recently discovered that women with endometriosis (the condition which very commonly occurs in women over the age of 40 where the secretory lining of the womb painfully proliferates) have significantly higher levels of PCBs in their bodies than women without the disease. Seventy years ago only 21 cases of endometriosis had been reported in the world. Now, there are over 5 million cases in the United States alone.

Plague of Plagues

What appears to be happening is that a strange and potentially highly dangerous marriage is taking place between the proliferation of oestrogen-mimicking chemicals in the environment and the rise in various oestrogens prescribed medically to women. It is out of this union that oestrogen dominance has probably developed. The oestrogens and progesterone in a woman's body must balance each other for a woman to remain healthy. In many of us they are becoming more and more out of kilter. As a result we are now seeing a widespread rise in many diseases and discomforts for which – with a strange irony – doctors are prescribing more oestrogen. (See page 47 for a few of the ways in which oestrogen dominance can manifest itself.)

Go to the Source

So potentially dangerous is oestrogen dominance that it is essential we communicate information about it both to other women of all ages and to our doctors. It is also important that we put pressure on our politicians and government leaders to increase control over what chemicals are allowed to be used in the world around us. Scientists throughout the western world are working to identify as many specific agents responsible for the increase in xenoestrogens in our environment as they can. However, we are constantly exposed to so many chemicals which exhibit an oestrogenic characteristic that it may turn out to be a task as complicated as finding the proverbial needle in the haystack. Some researchers suspect that ethynylestradiol (EE) – the primary oestrogenic compound in birth control pills – plays a big role as well.

EE in the urine of women on the Pill is able to pass through water treatment plants so it ends up in our drinking water. EE is a much more potent oestrogenic compound than oestradiol. To test the effect of EE and other oestrogens on wildlife, researchers incubated fish in aquariums which had dilute concentrations either of EE or oestradiol, the primary oestrogen in the whole of the animal kingdom. They found that even concentrations of EE as low as 0.1 nanograms per litre of water exert significant effects. Researchers concluded that EE is one of the most potent biologically active molecules. Since then, at the Fish and Wildlife Services in Atlanta, Georgia, in the United States, scientists have issued a prohibition on the use of oestrogenic chemicals, including pesticides, in more than a hundred wildlife refuges managed by the federal government.

As yet little of the information about the mounting effects of xenoestrogens and oestrogen dominance in women has even *begun* to filter down to the general public. Neither has it been made easily available to the busy doctors to whom the women suffering from PMS or menopausally related symptoms turn for help. For any woman keen to take control of her own reproductive destiny in terms of fertility, PMS, menopause and beyond, it is essential that she be aware of just how widespread the challenges of environmental chemicals has become.

Magnetic Powers

It may not be only chemicals in our environment which are capable of unbalancing hormones and undermining health and reproductive capabilities either. For many years there has been a recognition that the presence of certain electric energies, radio waves and electromagnetic fields seems to increase susceptibility to breast cancer. There are indications that they may also alter the development of male foetuses. Researchers have discovered, for instance, that prenatal exposure of animals to low frequency fields (15 hertz) can demasculinize males so that they do not mark their scent in the way normal mature males do. More than 20 years ago researchers at the University of Manitoba in Winnipeg exposed male rats to chronically magnetic fields, either while in the womb or just after birth and then monitored the results. Scientists discovered that when the rats were prenatally exposed they developed larger testicles, whereas if they exposed the animals as adults testicle size decreased. Like the good-guy oestrogens and the bad-guy oestrogens, some magnetic fields appear to be beneficial and some detrimental. So does exposure to light itself. Studies show that both can influence the secretion of a brain chemical which among its many other properties helps to regulate oestrogen concentrations in the animal's body. For the past quarter of a century researchers have wrestled with epidemiological data that tie together electromagnetic fields and cancer. They have had a tough time making sense of their findings since most low-frequency fields (associated with household electric currents, microwaves and radio waves) appear to be too weak to break the chemical bonds that would bring about the genetic changes typically associated with the production of cancer cells.

Then, in the April 1987 issue of the *American Journal of Epidemiology*, Richard G. Stephens of the Pacific Northwest Laboratory in Richland, Washington, published an interesting theory which scientists concerned about environmental influences on human health now take very seriously indeed. It goes something like this.

During the hours of darkness the pineal gland in the centre of the brain secretes a hormone called melatonin in direct response to the amount of sunlight which we are exposed to during the previous hours of light. It is a deficiency in melatonin production which produces the now widely publicized Seasonal Affective Disorder, or SAD, where some people become depressed during long, dark winters. Melatonin is also largely responsible for the experience of jet lag when we cross time zones. And, taken as a nutritional supplement, melatonin has shown itself useful in counteracting jet lag. Among its other attributes melatonin inhibits the body's production of both oestrogen and prolactin, the hormone that stimulates milk production. However, animal studies have shown that exposure either to electromagnetic fields or to light during the night hours can suppress the secretion of melatonin from the pineal. Stephens' work suggests that the chronic exposure to artificial lights which most of us in the industrialized world continually live with may be increasing our cumulative lifetime dose of oestrogen and also be increasing our risk of developing breast cancer.

Not long after Stephens published his theory, two

researchers at the University of Arizona in Tucson announced another important discovery which supports it. David E. Blask and Stephen M. Hill found that giving melatonin can directly inhibit the proliferation of human breast cancer cells in a culture. Even more important, the quantity of melatonin needed to do this is extremely small, comparable to the amount present in human blood at night. Blask believes that melatonin may have the ability to increase the levels of naturally occurring anti-oxidants in breast cancer cells which not only help protect against the development of cancer but heart disease too. Melatonin may even be capable of reducing the number of oestrogen receptor sites on breast cancer cells. Since it is oestrogen that feeds the growth of hormone-responsive breast tumours, increased melatonin may help decrease tumour growth. Meanwhile, at the University of California at Berkeley, scientists such as Robert Liburdy have shown that some magnetic fields can limit or block melatonin's ability to inhibit the proliferation of human breast cancer cells in a culture. Other researchers speculate that it may be the suppression of melatonin by electromagnetic fields and light which tends to promote cancer, especially breast cancer.

The whole melatonin issue is a particularly important one for menopausal women. First, the production of melatonin tends to drop as the body gets older. Many age researchers now believe supplements of melatonin have anti-ageing properties. One of the things menopausal women tend to suffer commonly from is wakefulness at night. It is a strange kind of wakefulness not treatable by ordinary natural tranquillizers such as valerian or passiflora. For such women, taking 15 milligrams of melatonin before bed can often make the difference between a night spent half awake and hours of blissful sleep. (See Never Come Morning, p. 338, for more information about melatonin.)

We shall probably be well into the twenty-first century before the devastating effects of the twentieth-century post-industrial environment can even begin to be tallied. Our wildlife was the first to send signals that something is seriously wrong. However, in the face of economic pressures from manufacturers of chemical products, governments may never be able to pass laws adequate to control the addition of new poisons to the rising sea of oestrogens around us. But there is a great deal that a woman who feels respect for the wisdom of nature and for her own body can do to protect herself now as well as to protect the world around her.

Chapter Four

Search for the Grail

Think of menopause and chances are you think of oestrogen. For menopause they tell us is simply an oestrogen-deficiency state. We are also led to believe that problems which arrive at menopause – from hot flushes to weird emotions – are the result of this oestrogen deficiency and are therefore fixable either by 'oestrogen replacement' or HRT. So deeply ingrained have such notions become in the industrialized world that to challenge them seems sacrilege. Yet challenge them we must if we are to tap into the power of the bloodless revolution.

Two main sex hormones dominate a woman's reproductive life – oestrogen and progesterone. To be healthy emotionally and physically so that menopause becomes a voyage of discovery instead of a living hell, they need to be balanced. In recent years we have been bombarded with information – and misinformation – about oestrogen but little has been said about the equally important role progesterone plays in female wellbeing. It is time to redress the balance, time we delved into the mysteries of oestrogen's silent partner. This is a task easier said than done. For the role of progesterone has been both neglected and misunderstood even by the so-called experts. The mysterious progesterone holds many secrets. Some are brand new, some long forgotten. They are secrets which can empower women.

Forgotten Hormone

An understanding of what progesterone is and how it works is central to the revolution in natural menopause. Among this hormone's many attributes is an ability to do what most medical science still considers impossible – *reverse* osteoporosis. Exciting as all this may sound, progesterone is not some miracle substance nor is it a new-fangled alternative to HRT.

It is simply a forgotten piece of the menopause puzzle. As such, the story of how progesterone's role in women's health has been discovered is an ideal jumping-off point for our journey into natural menopause.

For the past 15 years, while the high-powered medical world has been extolling the virtues of oestrogen drugs and HRT, John Lee, a country doctor in northern Carolina, has been diligently researching the actions of natural progesterone. When he began to apply his knowledge of this remarkable hormone, Lee discovered that women who use it are able to eliminate a myriad of menstrual and premenstrual problems as well as banish a litany of menopausal complaints for which conventional medical science still has no answers. In some cases natural progesterone has even shown itself useful in making barren women fertile. Lee and many other physicians and health practitioners in several countries of the world who use and recommend progesterone have watched it transform the lives of first hundreds, then scores of thousands of women.

A tall, soft-spoken man of Norwegian descent, John Lee retired from a busy practice as a country doctor five years ago to create more time for writing and research. Before that he had for many years been gravely concerned about the widespread phenomenon which scientists in the field of ecology are now reporting evidence of throughout the industrialized world. Chemical after chemical in our environment is capable of exerting an *oestrogenic* effect on the human body, thereby upsetting the delicate balance of hormones and exerting a detrimental effect on human health and fertility.

Bad News: Good News

It was Lee who a few years ago coined the phrase *oestrogen dominance*. He used it to describe a biological state in which the finely tuned balance between oestrogen and progesterone in a woman's body has been disturbed, often as a result of high levels of these mock oestrogens. So far oestrogen dominance is something about which the majority of doctors throughout the world remain ignorant. That is the bad news.

Happily there is good news too: oestrogen dominance is relatively easy to correct once you know how. And correcting it when it has occurred in the body brings enormous benefits to a woman's overall health.

Here are a few of the ways in which oestrogen dominance can manifest itself.

- When oestrogen is not balanced by progesterone it can produce weight gain, headaches, bad temper, chronic fatigue and loss of interest in sex – all of which are part of the clinically recognized premenstrual syndrome or PMS.
- Not only has it been well established that oestrogen dominance encourages the development of breast cancer thanks to oestrogen's proliferative actions, it also stimulates breast tissue and can in time trigger fibrocystic breast disease – a condition which wanes when natural progesterone is introduced to balance the oestrogen.
- By definition, excess oestrogen implies a progesterone deficiency. This, in turn, leads to a decrease in the rate of new bone formation in a woman's body by the osteoblasts – the cells responsible for doing this job. Although most doctors are not yet aware of it, this is the prime cause of osteoporosis.
- Oestrogen dominance increases the risk of fibroids. One of the interesting facts about fibroids – often remarked on by doctors – is that, regardless of their size, fibroids commonly atrophy once menopause arrives and a woman's ovaries are no longer making oestrogen. Doctors who commonly use progesterone with their patients have discovered that giving a woman natural progesterone will also cause fibroids to atrophy.
- In oestrogen-dominant menstruating women where progesterone is not peaking and falling in a normal way each month, the ordered shedding of the womb lining doesn't take place. Menstruation cycles become irregular. This condition can usually be corrected by making lifestyle changes and using a natural progesterone product, and is easy to diagnose by having the doctor measure the level of progesterone in your blood at certain times of the month (see Appendix to Resources, p. 513).

- Endometrial cancer (cancer of the womb) develops only where there is oestrogen dominance or unopposed oestrogen. This too can be prevented by the use of natural progesterone. Some of the artificial progestogens may also help prevent it which is why a growing number of doctors no longer give oestrogen without combining it with a progestogen drug during HRT.
- Waterlogging of the cells and an increase in intercellular sodium which predisposes a woman to high blood pressure or hypertension frequently occurs with oestrogen dominance. This can also be a side-effect of taking a progestogen. Progesterone usually clears it up.
- The risk of stroke and heart disease is increased dramatically when a woman is oestrogen dominant.

Like British scientist James Lovelock, father of the Gaia theory which views the earth as a living organism, John Lee is an *independent* scientist. He does not work for anyone. He is not a consultant to any drug manufacturer, cosmetic manufacturer or health-food company. Lee takes no money for the talks he gives to doctors, scientists and women's groups throughout the world and he has nothing whatever to sell. Blessed with down-to-earth common sense and a brilliant inquiring mind, Lee has spent decades searching for simple answers to complex questions. His area of greatest knowledge and expertise with regard to women's health is the use of plant-derived progesterone – a molecule which is chemically *identical* to the progesterone produced by a woman's body. As such, natural progesterone is very different in its actions and effects from the drug-based hormones now prescribed for contraception or HRT.

Mysteries of Mistletoe

John Lee's first encounter with plant-derived progesterone came almost by accident. In the late 1960s he was the editor of a bulletin for his local medical society. Obliged to produce an editorial each month, he was always on the lookout for interesting subjects to tackle. Stuck for copy for the December issue one year, and conscious that his deadline was approaching, Lee came across two interesting articles. One had appeared in the *Harvard Alumni Journal*. It concerned the origins of the Christmas custom of kissing under the mistletoe. This mysterious ritual, the article said, originated with the Celts although reasons for it remained unknown. The second article had appeared in the *Journal of the American Medical Association*. It was about a retired doctor who on returning to his birthplace in Texas met an old gypsy, a woman much celebrated in the community for her 'morning after' cures for pregnancy. The gypsy had told the doctor that her success came from the use of European mistletoe berries. Curious, the retired physician had gone to the trouble of having the European mistletoe berry analysed. He discovered that European mistletoe contains high levels of progesterone together with some other steroid hormones and glycosides including digitalis.

Lee became fascinated by the mystery. He knew that most of the information which we have about the Celts and their practices comes from the Roman historian Pliny so he went in search of what Pliny had to say. Pliny recorded the respect that the Celts had for the medicinal properties of the mistletoe plant. Lee discovered that the mistletoe's name translated means 'all heal' and that the Celts believed the plant to be sacred. Each year at the time of winter solstice their Druids would hold a week-long ritual in worship of the sun importuning it, instead of dying, to be reborn with a promise that spring will return. At this time of year they would give gifts to one another, feast, and drink deeply of hot mead laced with the holy mistletoe which had been carefully gathered in a white cloth that was never allowed to touch the ground. Then, with the usual restrictions on sexual behaviour lifted, they would party long and hard.

Sexy Progesterone

One of the major characteristics of progesterone is its ability to stimulate libido. Another is that when the level of progesterone in a woman's body has been relatively high and then falls abruptly (as happens naturally around day 26 to 28 of her menstrual cycle), this drop in the hormone triggers a flow of menstrual blood causing the lining of the womb to be shed. Lee reasoned that this was probably what happened with the Druids' mistletoe rituals. After a week of sacred orgying on progesterone-tinged alcohol any fertilized ovum was likely to be eliminated with the subsequent menstrual flow that would take place after the feast was over and all the progesterone-laced mead had been drunk. No one would get pregnant. No wonder the Celts looked on the plant as a gift of the gods. Now all that remains of their winter solstice ritual is our Christmas tradition that a man can still kiss a woman with impunity under the mistletoe.

Learning about the Celtic ritual and the mistletoe gave John Lee just the material he needed to write an amusing editorial for the Christmas issue. This he did, then promptly forgot about it all. After his editorial was published he received some interesting letters. From them he learned that mistletoe is not the only plant which contains phyto-hormones (plant-derived hormones) capable of producing shifts in female hormonal balance. There are over 5,000 known plants which boast either precursors to progesterone or oestrogens (precursors are chemicals which can easily be converted by the body) or hormones themselves. In fact it is from such plants that wise women's traditional healing repertoires for female complaints have been fashioned throughout history. Both the hormone progesterone and its plant source origins now began to intrigue John Lee. He wanted to know more but he had little time as a busy country doctor to pursue his curiosity. Time passed until, almost before he knew it, his 40-year-old patients had become 60-year-old patients, and, by the mid 1970s, Lee found himself faced with more and more women in his practice who were suffering from osteoporosis. Their spines were crumbling and their bones kept fracturing but he did not know what to do to help them.

Darkness at Noon

In 1976 – the heyday of oestrogen replacement in the United States – a general consensus conference was held at the world-famous Mayo Clinic. Doctors from around the world gathered there to decide that oestrogen – then the only hormone given for osteoporosis and menopause-related symptoms – should no longer be given on its own since more and more of the women on oestrogen replacement were developing cancer of the uterus (womb). Like many other physicians Lee found himself faced with a dilemma. The medical profession and drug manufacturers claimed that extra oestrogen was necessary to protect a woman from crumbling bones. But if this were true, then to stop osteoporosis and prevent fractured hips, Lee would either have to give oestrogen replacement and tell a woman that she might end up with cancer of the uterus as a result, or he would need to add one of the progestogens to the treatment. (Progestogens are drugs now commonly used with oestrogen as part of the HRT package.) But progestogens, Lee believed, carry a range of pretty ghastly potential side-effects of their own, including possibly an increased risk of breast cancer. It was a dilemma that nobody in medicine had ever been able to solve to the satisfaction of conscientious doctors wanting to do their best for women patients yet dissatisfied with current thinking on hormonal treatments. But let's pause a moment for a couple of important definitions before we continue with Lee's tale.

First Principles

Surrounding the word progesterone you will find many misunderstandings in both the medical and the lay world which take a bit of sorting out. For starters, the word progesterone tends to be used *erroneously* and *collectively* by doctors, researchers and the media alike to describe not the natural hormone itself (which Lee and others have now investigated) but rather one or more of the *progestogens* – these synthetic progesterone-analogues such as the widely used drugs Medroxyprogesterone acetate (Provera), Dydrogesterone

(Duphaston) and Norethisterone (Primulut). Together with one or more forms of oestrogen, progestogens – also called *progestins* or *gestins* – are incorporated into contraceptive pills and HRT. You will often hear doctors say that 'progesterone does this or that'. When you actually pin them down and get them to clarify exactly what they are talking about, ninety-nine times out of a hundred you find that the word is being used not to describe the natural hormone progesterone but rather one of these synthetic analogues.

The effects of natural and synthetic hormones on the body differ enormously. The synthetics do not match the body's chemistry so the body is not equipped to metabolize them properly. Taking a progestogen can inhibit ovulation in a menstruating woman – and can produce abortion which progesterone protects against. It can also suppress her body's production of its own natural progesterone and trigger other negative side-effects. You will find them listed at length in the manual your doctor refers to when prescribing drugs. Progesterone itself, on the other hand, has none of these. The use of synthetic progestogen in HRT can all too often aggravate some of the problems a doctor is trying to treat by making a woman moody, irritable and bad-tempered. Natural progesterone, by contrast, tends to make women feel calm and stable. A growing number of doctors and women who have used it in Europe and North America report that progesterone also banishes hot flushes, re-establishes fertility, eliminates PMS and reverses osteoporosis. But, since the natural hormone and the various progestogens so often get lumped together in common medical parlance, progesterone frequently gets blamed for negative effects which it doesn't cause. Meanwhile, doctors and women alike remain ignorant of the natural hormone's potential for good.

The Proliferator

And it is not only progesterone about which confusion abounds. Oestrogen too needs clarification. Although people commonly refer to oestrogen in the singular, this hormone is not a single compound like progesterone. It is a group of many different compounds each with different characteristics and actions. Oestrogen is the *collective* name used to describe all natural and artificial chemicals which are able to trigger oestrus – that is the release of an egg in a woman. Oestrogen is secreted primarily by the ovarian follicles of menstruating women. During pregnancy it is also secreted by the placenta. To be absolutely accurate, there is no such thing as oestrogen, but the word is used to describe many compounds – found in nature, in our foods and in our bodies as well as made synthetically either in the form of hormone drugs or petro-chemical derivatives – which exert an oestrogenic effect on the body.

The oestrogens are also responsible for the development of a woman's secondary sex characteristics. After puberty, together with progesterone and a few other steroid hormones, oestrogen or, more properly stated, *the oestrogens* help regulate menstrual cycles, building up the endometrium or womb lining during the first half of each cycle. Many women have been taught that after menopause a woman's body stops making oestrogen. This common error ultimately leads to an even greater untruth – that menopause is an 'oestrogen deficiency disease'. The truth is that even after menopause oestrogen is still made in a woman's body, only in smaller quantities.

The Protector

Antagonist to the collective 'oestrogen', progesterone is the name for a *single* steroid female hormone – one specific molecule – made by the corpus luteum. The corpus luteum is the yellow granular mass in the ovary formed each month after an egg has been released. Where oestrogen is the major female reproductive hormone during the first half of a woman's menstrual cycle while the endometrium is proliferating, progesterone is the most important hormone during the second half. Not only does progesterone help make other hormones, it is important for countering stress and immunity and is concerned almost entirely with holding on to the endometrium in final preparation of the lining of the womb for pregnancy.

Progesterone does this by promoting changes in the womb lining that makes the uterus ready for implantation by a fertilized egg. When a woman is pregnant the placenta takes over her body's production of progesterone which now increases ten or twenty fold – sometimes more – above the level of progesterone produced before. Progesterone during pregnancy helps the womb hold the foetus safely until a baby is ready to be born. Women who habitually miscarry often do so because their bodies do not produce enough progesterone especially during the early stages of pregnancy. Progesterone, and plants containing other chemicals from which the body can make this hormone, have been used throughout history to arrest threatened miscarriages. Midwives and wise women have relied on wild yam and other botanicals, which are rich in phyto-chemical precursors to progesterone, in the treatment of pregnant women who are experiencing breakthrough bleeding. It is also the high level of progesterone synthesized during pregnancy that makes many women feel and look so well during the last few months before birth – often better than at any other time in their lives.

By the time of the Mayo conference in 1976 it had been well established that giving excess oestrogen as 'oestrogen replacement' to women with a history of breast cancer was highly dangerous because in some women the proliferative character of oestrogen reactivated cancerous growth. Progesterone on the other hand has no known negative side-effects. Progesterone is an important compound in the body for another reason too: from it the body derives more than a dozen other important hormones – including the oestrogens themselves. More about this in a moment but for now let's go back to Lee's story.

Mission Impossible

John Lee had a number of osteoporosis patients with a history of breast cancer. He believed that for them oestrogen was absolutely contra-indicated since it could stir up metastases, causing the cancer to recur. There seemed to be no way out. Treating their osteoporosis the accepted way by giving oestrogen meant exposing these women to the possibility of more disease – something he did not feel right in doing. Then, in 1979, while he was wrestling with these issues, John Lee heard a talk given by another of the trailblazers in the menopause revolution: Dr Ray Peat.

An outspoken and tireless investigative biochemist at Black College in Oregon, Peat had spent years studying the effects of progesterone on the human body. His research had taken him back to studies carried out half a century earlier – long before the Pill and HRT became big business and the investigation of the natural hormone had been replaced by studies into its drug-based analogues. In the lecture Peat pointed out that the medical profession had virtually forgotten that natural progesterone exists. He said that progesterone is easy to obtain without a prescription and that it can be derived from many plants. Unlike the progestogens, progesterone has no negative side-effects, said Peat. It is even included in the formulas of certain cosmetics because it is so good for the skin. It is time, insisted Peat, that doctors included progesterone in their thinking about how to manage the treatment of women patients. Peat's words rang bells for John Lee. Lee contacted the biochemist and asked for all his research references. Later, ploughing through scientific papers, Lee discovered that Peat was right. There had indeed been masses of research into the uses of natural progesterone right from the early 1900s up to around 1960. After that, with the development of the synthetic progestogens, little further research or clinical work was carried out with the natural hormone – except in Britain.

British Breakthrough

Back in the 1950s pioneering British gynaecologist Dr Katherina Dalton first identified premenstrual syndrome (PMS) and coined the phrase. In fact, she was herself a victim of it. Having suffered terrible migraines associated with her menstrual cycle, Dalton discovered that many of the symptoms associated with PMS could be alleviated when progesterone was given by injection. She chose to experiment with progesterone because she noticed that her migraines disappeared during the final months of her own pregnancy when progesterone levels in the body soar. Dalton published her first reports as far back as 1953. Although she had to fight hard to have PMS accepted as a genuine condition requiring medical attention, she was able successfully to treat some women with natural progesterone.

Progesterone is not always easy to take. Dalton's methods involved regular injections of relatively large amounts of the hormone. This can be costly and inconvenient and in a few cases, according to Peat, can lead to a serious reaction at the injection site in part because the solvents used for the injectable progesterone are unfriendly to the body. So a few doctors experimenting with the use of the hormone changed to using progesterone suppositories. But they too can be cumbersome and frequently do not absorb easily, yielding at times as little as 5 per cent of the hormone present. Progesterone can also be taken orally. After all, mother's milk contains significant quantities of progesterone. This is an important ingredient in breast milk for progesterone makes a considerable contribution to the health of a baby's developing endocrine system. Later on a few doctors began to use an oral pill filled with powdered micropulverized progesterone but some were disappointed with the results. They claimed that progesterone, in oral form, tends to be converted into a water-soluble metabolite which is mostly excreted.

However, most progesterone given by mouth is first digested in the small intestines then passed through to the liver. One of the liver's tasks is to filter out and dispose of excess hormones and, once there, oral progesterone is converted into a water-soluble form and put back into the digestive tract. Here it blends with other chemicals and much of what remains of the hormone can be excreted instead of absorbed. To overcome this 'first-pass' phenomenon in the liver, oral progesterone has to be carefully 'packaged'. Even so, it can be hard to give small doses of the hormone by mouth and be sure about absorption, although some doctors still use larger quantities of progesterone in this form with good results. (It is worth remembering that the major success of the contraceptive Pill only happened because scientists developed a form of hormones which would be absorbed by the digestive system without being destroyed in the process.)

After much experimentation with various forms of the hormone the most successful and now the most widely used has turned out to be *transdermal* progesterone. Progesterone in a cream is applied to the skin which readily absorbs it and it is then distributed throughout the body. This form of the hormone can be derived from plants – most commonly from the wild yam.

Down in the Valley

The first progesterone which scientists experimented with had been derived from animal sources – mostly pig. It was therefore expensive. However, the exact same molecule you find in a woman's body can easily be made from plant sources. Plant-based hormone can be derived from *steroidal saponins* – compounds which are found in some foods – such as beans or yams as well as in many other herbs and wild plants. Many saponins resemble cholesterol, cortisone, oestrogen, progesterone and vitamin D. As such they are capable of acting as *exogenous* steroids (meaning from a source outside the body), helping to regulate the body's steroid hormonal actions as well as to protect it from the negative effects of stress. Some plants which boast hormone-regulating abilities are also *adaptogens*. This means they are capable of strengthening an organism's 'non-specific resistance' to ageing, illness and fatigue. These include many 'rejuvenating' plants such as ginseng, damiana and sarsaparilla – all of which are capable of enhancing the body's ability to adapt itself to all forms of stress while at the same time normalizing its biochemical activities. There are also literally thousands of plants which contain phyto-hormones or precursors to the body's natural hormones. They include liquorice, black cohosh, blue cohosh, squaw vine, false unicorn root, fenugreek and wild yam. One of the most important plants of all for women's health is the wild yam. One might call it the mother of progesterone, and among progesterone's many beneficial properties is an ability to balance excess oestrogen in the body thereby helping to protect against its side-effects, including cancer of the womb. Perhaps progesterone, reasoned Lee, would offer his osteoporosis patients on oestrogen replacement the protection they needed without the side-effects implicit in giving a synthetic progestogen.

Leap in the Dark

John Lee had spent some time gathering Ray Peat's references. He had also discovered many new ones too. He found that everything Peat had said about progesterone seemed to be true. It has hardly any side-effects and as far as its benefits were concerned they turned out to be far more than Lee had ever imagined. Progesterone helps the thyroid hormone do its job properly for instance. It protects against the oedema which excess oestrogen can cause and against the retention of sodium which results in waterlogging. It also helps keep cell membranes intact so they are not easily damaged by viruses or toxic substances from the air we breathe, the water we drink and the food we eat. Progesterone even exerts anti-ageing effects on skin. It is a natural anti-depressant and can restore lost libido. All of this sounded pretty good to Lee, so he suggested to his women patients who suffered from osteoporosis – whether or not they were taking oestrogen replacement – that they go to their pharmacy or their health food store, buy a jar of progesterone cream and try it for themselves.

About that time a new technique for measuring bone mineral density had been developed. It is called photon absorptiometry. Photon beams pass through skin and soft tissues but are reflected back by bone. The number of reflected photons can be counted as an indication of the density of bone mineral. The new technique enabled a technician to measure the bone mineral density of any woman to within 96 to 98 per cent of absolute accuracy. It was a real breakthrough. Methods in use before the 1980s were highly inaccurate. X-rays, for instance, besides subjecting women to doses of radiation, are not able to show a radiologist the degree of bone loss until it exceeds 30 per cent. And if a woman has a 30 per cent bone loss she already has a terrible risk of fracture.

Lee not only wanted to see what effect topically applied (i.e. on the surface of the skin) progesterone would have on women, he wanted accurate objective measurements of how progesterone, used regularly, would affect osteoporosis. So he persuaded his women patients to have bone mineral density tests done in this new way. He took measurements of bone mineral density before they began using progesterone cream and then again at intervals afterwards, and he kept extensive records of changes observed. All a woman had to do, in addition to taking a few vitamins and minerals, watching her diet and getting a bit of exercise, was to rub a little of the progesterone cream on to her skin once or twice a day. To Lee's amazement, six months to a year later not only had progesterone been able to protect these women from further bone mineral loss, it had actually *improved* the state of their bones.

Lee's discoveries about the reversal of osteoporosis using progesterone are rapidly changing the whole face of women's natural health care. For such improvement had never in medical history been recorded before. What had been already established was that oestrogen supplementation could *slow* bone loss to some degree by preventing some of the breakdown of old bone. But oestrogen can do nothing to create new bone once mineral loss has taken place. Progesterone can. John Lee's discovery took place more than ten years ago. Since then information about Lee's clinical studies using progesterone has been published in *The Lancet, International Clinical Nutritional Review,* and *Medical Hypothesis* as well as in many other journals, magazines and even in a few books. Still, however, John Lee's findings remain virtually unknown in the mainstream medical community. As yet, too, far too few women know enough about it all to be able to put progesterone to work to improve their own lives.

The Colour of Money

One of the closest molecular relatives to progesterone is the plant saponin known as diosgenin – well supplied by nature in the wild yam root. In a laboratory, this phyto-chemical is easily converted into progesterone – the exact same molecule you will find in your body. By further conversions it can also be changed into any number of other molecules, both into those which are molecularly identical to the body's own hormones and also into synthetic unique molecules which can be sold as drugs. In fact diosgenin is used by many pharmaceutical manufacturers to synthesize their hormone drugs. Drug companies have access to thousands of acres of wild yams from which they make their products. But why, John Lee asked himself, would pharmaceutical manufacturers forgo a perfectly natural hormone like progesterone, which is chemically identical to the body's own hormone and which offers all these benefits with no problems of safety and no negative side-effects, choosing instead to market products which are synthetic and which because they are foreign to the body carry potentially serious side-effects?

One reason comes to mind. Progesterone cannot be patented. Patent law lies behind the continuing insistence from the medical-industrial complex that drug-based HRT is the treatment of choice for just about every perimenopausal, menopausal and postmenopausal complaint you can imagine. Once you have synthesized a compound in the laboratory – once you have created a unique molecule – one which is not found in nature, you have a new *drug*. You can put a patent on it and you can *own* it. As soon as a company patents such a compound they can control its sales and its prices so nobody can undersell them. In fact nobody else can sell it at all for a number of years. This is what the pharmaceutical business is all about. And a very big business it is, with enormous profits.

Selling drugs is a very different kettle of fish to selling herbs, nutritional supplements or a generic hormone like progesterone. With a generic therapeutic substance such as vitamin C, vitamin D or natural progesterone, a company can sell it but it will never be able to acquire a patent on it since these are all compounds obtainable from nature and anybody else can sell them too. To do further medical research on a new use for a compound like progesterone would cost in the hundreds of thousands – as much as the research into a new drug does. If any pharmaceutical manufacturer were to undertake such research and spend the huge sums of money necessary to establish that progesterone is beneficial, the money they invested would be largely wasted because their competitors could then produce the same product and reap all the financial benefits without ever having spent a penny. So naturally pharmaceutical companies who manufacture contraceptives and HRT drugs choose instead to grow massive quantities of the Mexican wild yam, extract its diosgenin, turn it first into progesterone, then, by altering the molecule further, produce a unique and patentable synthetic drug. In fact, the seven most common progestogens used in the Pill and HRT are all synthesized either from the 21-carbon nucleus of progesterone or from the 19-carbon nucleus of the male hormone nortestosterone. Meanwhile natural progesterone never has been produced in a major way by a large drug company. For it will never be a patentable commodity from which a pharmaceutical manufacturer can derive big profits.

Pale Mimics

Although progesterone and the synthetic progestogens can both be made out of diosgenin taken from the Mexican wild yam, they have little in common in most of the actions they exert on the body. Both can sustain the lining of the womb – the secretory endometrium. Both also appear to offer some protection against cancer of the womb to a woman being given oestrogen replacement drugs. Beyond that, the synthetics differ as dramatically from the real thing as night from day. Where the natural hormone given during pregnancy protects the development of the foetus and is used to guard against miscarriage, medroxyprogesterone – a commonly used progestogen – carries a warning that its use during pregnancy may increase the risk of early abortion as well as birth defects. Dosage of synthetic hormones when they are given as HRT needs to be carefully controlled since, unlike natural progesterone, they become more toxic the more you take. By contrast, progesterone is safe regardless of dose. Although by now thousands of women have used natural progesterone for many years, doctors with expertise in its use have not found it to be toxic at any levels. Ray Peat confirms these findings from animal studies: 'Animals are generally more sensitive to progesterone than humans are,' he says, 'and in animals no toxic level has been found, except that in the highest doses it is anaesthetic. In humans, even this effect has never been reported in the medical literature, and it is clearly anti-toxic in nature. Besides preventing acute poisoning of many kinds, it also reduces the incidence of birth defects and cancer.'

Yet because of the confusion over the definition of progesterone, and the fact that the word is so frequently misused, even many doctors learning about the side-effects of the progestogens wrongly assume that they also apply to progesterone. You can still hear so-called experts in women's health claim that natural progesterone is dangerous – that it causes dangerous irregular bleeding or migraine, depression, weight gain, painful breasts and leg cramps – when in fact not one of these things is true. Even many of the library and computer references to research and clinical studies refer to the dangers of 'progesterone'. However when you go back to the papers themselves and look carefully to see what researchers were actually using, without exception you find that what in the references has been called 'progesterone' turns out not to have been the natural hormone at all but one of the synthetic progestogens. This is a major reason why the majority of doctors remain ignorant of progesterone's power.

Women using a progesterone product consistently report a sense of increased energy and wellbeing both mentally and physically. However, the official product information on Provera, issued to doctors by its manufacturer Upjohn, contains a list of contra-indications and adverse reaction warnings wide-ranging enough that were prospective women users to read it while sitting in their GP's waiting room, many, I suspect, would have some very searching questions for their doctor (see pp. 428–429).

From the Horse's Mouth

Since his first successes with the natural hormone John Lee has recommended progesterone in cream form to hundreds of doctors and thousands of women. But it is primarily the women themselves who pass on the good news to one another by word of mouth. It is also they who have reported back to Lee and other professionals on the hormone's remarkable effects. Like the French surgeon Michel Odent, who claims he learned about childbirth by watching women give birth and listening to what they could tell him about their experience, Lee has learned most of what he knows about progesterone from women themselves. Many using the cream have found their hypothyroidism disappeared as their bone densities went up. Aches and pains in the body also often vanish. Women report they feel calmer and stronger and their skin improves. It was also from women using progesterone cream that Lee learned about a phenomenon called *oestrogen rebound* (see p. 441).

When you first use a progesterone cream it can make you temporarily more sensitive to the oestrogens in your body so for a short time symptoms such as breast tenderness can get worse. This is because oestrogen and progesterone, while antagonistic in some actions, are synergistic in others. Alter the level of one and you affect the actions of the other. This means some women get temporary breast swelling, tenderness or other signs of excess oestrogens right at the beginning of using progesterone. These symptoms soon pass as the oestrogen dominance disappears and the system rebalances itself. Lee also discovered from working with his patients that the presence of adequate progesterone in a woman's body means that her need for oestrogen is automatically reduced. So, Lee believes, if a doctor decides to give progesterone to a woman on oestrogen replacement he will need to cut her dose of oestrogen in half or more. She will then get all the benefits of oestrogen replacement – but in a much lower (and much *safer*) dose. Most women taking progesterone, however, find they need no extra oestrogen at all since progesterone can be converted into oestrogen by the body.

Lee observed that a simple progesterone cream rubbed on a woman's body eliminated the excess facial hair which some women develop as they get older and the weakened nails and loss of hair from the head which others experience postmenopausally. Many of his women patients reported that after using the cream the hair on their heads grew thicker. He learned too, that women who before had relied on diuretics to prevent water retention usually didn't need them any more. Progesterone is a natural diuretic. He found frequently that women with high blood pressure no longer needed to take their hypertension medication. Many women on thyroid medication no longer need treatment either since progesterone makes the body's use of its own thyroid much more efficient.

The Champions

Now that John Lee has retired he continues to learn more and more about progesterone from doctors, biochemists and – still most important of all – the women who use it. They come to him for information, for help and to share knowledge about diet, lifestyle changes and other factors which can help revolutionize the lives of menstruating women as well as their menopausal and postmenopausal sisters. Lee frequently receives letters and phone calls from medical colleagues who, coming upon the wonders of natural progesterone for the first time, are astounded. 'My God, it works!' reported one doctor from New York City. She had pooh-poohed the whole idea of using a progesterone cream when a patient first told her about it. 'First of all you can't absorb hormones through the skin,' her doctor had argued. Then she said, 'Anyway, you can't get proper hormones from a wild yam.' Her patient pointed out that this is exactly where many major pharmaceutical companies get theirs – by growing wild yams from which they derive progesterone which they then sell to other pharmaceutical manufacturers for use in making synthetic progestogens. 'Well I just don't think it will work,' insisted the doctor. 'Do you mind if I try it for three months?' asked her patient, a woman who had fibrocystic breast disease, ovarian cysts and endometrial thickening together with fibroid tumours. The doctor agreed, 'OK, you can do it for three months. But if the tests show any positive results, I will personally eat the report.'

The patient used the progesterone for three months. Her fibrocystic breast disease vanished. The ovarian cysts went away and the fibroids shrank by 18 per cent – all of which showed up clearly on sonograms and mammograms. Delighted, the woman rang John Lee to report her success and to tell him all that had been said. Lee asked, 'What are you going to do?' The woman replied, 'I'm just on my way to my doctor's office. I am going to sit there until she eats the medical reports.'

Living in Time

It is in many ways not surprising that most of the medical profession remains ignorant about the powers of progesterone. In the last half of the twentieth century scientific and medical knowledge is changing so rapidly that it is almost impossible for anyone to keep up with what is taking place. John Lee recalls that, when he attended the twentieth class reunion of his medical school, the University Dean told doctors in attendance that the half-life of what is now taught in medical schools is only about ten or fifteen years: ten or fifteen years after a doctor leaves medical school half of what he has been taught will be found to be wrong in one way or another. The Dean said he had known at the time they graduated from medical school that half of the things that they had been taught would turn out to be wrong. The problem was nobody could tell which half. 'Next year, when I attend my fortieth class reunion,' muses Lee, 'I suspect he will say that the half-life of medical information is down to six or seven years because of the accelerated rate at which things now change.'

So when you ask your doctor what he thinks of natural progesterone don't be surprised if he doesn't know what you are talking about, or if he makes the mistake of confusing the natural hormone with synthetic progestogens, or if he lumps them all together as 'progesterone'. And reporters in the media and writers of books on women's health can sometimes be as uninformed as scientists and doctors. For instance, after wrestling with the whole question of progesterone and its synthetic analogues, Gail Sheehy, author of the well-known book on menopause *The Silent Passage*, admitted to being so confused about names that she decided to call all of them 'progesterone' throughout the book – even though most of what she has written refers not to progesterone but to the synthetic progestogens.

Given progesterone's ability to enhance women's health it might be easy to fall into the trap of believing it to be some kind of miracle cure-all which will solve your problems while you go on living a stressful life that doesn't feed your soul, swigging back the gin, smoking like a chimney and going on and off crash diets. It most certainly will not. Although it is central to the bloodless revolution, progesterone is but one important piece in the natural menopause puzzle. For this natural hormone to yield up the finest it has to offer a woman in terms of enhanced health and emotional wellbeing, it needs to be joined together with all the other pieces as well – specific nutrients which facilitate progesterone working in the body fully, and the use of specific herbs and plants and brain-enhancing metabolites as well as the best that leading-edge energy medicine can bring. Finally it needs to be placed within a much larger context that examines not only an individual woman's health but her relationship to her own deepest values, to the environment in which she lives and to the health of the planet. All of these things must work together to help women make menopause a true passage to power. None the less, given all that natural progesterone has to offer a woman, one big question arises. Why should any woman need progesterone anyway? In search of an answer we need first to examine the whole process of hormone cycles in a woman's body going back to long before menopause arrives.

Chapter Five

Cycles of the Moon

Like the moon's waxing and waning or the snake which sheds its skin to be born anew, woman is a cyclical creature. Both the fecundity of the moon and the snake's bondage to the changes of life through time are endemic to her nature. They are, in fact, so much a part of our make up that seldom do we stop to think about them. Yet both depend upon the almost infinitely complex multiple interactions of hormones within our bodies. In short, hormones matter a lot. An awareness of the profound influence they exert on a woman's health and emotions is essential to making menopause a passage to power rather than a source of misery. So complicated are the interactions between hormones in the human body that many are still not understood by science. But bear with me while we explore the basics. Some of what follows may sound a bit like one of those children's manuals on sex but it really is important to understand how the main steroid hormones in your body act and interact if you are to maximize your health and make of menopause an adventure instead of a catalogue of miseries.

Spiritual Interface

So central are hormonal events to how women think and feel that it would be no exaggeration to say the female endocrine system is an interface between body and spirit. Even our hopes and dreams are echoed in surges of hormones and in their shifting patterns – much as chords and rhythms develop into the themes and movements of a symphony. Changes in hormonal balance from day to day – even from moment to moment – can not only alter the way you feel emotionally, they can even affect your view of reality. Whether you see life as a challenge to be met or a source of constant misery and disappointment can also be reflected in hormone shifts. This is why hormonal imbalances create such emotional and spiritual agonies in women such as those associated with PMS or menopausal symptoms.

The psychic and spiritual aspects of a woman's hormonal interactions are all too often forgotten living within the confines of the mechanistic thinking that rules our society. Instead of recognizing the changes in mood and personality as natural to any cyclical creature, we tend to think we should always be the same – always rational, reliable, reasonable and steady. Meanwhile synthetic hormones continue to be doled out to us from puberty onwards, with no respect for a woman's cyclical nature and little concern for the long-term consequences these chemicals can have on our health and emotions. There is, I believe, far too little awareness of the way in which the use of one or two artificial hormones year after year may not only undermine our long-term health but can also affect a woman's ability to fulfil her potential and may even impede her spiritual development.

I Excite

The word hormone comes from a Greek word, *hormao*, which means 'I excite', and this is exactly what hormones do. They are messenger chemicals made in minute quantities in the brain or in special endocrine glands such as the thyroid, adrenals, pancreas and ovaries – sometimes even in fat cells – and then carried by the bloodstream to distant parts of the body where they control, activate and direct the ever-changing system and organ functions, urges and feelings which *are* you. Your body is continually creating new hormones out of amino acids, peptides and cholesterol in the presence of certain vitamins and minerals – all in response to its specific needs. Hormones are also continually being destroyed – that is metabolized and removed from your system – as your need for one or another of them changes. All this happens in much the same way that a theme or cadence in a piece of music gives way to the next. So rapidly can hormonal shifts take place and so closely interwoven is the endocrine system with your thoughts, feelings and external events, that measurements of oestrogen or progesterone levels can differ drastically when taken only an hour apart.

Hormones perform many tasks. Some help produce or store energy, some trigger growth, or balance blood sugar, some affect your water balance, others your metabolic rate. Still others regulate respiration, cell metabolism or neural activity. It is the task of the steroid hormones – from the oestrogens and progesterone to the anti-inflammatory cortisol and hormones which affect brain and mood – that we are mostly concerned with here. They are nature's servants for regulating sex and reproduction as well as for balancing brain chemistry and helping the body handle stress without succumbing to illness. Although they are only produced in small doses, steroids pack a big wallop. Each is highly specific in its actions. Each hormone will only excite the particular cells it is designed to affect.

A molecule of a certain hormone – take progesterone or DHEA – has a unique shape. It will be ignored by all receptor molecules (keyholes on the cells) as it travels through your body until it is at last recognized by the particular receptor molecule with which it is meant to connect. Into this receptor site in cells, and into it alone, the hormone molecule fits perfectly, just the way a key does in its lock. So powerful are a hormone's actions that your body only needs to make minute quantities of each as they are required. For instance, at any moment there may be as little as one molecule of a particular hormone to every fifty thousand million other molecules in your bloodstream. This is how powerful hormones can be and why giving relatively large quantities of synthetic hormones can be potentially so damaging to the body. The body's production of hormones and the way in which the relationship between them is continuously adjusted relies on complex interactions involving your pituitary (a tiny gland at the base of your brain) and your hypothalamus, often called the master gland, as well as other glands such as the adrenals.

Let's look at the hormonal symphony which is played between the major sex hormones oestrogen and progesterone – not in your forties or fifties when you are most likely to be faced with symptoms that can cause you grief, but long before. For it is how you live during the menstrual years – the way you eat, how you use your body, and the decisions you make about what medications you take or don't take – that sets the stage for a trouble-free natural menopause.

Moon Cycles and Ovarian Rites

Only since the late nineteenth century have women's menstrual cycles – the *menses* – been investigated scientifically. The name menses also comes from a Greek word meaning month. It in turn is derived from an even older word meaning moon. Quite literally the menses is the period of waxing and waning between one new moon and the next. Once menstruation begins at puberty which is a woman's first rite of passage, the ebbs and flows which her body goes through each month are the stuff of which the second movement in her life's hormonal symphony is made. This part of her life has one principal goal – childbearing. And its success depends greatly upon the two major steroids – the oestrogens and progesterone – working in close communication with her body's chief control centres, the pituitary and hypothalamus.

The hypothalamus is the control centre. It balances and oversees biochemical and energetic changes throughout the body. The limbic system in which it sits is the most primitive part of the brain. It is the part which deals with emotions and with our sense of smell, with our passions and with all the unconscious interfaces that take place between mind and body. The actions of the limbic system lie beneath the level of the thinking mind. This is one of the reasons that the hypothalamus is often referred to as the 'seat of emotions'. When excited, the hypothalamus triggers desire – for food, for water, for adventure, for sex. Its actions can also be influenced by inhibitory thought patterns. In a woman frightened of becoming pregnant, for instance, the fear itself – via the hypothalamus – can dampen sexual desire or even disrupt menstrual cycles so she remains barren.

The hypothalamus even reacts to bodily changes that take place as a result of meditation. Its activities are influenced by spiritual practices which is a major reason why women who meditate regularly tend to develop greater emotional balance, as well as why repeated experiences of joy or stillness can dramatically improve various female complaints such as PMS and hot flushes in both menstruating and menopausal women.

Sacred Cycles

There are three main branches of the female endocrine system involved in menstruation. The first is the control centre, the hypothalamus. It releases hormones with complicated names that you certainly don't need to remember, including gonadotrophic hormone (GnRH). The second branch is the anterior pituitary which releases follicle-stimulating hormone (FSH) and luteinizing hormone (LH) – both of which are secreted in response to GnRH from the hypothalamus. The third branch is made up of the oestrogens and progesterone which during a woman's non-pregnant childbearing years are secreted by the ovaries in response to FSH and LH. What is important to understand is just how complex and interlaced the actions of these hormones are.

All the hormones released during a menstrual cycle are secreted not in a constant, steady way but at dramatically different rates during different parts of the 28-day period, a cycle which like everything else in the natural world involves birth, maturation and death, only to lead to new birth again – in this case the egg a woman's body produces. Menstruation itself is simply the elimination of the thickened blood and blood-filled endometrium in the womb – the lining developed in preparation for a possible pregnancy. When a pregnancy does not occur this lining is shed at monthly intervals under the control of oestrogen and progesterone with a little help from their friends GnRH, FSH and LH. When ovaries are not stimulated by the gonadotrophic hormones from the pituitary they remain asleep, as they were during childhood and as they become again after menopause.

For the first eight to eleven days of the menstrual cycle a woman's ovaries make lots of oestrogen. It is oestrogen which prepares the follicle (a small excretory sac or gland) for the release of one of the eggs. The word *oestrogen*, like the hormones produced in a woman's body which belong to this family – oestrone, oestradiol and oestriol – comes from *oestrus*, a Greek word meaning frenzy, heat or fertility. It is oestrogen which proliferates the changes that take place at puberty – the growth of breasts, the development of a girl's reproductive system, the reshaping of a woman's body.

Each girl baby is born with all the primary follicles she will ever need. At the time of puberty a girl's ovaries contain about 300,000 of these follicles. And while each woman only produces one or two fully developed eggs each month, somewhere between 100 and 300 follicles have to start developing in order for one to become fully grown. This is why a woman can lose between 100 and 300 follicles a month. However, since she started with 300,000 she will have enough to last all her reproductive life.

On day one of each monthly cycle – that is the day of the onset of menstruation – hormones trigger a group of ovarian follicles, causing accelerated growth in the cells surrounding them. As cells around the eggs grow they secrete fluid which contains a high concentration of the oestrogen oestradiol to bring about many other changes, developing the potential of the egg so that it becomes capable of being fertilized by the male sperm.

It is not only the oestradiol secreted by the follicle which brings about the maturation of the egg. The interaction of this hormone with other reproductive hormones helps the process along until after a week or more when one of the follicles outgrows all the rest. This is the one that will become the female egg ready for impregnation, and so the final follicular growth can be completed and *ovulation* occur – that is the release of the egg into the fallopian tubes for its journey down into the uterus. Ovulation takes place, usually around the fourteenth day, in the middle of your cycle.

Enter Progesterone

The rate of oestrogen secretion begins to fall on about day thirteen, one day before ovulation occurs. As small amounts of progesterone begin to be secreted very rapid growth of the follicle takes place. Beginning with this secretion of progesterone ovulation occurs too. During the first few hours after the ovum has been expelled from the follicle more and more rapid physical and chemical changes take place to the egg in a process called luteinization. At this stage – known as the *luteal stage* of a woman's cycle – the follicle becomes known as the *corpus luteum* or yellow body. The cells around the follicle begin to secrete larger quantities of progesterone as the level of oestrogen decreases. Some of the cells around the follicle become much enlarged. They develop inclusions of lipids or fats which give them their distinctive yellow colour. From now on development becomes rapid until seven or eight days after ovulation when it peaks.

Ovulation changes the whole ball game. No longer is there a need for further build up of the womb lining. The challenge now is to hold on to the secretory endometrium and to render it capable of nurturing a fertilized egg long enough for it to grow into a baby. That is progesterone's task – and remember that progesterone is only secreted when you ovulate.

The corpus luteum which forms each month is a tiny organ with a huge capacity for hormone production. It releases large quantities of progesterone plus some oestrogen which cause a feedback decrease in the secretion of pituitary hormone, so that no new follicles begin to grow. But as soon as the corpus luteum degenerates at the end of its twelve-day life – which is about the 26th day of the female sexual cycle – this lack of feedback triggers the anterior pituitary gland to secrete several times as much FSH, followed a few days later by more LH as well. This in turn stimulates the growth of new follicles to begin the next ovarian cycle. And at the same time, a fall in progesterone and in oestrogen secretion triggers menstruation.

Peaks and Falls

From day one until about day thirteen of a woman's menstrual cycle the level of progesterone in her body is very, very low. Yet at the point at which a follicle is released it continues to rise dramatically until day 21 to 23 when it begins to fall again to its lowest level as menstruation begins around day 28. In addition to maintaining the endometrium and shifting down activity in the other ovary, the progesterone provided each month travels to other parts of a woman's body to fulfil other roles. It protects her from the many negative effects of oestrogen dominance by balancing the oestrogen in her body. Progesterone also brings surges of libido. You still hear a few experts say that oestrogen increases libido. But think about it. Which hormone would you rely on for sex-drive – oestrogen which is present *before* the egg is made, or progesterone which comes *after* the egg is released and is ready for fertilization? Libido increases with progesterone surges.

When this rhythmic cycling of oestrogen and progesterone during each lunar month gets out of sync (and many things in modern life can cause this), then all sorts of things can go wrong – from infertility to PMS, depression, bloating, endometriosis and fibroids. For the oestrogens and progesterone each have their characteristic roles to play and for a woman to be healthy they must balance each other.

The Last and the First

So do all the other steroids. This group of hormones to which cortisol, aldosterone, progesterone, DHEA, testosterone and the oestrogens belong is intimately involved in how you feel both physically and emotionally as well as how rapidly your body ages. Steroids have a characteristic molecular structure which resembles cholesterol, from which they are all ultimately derived. Cholesterol is the vital fatty substance that has had such a bad press in recent years but which is absolutely essential to life. Out of each steroid hormone made from cholesterol yet another and another can be made in a knock-on effect. For instance, pregnenolone is the steroid manufactured directly from cholesterol. It in turn becomes a precursor to progesterone as well as to many other hormones (see diagram on opposite page).

Natural steroid hormones such as progesterone made by biosynthesis in your own body have a remarkable capability to act as precursors. In other words they are capable of being

Pregnenolone   17α-hydroxypregnenolone   Deyhydroepiandrosterone   Androstenediol

Progesterone   17α-hydroxyprogesterone   Androstenedione   Testosterone

11-deoxycorticosterone   11-deoxycortisol   Estrone   Estradiol

Corticosterone   Cortisol   Estriol

18-hydroxycorticosterone   Aldosterone   Steroidogenesis pathways

Every hormone in the shaded area can be made by your body from progesterone. If you don't have enough progesterone then you may not be able to produce enough of the anti-inflammatory hormones such as cortisol, as well as other hormones which affect brain and mood. (From Natural Progesterone *by John Lee MD, BLL Publishing, 1993.)*

turned into other hormones further down the pathways as and when your body needs them. Progesterone is the mother of many other hormones. It can eventually be turned not only into various oestrogens but also into cortisol (the anti-inflammatory hormone) and into other steroids such as corticosterone or aldosterone with equally important jobs to do. All of these conversions happen through slight alterations in the shape of a molecule thanks to the actions of enzymes, each of which carries out a specific task. But these conversions can only take place if the molecules on which the enzyme is acting 'fit' precisely. All of these changes which take place through the magic of enzymes occur in the presence of vitamin and mineral co-factors such as magnesium, zinc and B6 which catalyse each enzyme reaction. Like the menstrual cycle, they too are carefully modulated by elaborate feedback mechanisms. The names and chemical transformations from one steroid to another are not important to remember. Again, what is important is that you get some sense of just how complex hormone synthesis and interactions can be and how important it is to have sufficient co-factors as well as 'primary' hormones such as pregnenolone and progesterone to be able to synthesize others. A rich hormonal symphony? Immeasurably. Yet all this still does not take into account the myriad pathways by which these steroid hormones interact with other hormones or master central mechanisms within the hypothalamus and pituitary or psychoneuroimmunological pathways by which hormones affect our emotions and emotions our hormones.

Sabotage

It is in coming face to face with the rich textures of such hormonal symphonies that the synthetic progestogen drugs can come a cropper. When you look at the structures of their molecules, you find that although they resemble the body's homemade hormones their shapes have been altered slightly by adding extra atoms here or there at unusual positions. It is this that has enabled them to qualify as patentable drugs.

However, unlike the natural hormones (which they attempt to mimic and which not only fulfil their own functions by binding with their own receptor sites but also act as precursors for a myriad of other hormones with other important jobs to do), the progestogens are *end-product molecules*. They are also completely foreign to the living body. Unlike nature's own steroids they cannot be augmented or diminished as necessary to maintain balance and to keep the body's hormonal symphony flowing smoothly. They also cannot easily be eliminated when their levels get too high. Like the xenoestrogens in our environment, although the synthetics can still bind with the receptor sites of the hormones they are made to mimic, they don't fit as well as the homemade steroids do into the enzymes meant to act upon them. This means they are not under the watchful eye and control of these enzymes, nor of the body's self-regulating capacities. This is why drug-based oestrogens and progestogens in contraceptives and HRT cocktails can significantly disrupt a woman's normal hormonal cycles by introducing foreign elements into her body. They also virtually wipe out the moon cycles to which a woman's natural fertility and spiritual balance are inexorably bound from puberty onward. So, although in the short term they may do a job such as provide birth control or quell heavy bleeding or hot flushes in a menopausal woman, in the long run they only sabotage hormone balance.

Friends and Lovers

Quite apart from their biochemical actions, rather like people, hormones have characters with highly individual personalities. To the biochemist the 'personalities' of the oestrogens and progesterone will always remain a mystery. The biochemist is interested in nothing beyond their molecular configurations. But many women come to know these personalities well – by allowing intuition and instinct to be their teachers. When progesterone is surging through the body a woman can feel high. Provided her body is producing enough of this steroid she is likely to feel great. Your senses are keen when progesterone is running. Smells smell sweeter – or more horrible. Touching, sensing, tasting, hearing are all richer experiences than usual. In the presence of progesterone women have a desire to *do* something, to create something, to work in the garden, to dance or sing a song, or make love. Sometimes progesterone surges can feel like falling in love. This can happen during the luteal phase of the menstrual cycle after ovulation when the follicle turns into the yellow body or corpus luteum but it becomes far more intense when you are pregnant. It is a high level of progesterone that makes a woman feel on top of the world during the last months of pregnancy. At this time the placenta churns out an amazing 300 to 400 milligrams per day of the steroid. During the luteal phase of your menstrual cycle it will have only been producing 20 milligrams or so a day.

I suspect that among those women who seem to get pregnant over and over and who so love the whole experience, you are likely to find high progesterone levels. You also find them in women who have trouble-free menstruation. Sadly the opposite is true too. When progesterone is low – as it is in a growing number of women who have become oestrogen dominant – women never seem to feel well even during pregnancy. Many have all sorts of trouble with their female organs and cycles including PMS – sometimes from puberty right through to death.

When Oestrogens Flow

The oestrogens have quite a different character. When oestrogens peak in the menstrual cycle just before the 'fall' of ovulation a woman feels less independent. She is more willing to adjust herself to the needs of others. When the oestrogens are running, women like to attract a mate not so much to draw him into her body as to comfort, admire and care for her. Her ovaries seem to be smiling – 'Whatever you want, I'm happy to give' they seem to say. A few women who by nature are high oestrogen producers feel quite dependent on others for approval, and for the definition of their being. While such an experience can be lovely and make a woman feel highly 'feminine' it can also go too far. However, in these women, when menopause finally arrives and oestrogen levels drop dramatically, often they find to their surprise and delight that for the first time in their lives they feel complete in themselves – as though they don't need anybody else to validate their lives. Provided they are otherwise well, menopause can be sheer joy in the sense of freedom it brings to these women, once they get over the shock of being such a 'different person'.

From a biological point of view there are many important actions that progesterone and oestrogen exert upon the body and psyche. Since these are little known among women and doctors alike it is worth looking at a few (see below).

Effects of Progesterone	Effects of Oestrogen
Increases libido	Decreases libido
Prevents cancer of the womb	Increases risk of womb cancer
Protects against fibrocystic breast disease	Stimulates breast cell activity
Helps protect against breast cancer	Increases risk of breast cancer
Maintains the lining of the uterus	Proliferates the lining of the uterus
Stimulates the building of new bone	Slows down the resorption of old bone
Strengthens skin	Thins skin
Is a natural diuretic	Encourages salt and water retention
Anti-depressant	Can produce headaches and depression
Encourages fat burning and the use of stored energy	Lays down fat stores
Normalizes blood clotting	Increases blood clotting
Concerned with procreation and survival of the foetus	Concerned with the development and release of the egg
Precursor to important stress hormones	End-molecule steroids

The reproductive hormonal menstrual cycle of a woman between puberty and the menarche is a superbly ordered natural work of art. It becomes so much a part of our lives that unless we have some particular difficulties with PMS or fertility we hardly give it any thought. Not, that is, until things begin to alter. Once they do – in most women some time between the age of forty and fifty – they usually change gradually until finally a woman senses that something deep in her being has shifted. Such feelings herald the coming of menopause – the third phase of a woman's life.

Chapter Six

Crazed Woman

There are many bizarre ironies surrounding HRT. For example, despite all the glossy pamphlets and pro-HRT articles in newspapers and women's magazines, most women – including those who actually take HRT – are enormously ill-informed about what it is and why they are taking it. In one national opinion survey of over 1,000 women on the treatment most claimed that they were taking it in order to help them stay young and sexually attractive, something which it most decidedly does not do. Only 3 per cent of the women polled were the least concerned that it might reduce the risk of a heart attack (the reason for which it is currently being aggressively marketed), while two-thirds did not even know the cause of menopause. No wonder there are so many crazed women trying to make sense of it. Let's look at HRT, how it came into being, and what is being claimed for it by whom.

Just what is HRT anyway? Based on the assumption that menopause is not a natural occurrence in which hormonal changes take place in a woman's body, but an oestrogen deficiency disease – much as hypothyroidism is a thyroid deficiency disease – HRT is an attempt to restore hormonal 'normality' by *replacing* the hormone or hormones that are deemed to be missing in perimenopausal, menopausal and postmenopausal women. HRT comes in four presentations – tablets, implants, creams and patches. Tablets are most commonly used in three- or four-week packs. Creams are sometimes described for women whose main difficulty is either vaginal itching or dryness or inflammations of the urinary system. Patches are put on like plasters, generally to the lower abdomen, and then changed every three or four days. HRT also comes in four main forms:

- giving oestrogen alone, which is called *unopposed oestrogen.*
- *opposed sequential therapy* where oestrogen is given for a period followed by a shorter period where a progestogen is given.

- *opposed continuous combined therapy* where both oestrogen and a progestogen are given at the same time.
- giving a *progestogen alone.*

Within each category there are numerous drugs in different combinations which a doctor can choose from. For an unopposed oestrogen regime, for instance, he might use conjugated equine oestrogen in doses of between 0.3 to 1.25 mg a day, or oestradiol valerate in a dose of 1–2 mg a day, or an implant of micronized oestradiol or some form of transdermal oestrogen. If he decides to give opposed sequential therapy he might choose transdermal oestradiol together with norethisterone acetate, or conjugated equine oestrogen together with medroxyprogesterone acetate, or oestradiol with norethisterone acetate and so on. The possibilities are many. Each drug company promotes its own packages and each doctor has his or her favourite treatment programme.

Hobson's Choice

Because there are many unpleasant as well as dangerous side-effects to the hormones used in HRT, and because such problems as the development of endometrial cancer have been shown to be directly related to the levels of oestrogen a woman is given, most doctors try to use as little of the drugs as possible to get results. After all there would seem little purpose in putting a woman on oestrogen for 20 years in an attempt to protect her from osteoporosis if she ends up developing cancer of the womb in the process. But any doctor prescribing HRT is faced with a delicate balancing act in which there are many unknowns. For each drug used in any of these combinations of treatments will affect different women in different ways and each drug has its own list of characteristic possible side-effects.

In Britain, as in many industrialized countries of the world, the popularity of HRT is still growing. In a recent four-year period the number of British women choosing to take hormones more than doubled. In 1990 only 9 per cent of postmenopausal women took HRT, but by 1993, 18 per cent did. Pharmaceutical companies hope by the millennium to have more than 50 per cent of menopausal women in Britain on HRT. Many doctors insist that HRT is likely to be 'the most important advance in preventative medicine in the western world for half a century'. They proselytize that it is through taking hormone drugs that postmenopausal women are going to be able to safeguard their bones and hearts. So powerful is the HRT rhetoric and so widespread has this message become that, as American physician Christiane Northrup, author of *Women's Bodies, Women's Wisdom*, says, 'By combining so-called medical "fact" with fear, an entire new generation of women is being brainwashed that ERT [HRT] is the gold standard – "Don't leave menopause without it." The current "medicalization" of menopause has been so successful that most women's own menopausal wisdom and trust in their bodies to remain healthy during this natural life-stage is almost nonexistent . . . The rare woman who wants to get through menopause *without* oestrogen replacement now has to fear that she may not be making the right choice. She doesn't get the cultural seal of approval that she would get if she were on ERT.'

Despite the impression created that HRT is both a miracle of modern science and an essential treatment for menopausal women, there is much evidence that once the immediate flush of excitement over a new treatment and all the promises it carries is over, women's experience of HRT does not back up these assertions. A recent Swedish survey of the university town Linkoping has shown that there, as in other countries such as New Zealand, 49 per cent of the women who go on HRT stop taking the drugs within a year. Many starting on HRT initially experience a kind of euphoria, primarily because the one thing that oestrogen replacement gets rid of almost immediately is the hot flushes that may have been disturbing sleep and contributing to exhaustion. Many women report that a few months later their experience of HRT has worsened dramatically because of side-effects like mood swings, decreased control over the bladder, fatigue and headaches. The most common side-effects which women complain of are migraine, depression, bleeding, water retention, increased blood pressure, weight gain, thrush, breast problems, varicose veins and chest pains. Some researchers believe that the depression that frequently follows in the wake of HRT may to some extent be a result of disappointment at its not having lived up to expectations. According to a British study, among the reasons women give for giving up HRT are these: about half stop taking it because of side-effects, about one-fifth because they are advised to do so by their doctors, and about one-third either because they are afraid of long-term consequences such as cancer or because HRT has shown itself to be ineffective in helping them.

Chemical Addictions

For some women addiction is the worst problem that arises on HRT. Researchers S. Bewley and T.H. Bewley recently reported in *The Lancet* that oestrogens like other drugs which are potentially addictive and abusive, have the potential to cause symptoms of both tolerance and withdrawal. Advocates of HRT strongly deny that this is so. Other researchers have established that the use of oestrogen implants can result in a build-up of what is called *supraphysiological* oestrogens in the body of a woman receiving HRT and lead to a diminished responsiveness (known as *tachyphylaxis*) to increasing amounts of physiologically active substances. It is a phenomenon which hormone drugs appear to share with other drugs already known to be addictive.

There is another issue in relation to the use of Premarin – whose name gives clear indication from where it is derived (PREgnant MARes urINe) – that women and animal rights groups object to. They are troubled by the conditions under which the horses used to collect the hormone are held. In a recent editorial in *Townsend Letter for Doctors*, American physician Alan R. Gaby MD writes 'the way the horses are treated in the production process is anything but "natural". To produce the drug, horses are impregnated, then fitted with a rubber collection device so that all of their urine can be collected . . . the mares are then forced to stand on concrete floors in stalls measuring just 8 feet long and 3½ feet wide for most of their 11 month pregnancies. This is because allowing the mares to roam about in the pasture might result in the loss of precious urine, which is worth $17 a gallon to Wyeth-Ayerst Laboratories, the makers of Premarin.' The horses' physical confinement makes it virtually impossible for them to turn around or even to lie down properly, according to the American animal rights organization PETA – People for the Ethical Treatment of Animals. This, they claim, results in some of the mares becoming crippled while occasionally an animal dies. Soon after giving birth, say PETA, the foals are taken from their mothers who are impregnated yet again. Some of the foals, they say, are killed immediately, others are fattened and slaughtered or retained to replace the burnt-out mares from which they came.

Risk-Benefit Assessments

It is very hard to sort out the benefits that are quoted by HRT supporters from the risks. Proselytizers for HRT often refer to follow-up studies done on American postmenopausal women who took oestrogen a decade or more ago. They are all studies which are highly prone to bias since the women studied tended to come from a higher socio-economic group and as such were likely to be healthier in the first place than women from the lower socio-economic groups. When it comes to looking at the effects of hormone treatments it has always been difficult to do randomized studies – that is studies in which women enter a trial without knowing whether or not they will be put into the group which will take HRT or the control group which will not. Women just won't go for it. When it comes to examining the results of studies which have been carried out it is important to remember that the hormonal mixtures being prescribed now differ tremendously from the formulations that were used in the 1960s, 1970s and 1980s. We really have no way of quantifying what the long-term effects of HRT are on women's health.

None the less, medical and commercial apostles for HRT continue to back up their assertions by referring to all sorts of follow-up studies of American postmenopausal women on oestrogen. One major thing that they claim now is that HRT can decrease a woman's risk of suffering a heart attack or stroke by 50 per cent as well as reduce the chance of fractures from osteoporosis. Before going any further it is important to take a look at what they are claiming. Fifty per cent sounds a lot and makes you think of 50 out of 100 women are going to be safer if they take HRT. This is not the case. What is really being claimed does not amount to much. Statistics show that, in general, women between the ages of 65 and 75 in industrialized countries have a 6 per cent relative risk of heart disease. Translated into real people this means that 6 out of every 100 women are at risk of having heart problems at some time in their lives. A 50 per cent reduction in the number of women at risk would mean that instead of 6 women out of every 100 running the risk of heart problems this figure is reduced to 3 women per 100 – a long way from the 50 out of 100 women that is commonly perceived when 50 per cent reductions in risk are talked about.

The force of the assertions about the ability of various forms of HRT to give a woman long-term protection against degenerative diseases, the complacent manner in which they are made and the way they are attributed to numerous frequently cited studies, often bear little relationship to the facts stated when you scrutinize closely the studies quoted and the overall conclusions drawn from them. For instance, the study most often cited to back up the assertion that HRT protects against heart disease was carried out in the United States on 48,470 nurses and reported in 1971. It mentions a decreased risk of major or fatal heart disease in oestrogen users. When you look closely at the coronary risk factors of the study you realize that the decreased cardiovascular disease among HRT users is likely to have little to do with the HRT these women were taking but a great deal to do with the fact that they came from a self-selected group of healthy women with less severe vascular risk to begin with, and that the women studied, unlike the general population, all had a continued commitment to preventative medicine in general. Carol Ann Rinzler, author of *Estrogen and Breast Cancer: A Warning To Women*, describes this phenomenon well when she says: 'It might look as though estrogen kept a woman healthy when in fact it was just the other way around: healthy women took estrogen.'

Meanwhile the believers in oestrogen drugs seem occasionally to behave like ostriches – burying their heads in the ground and ignoring the fact that oestrogen in the contraceptive pill has already been credited with thrombosis in women who smoke or already have heart disease. So the effects, if any, of HRT on coronary heart disease and its prevention remain uncertain. Meanwhile there is also conflicting evidence about the relative risk of stroke in women being given HRT.

As far as the role of hormone drugs is concerned in relation to osteoporosis, data from a number of randomized trials have shown that oestrogen drugs can indeed reduce the rate of decline in bone density after menopause. This is a result of the fact that oestrogen slows down the rate of bone resorption. However, unlike natural progesterone, oestrogen can do nothing to build new bone and the small benefits which it can confer are only maintained as long as the HRT is continued. Once HRT is discontinued, then bone density is lost at a similar rate to that which happens in women on a western diet without adequate exercise or adequate progesterone during menopause.

Most important of all, after all the studies are cited and all the positions aggressively defended, it is essential to remember that what is most frequently obscured by the medical-industrial complex in their claims for HRT is that a woman's lifestyle is far more important in protecting her from cardiovascular disease and osteoporosis than giving hormone drugs could ever be. The discrepancy is wide between what is claimed for HRT and what it delivers not only in these two areas but in many others. It is an excellent example of just how irrational the so-called rational assessments of HRT have become. There is also something ironic in such inconsistencies, especially considering the way in which women themselves have for many years been accused of being irrational by the male-dominated medical profession. But then the history of drug-based hormone treatments is full of inconsistencies.

History Speaks

As far back as the 1930s scientists knew that oestrogens will produce abortion even when given in small doses. When given early enough they will also prevent implantation of fertilized embryos. It was also known that oestrogens could cause various forms of cancer in animals. And as early as the 1940s scientists were aware that progesterone was capable of protecting against many of oestrogen's toxic effects including its abortifacient actions. But until the mid-1940s chemists assumed that progesterone's activity was very narrow. In the words of Carl Dyerassi, who reported on 'The Making of the Pill' in *Science*, they believed 'that progesterone's biological activity was extremely specific and that almost any alteration of the molecule would diminish or abolish its activity.' As a result, any interest drug companies might have had in progesterone was overridden by commercial interests since it is only possible to profit from patentable substances and you can only patent something which has been chemically modified to produce a unique molecule.

In the 1950s the search was on for chemicals which would prevent ovulation and could be used for birth control. Chemists discovered that there are many chemicals which have oestrogenic actions. Out of this discovery the contraceptive pill was born. It created a gigantic market. Ten years later, having developed the technology of using oestrogens in contraceptives, it was only logical for pharmaceutical manufacturers to look towards wider markets for their applications. New Zealand health-educator Sandra Coney describes the way in which it all happens: 'Medicine can create diseases to provide a market for new products developed by the pharmaceutical industry. There are two alternate scenarios in the development of drugs: biomedical scientists can go looking for a cure for a known illness, such as cancer; but new compounds are sometimes synthesized in the laboratory without anyone being initially clear what purpose they can be put to. The end result is a drug in need of a disease. The more broadly the disease can then be defined, the greater the treatable population and the greater the potential sales. Well people and others experiencing social problems are obvious targets.' Once oestrogen drugs and delivery systems had been developed as contraceptives the next logical step for drug manufacturers was to find a new use for them. The menopausal woman, standing poised at the threshold of profound changes in physical and spiritual life, was ideal.

Hidden Persuaders

Until the 1960s medicine was not much interested in the menopause. It was something which women patients were told they would simply have to put up with. Then as the *psychotropic* (mind-altering) drugs began to hit the market, medical journals became littered with advertisements for Librium and Valium as treatments for 'women's complaints' – from crying jags, to lethargy, anxiety, insomnia and depression. These drugs were then toted as 'cures' for the 'symptoms' of menopause and doctors began to write prescriptions for them. It was not long before the use of oestrogen followed suit, thanks largely to three forces: first, a book called *Feminine Forever* by New York gynaecologist Robert A. Wilson MD, which made oestrogen drugs sound like the best thing ever; secondly, women's magazines which carried articles on this newly discovered magic bullet treatment which was to keep women young for ever; and thirdly, massive promotions and advertising by pharmaceutical companies.

Wilson's book represented 'oestrogen replacement' as a kind of youth pill that would save poor fading women from the horrors of age. The crusade which he launched almost single-handedly to rescue women from what he termed the 'living decay' of menopause has all the hallmarks of a fundamentalist religion. He spoke of the 'tragedy of menopause' which often 'destroys her character as well as her health'. Wilson's message is clear – that menopause is a hideous disease with disastrous consequences. And only oestrogen carried by the noble White Knight of medicine is able to save her from its clutches. Wilson's paternalistic desire to prevent the ageing woman from becoming 'redundant' by making her 'feminine forever' has echoes of the very worst of cosmetic marketing about it. 'The unpalatable truth must be faced,' says the good doctor, 'that all postmenopausal women are castrates . . .' Wilson obviously felt it was his mission to identify the 'serious consequences' of the loss of oestrogen which happens to a woman at menopause. According to Wilson they include heart attacks, osteoporosis, tough, dry, scaly and inelastic skin, 'atrophic' breasts and shrivelled genitals. As Sandra Coney says, 'There is something unpleasantly voyeuristic about his desire to ensure that all women are walking around with plump juicy genitals. Wilson's views as a man determined his clinical judgement. He was the Hugh Hefner of Menopause.' A lot of Wilson's rhetoric reads like something out of Monty Python. By now it has lost whatever Pythonesque humour it may once have had. After 30 years of propaganda based on such nonsense, it now reads more like a blueprint for fear which we are still being sold.

In 1963 Wilson founded a private trust known as The Wilson Foundation for the sole purpose of promoting the use of oestrogen drugs. Its funding of $1.3 million came from the pharmaceutical industry. Each year Wilson received money from pharmaceutical companies including Searle, Wyeth-Ayerst Laboratories and Upjohn, all of which made hormone products which he claimed were effective in *treating* and even in *preventing* menopause. Since then Wilson's foundation has become very much the prototype for similar organizations in industrialized countries which continue to further the sale of HRT usually under the banner of saving women from post-menopausal agonies. Then it was more loss of femininity, neurosis and haggard shrivelled skin that was threatened. Now it tends to be osteoporosis, stroke and coronary heart disease. The words may change but the message remains constant: mid-life women need hormone drugs to rescue them from the horrors of menopause.

Comedy of Errors

Now, more than 30 years on things have changed. In the 1970s it became known that oestrogen used in the way Wilson had pioneered it – *unopposed* – had led to a tenfold increase in cancer of the womb. First warnings about HRT were substantiated by two articles published in the *New England Journal of Medicine* followed by a third which appeared in 1976. An editorial in *The Lancet*, 'Dangers of Eternal Youth', made the bizarre makeshift suggestion that women who wanted to continue on HRT should have hysterectomies since no woman could get cancer of the womb if her womb had been surgically excised. Other scientific articles around the same time linked oestrogen replacement with gall bladder disease, with the increased development of fibroids and increased frequency of breast and ovarian cancer. Overnight, oestrogen replacement lost its glamour with both doctors and the patients who had been using it. The United States Food and Drug Administration (FDA) demanded that all oestrogen medications carry a package insert warning of its dangers as well as back-pedalling their sale as a 'youth pill'. But with the backing of the American Medical Association – which is *supposed* to be an independent body – United States drug manufacturers went to court in an attempt to resist printing the package inserts. Their main argument was that such information would unnecessarily 'frighten women'. Before long the first studies indicating that oestrogen replacement is associated with reduced fractures from osteoporosis brought hope to drug manufacturers who were trying to pick up the pieces left by the cancer scares. Yet many doctors were afraid to use unopposed oestrogen because of the link with uterine cancer.

So in 1976 Wyeth-Ayerst Pharmaceuticals hired a top American public relations firm to help refocus their marketing of Premarin, taking it away from the eternal youth image towards a product used for the prevention of osteoporosis and heart disease. Their advertising was altered. The pharmaceutical companies as a whole also came to the rescue by altering the 'product' they were selling – unopposed oestrogen. By adding one of the newly developed progestogens such as Provera they were able to come up with a new 'product' – a cocktail of hormone drugs which (they insisted) would reduce the risk of oestrogen's overstimulating the womb lining and causing cancer. Some also started referring to hormone treatments not so much as ERT (Estrogen Replacement Therapy) but as HRT. A new product. A new name. A new image. Over the next 15 years hormone manufacturers funded study after study and publicized the findings to doctors and the press in an attempt to demonstrate the benefits of HRT.

Sweet Talk

To some extent the relaunch of HRT has been a successful project. Some women are reassured by the calm, rational voice of such books as the British publication *The Amarant Book of Hormone Replacement Therapy*, offspring of the Amarant Trust, which relates that, 'There was a scare in 1975 that HRT "caused" cancer, but at that time oestrogen was used by itself, without the added progesterone . . . What doctors had not realised then was that progesterone was needed as well to induce the womb to shed the lining and so prevent the build up.' Its authors, Gorman and Whitehead, go on to explain that the new 'opposed therapy' produces a monthly bleed which they define as a safe 'normal period'. They reassure their readers that so successful has the campaign to promote HRT been in some countries that certain gynaecologists now claim that *all* postmenopausal women need HRT in order to reach their health potential. To other women, however, such rhetoric seems reminiscent of TV advertising for washing powders. The same book also speaks of 'long-suffering husbands' as a result of their wives 'letting themselves go', wives 'looking hot and bothered' and wives who have 'gone off sex'. It concludes that men should encourage their wives to see a doctor since 'it may save your marriage' and insist that for over a third of a woman's life she is living in a state of oestrogen deficiency. 'HRT is the greatest treasure of a middle-aged woman's life,' claim its authors. With HRT, they promise, a woman can have 'reached fifty but feel like twenty'. Meanwhile, doctors, unaware of how lifestyle alterations, the use of botanicals and natural progesterone can transform the health and energy of women in mid-life, are beginning routinely to warn women of the dangers of *not* using HRT. And journalists, fed information by supposedly independent organizations, which are in fact largely funded by pharmaceutical manufacturers, conclude in articles published in such papers as *The Guardian* that: 'Once the only cure for the menopause was said to be death . . . now there are other options.'

Cancer Scares

According to recent research, what women seem to worry about most in relation to HRT is that it may increase their risk of cancer, especially endometrial cancer, but breast cancer too. There is much evidence that hormone supplementation does indeed increase the risk of some cancers. As far back as the mid-1970s epidemiologists remarked that endometrial cancers were rising at an alarming rate. The culprit was identified as unopposed oestrogen which encourages the proliferation of the womb lining. This is why most doctors today add a progestogen to their oestrogen replacement. However, it is not even known whether or not adding a progestogen to the HRT cocktail may be wiping out any postulated benefit which oestrogen replacement may offer as a protection from heart disease. This is an example of how incomplete the highly vocalized research into the supposed benefits of HRT may be. As far as the effect of taking oestrogen on the development of breast cancer in postmenopausal women is concerned, Elizabeth Barrett-Connor of the University of California at San Diego concluded, as have others, that taking oestrogen for five years or more increased the risk of breast cancer by as much as 50 per cent. Meanwhile, many other scientists, including Kay-Tee Khaw, Professor of Gerontology at the University of Cambridge and editor of the scholarly book *Hormone Replacement Therapy*, suggest that adding a progestogen may actually compound the risk.

Forgotten Oestrogen

Amidst all the arguments, confusion and disagreement over HRT there are two benefits which it undeniably brings to the few women who are genuinely very low in oestrogen after menopause and who can therefore benefit from supplementary oestrogen. These lie in the ability of this important female hormone to relieve vaginal dryness and to stop hot flushes.

What is usually forgotten is that oestrogen is not the only way of eliminating either symptom. Neither is it necessarily the best way for most women. For the majority of women, who in the western world tend to be oestrogen dominant, adding more oestrogen drugs only serves to mask the underlying hormonal fluctuations taking place in their bodies which involve the hypothalamus – triggering hot flushes while further increasing oestrogen dominance. And although hot flushes do not usually respond to the use of natural alternatives as rapidly as they do to oestrogen drugs, they do respond well, frequently bringing permanent relief with no side-effects (see Field and Forest, p. 346). Similarly, a natural progesterone cream or oil used regularly both on the body and in the area of the vulva and inside the vagina itself is usually enough to clear vaginal dryness, itching, irritation and the thinning of vaginal tissue, in the vast majority of cases within a few weeks. For that matter a good cream based on comfrey is usually enough to do the trick for most women. For the very small number of women to whom such actions don't bring relief a small amount of oestrogen used for a while will bring relief. But what kind of oestrogen?

All oestrogens are not created equal (see p. 109). Oestrone (E1) and oestradiol (E2) are highly stimulating to breast tissue and, like the artificial oestrogens used in HRT and the xenoestrogens in our environment, have been implicated in breast cancer. By contrast the third oestrogen which the body makes, oestriol (E3), being a weak oestrogen, has actually been shown to inhibit the development of cancer in animals and may help protect from it in women. At the beginning of HRT there were few alternatives to artificial oestrogen drugs. Now less carcinogenic forms of oestrogen, such as oestriol itself or what is known among doctors who favour natural methods of helping women deal with menopausal difficulties as *triple oestrogen*, are available. An invention of American physician Jonathan Wright, triple oestrogen is made up of 80 per cent oestriol with 10 per cent each of oestrone and oestradiol. It is available in the United States through compounding pharmacies (see Resources, p. 505) and can be ordered by doctors outside the US on prescription. So can excellent vaginal creams containing high levels of the safer oestrogens – oestrogens which are chemically identical to the hormones secreted by a woman's ovaries. In the rare cases when small amounts of oestrogen are needed temporarily as part of a woman's bloodless revolution such products have become the treatments of choice by doctors who take a natural approach to the treatment of menstrual and menopausal problems.

As far as getting off HRT, if you are already on it and dissatisfied, this is not a difficult thing to do (see Magnum Force, p. 425). It should be done slowly, and it is best carried out with the help of a physician or health practitioner knowledgeable about the techniques and products which form a part of the natural menopause revolution.

In Praise of Straight Talk

The one thing on which almost everyone seems to agree is that women should have the right to make an informed choice about whether or not to use HRT. However, becoming informed enough to make that choice is another matter. Most 'educational' materials readily available to women on HRT which purport to present objective information are in truth a travesty of objectivity. Under the guise of rational language, these publications lay out all the supposed benefits HRT offers, sometimes in rather patronizing language. The average woman wanting to inform herself about the pros and cons of treatments available to her through her doctor has little access to *real* information and is unlikely even to know where to go to get it.

Some excellent stuff has been written that does give the facts. Books like Sandra Coney's *The Menopause Industry*, and Gail Vines' *Raging Hormones*, for instance. Often such books have received little publicity since even much of the press has been indoctrinated into the value of HRT and books like these challenge it – sometimes in highly technical terms. They also demand an intellectual commitment to the search for information on HRT that many women have neither the time nor the inclination to carry out. There are also some excellent official reports such as 'Hormone Replacement Therapy', a report to the National Advisory Committee on Core Health and Disability Support Services in New Zealand, published in 1993, and some well-researched papers produced with the support of women's groups, such as the highly erudite and hard-hitting 'Disempowering Mid-Life Women: The Science and Politics of Hormone Replacement Therapy' by Renate Klein and Lynette J. Dumble from the Women's Studies International Forum in Australia in 1994. But, unlike the slick little booklets available in every doctor's office, the paperback books, and the 2,500-word reassuring articles informing women about the latest benefit of HRT readily available in the general press, few women as yet have access to them.

Stepford Wives Revisited

As Klein and Dumble say of HRT, 'Given the fact that millions of [peri]menopausal women are advised to use this therapy, we believe that this amounts to nothing less than "drugging" healthy women and furthermore does this without even informing them of the possibility of addiction.' It is a sentiment with which I heartily concur. They continue, 'We reject the view that menopause is a disease and believe it to be extraordinarily unethical to risk drug dependence in healthy women. Mid-life women have arrived at an important point in their lives where many of them feel the time has come to focus on their own needs and interests. By medicalising the menopause and administering addictive drugs, this empowering process of self-determination is threatened . . . HRT has the potential to *disempower* mid-life women . . . another form of medical violence against women.'

One of the interesting issues surrounding the whole question of HRT, and yet another strange irony, lies in the way some feminist groups view it. An important question in the future will be whether or not feminists take the lead in exposing the way in which mid-life women are being disempowered or whether they, too, become pawns in the hands of profit-orientated pressure groups? McCrea and Markle investigated the attitudes of feminist groups on both sides of the Atlantic. They came up with some fascinating observations about the differences. In the United States as long ago as the late 1960s feminists had begun to challenge the notion that menopausal women are suffering from a deficiency disease which needs treatment. They presented menopause as a normal event in a woman's life and in doing so attempted to remove the stigma that has surrounded it ever since Robert A. Wilson first issued his warning that a woman's worth ends in mid-life. American feminists pointed out that to take the standard view of menopause is to acquiesce in the belief that menstruation, like menopause itself, is a physical and emotional handicap rendering women incomplete in comparison to men. Out of such thinking a number of active American, Canadian, Australian and New Zealand women's health and consumer groups have developed who have become highly vocal in their opposition to the use of hormone drugs.

'Many long-time feminists are approaching mid-life,' say Klein and Dumble. 'Will we personally resist HRT and politically expose the extraordinarily paralysing consequences if millions of women at the prime of their lives and ready to challenge the world instead become the Stepford Wives of the 1990s: rigid in their "happy" state, heterosexually active because they must, running from mammography to bone density test to endometrial biopsy, coping with migraines, hypertension and weight gain; stressed out from surviving the cancer scare which resulted in a breast biopsy – all from a drug for the prevention of osteoporosis and heart attacks which they might never get?'

By contrast in Britain and some other western countries, with the exception of Germaine Greer who has put together a powerful case against HRT, many feminists have campaigned enthusiastically for hormone treatments. Together with consumer groups they have tended to view HRT as something they believe British doctors are denying women the right to – too often, they say, by insisting that the problems women have around the time of menopause are figments of an overactive imagination. As Gail Vines, author of *Raging Hormones*, says, 'American feminists have tried to show that differential socialisation, not biological difference, accounts for women's inferior social status. In Britain, on the other hand, feminists tend to be more closely aligned with the socialist movement, and have tended to see the roots of women's oppression in the structure of capitalist societies and so to give the biological debate less priority.' But, as McCrea and Markle point out, 'it has been individual feminists and not a whole social movement who have militated for ERT [HRT] in Great Britain'.

A major problem with all the talk about HRT is that it has stolen the whole woman's health agenda by taking attention away from the real issues about women's health. The crux of preventing heart disease and osteoporosis lies not with HRT but in making lifestyle changes – particularly and especially to diet. Our bone fracture rates in the West have been increasing dramatically so that both men and women have three times more hip fractures now than were experienced in the same age group some 30 years ago. It is important that we don't become so focused on looking for 'magic bullets' that we beg the real question of how far-reaching an effect lifestyle change can have on women's lives.

Of major importance in the success of the bloodless revolution and the rate at which it is carried out is the attitude that feminists and women's groups take to it. It is essential that they, like all women, become aware of the work of its trailblazers so that we can make the best possible use of all the information, techniques and substances now available to us. Important, too, is our finding ways to reconnect with the energies of instinct and deepening our awareness of the powerful and life-enriching archetypes of menopause. All of these things are here to help each one of us. Until HRT or some other 'magic bullet' is able to promise that kind of freedom and fulfilment it is of minor importance.

Chapter Seven

Dark Gods

Cancer is probably the most serious disease affecting women. Certainly it is the most terrifying. We are continually being urged by the medical profession to guard ourselves against death from breast, cervical and womb cancer by getting regular mammograms and Pap smears. We are bombarded with information from the media about the dangers of breast cancer. Yet, instead of equipping us so that we can take action to make cancer's appearance in our own lives less likely, most of the information we receive day to day about the illness fills us with the kind of fear that makes it difficult to sort out the facts from the fantasies. Each woman responds to fear in a different way. For some, fear of cancer has them booking regular appointments at well women clinics. Others hope against hope that the cancer terror will pass them by. Even the words we use to describe someone who has the illness – a cancer *victim* – give to the illness a power which it does not deserve. Meanwhile the threat of cancer – both real and imagined – continues to disempower us.

The Perils of Protection

Ask most medical experts about what you can do to best protect yourself from dying from some form of female cancer and they are likely to tell you that early detection is the answer. The theory is that the earlier you detect cancers the better your chances of survival. Breast cancers are diagnosed through a combination of sonograms, aspiration of lumps, physical examinations, mammograms and, if necessary, surgical biopsy, where a piece of tissue taken from the breast is removed and examined under the microscope. A mammogram is an X-ray taken of the breasts which is used to diagnose breast cancer at its earliest appearance – supposedly before it can be felt by a physical examination. It is standard medical procedure in most countries to have mammograms taken of the breasts of women who can afford it every year or two.

Some interesting research came to light as the result of the largest study of its kind ever carried out in Canada. The Canadian National Breast Screening Study followed the fate of 89,836 women between the ages of 40 and 49 for an eight-year period during which half of them were given mammograms every year to eighteen months while the other half were only examined physically. To the amazement of the researchers, when all the results were tallied, they discovered that deaths among the women who got regular mammograms were significantly higher than those who had none. When finally the results were published – which incidentally did not happen until a full four years after the study was completed – the National Cancer Institute finally announced that the increase in death from breast cancer was 52 per cent. In simple terms this means that you are half again as likely to die of the disease if you do get regular mammograms than if you do not. Unlike much of the research that appears unheeded by the general public, this report made the headlines. 'Breast Scans Boost Risk of Cancer Death' announced the headline in an article that appeared in *The Times* on 2 June 1991. It then went on to announce that 'Middle-aged women who have regular mammograms are more likely to die from breast cancer than women who are not screened, according to dramatic new research.'

Another common notion about breast cancer is that the earlier it is detected and surgery is performed the better your chances of survival. This, too, appears to be untrue, as Petr Skrabanek reported in *The Lancet* as far back as 1985. 'There is no evidence that early mastectomy affects survival. If the patients knew this, they would mostly likely refuse surgery.' At the University of California at Berkeley, Professor Hardin Jones, whose expertise is in the areas of medical physics and physiology, had reported to the American Cancer Society more than fifteen years before that every serious attempt to relate early treatment to survival has been unsuccessful. Jones studied many reports that looked at detection and survival and found that those subjects chosen for treatment for cancer tended to be patients who were considered capable of being cured by operations while the inoperable or terminal patients tended to be lumped together as part of the untreated control groups. When he had made adjustments in the statistics to take this into account, Jones concluded that, 'My studies have proven conclusively that untreated cancer victims actually live up to four times longer than treated individuals.' That was more than a quarter of a century ago yet Jones' investigations, like those of other researchers since then, have gone largely unheeded.

Mammogram Miasma

Not only are mammograms not a cure-all for breast cancer, a clean mammogram is no real guarantee that you *do not* have a cancer developing. Mammograms are capable of missing its presence altogether in between 10 and 15 per cent of all cancers. They are also open to a great deal of confusion and interpretation since reading them is not an exact science but an art dependent upon the competence and judgement of human beings.

There is a great deal of fear in women which tends to surround the whole practice. American specialist in internal medicine Dr H. Gilbert Welch, a senior researcher at the Department of Veterans' Affairs in White River Junction, Vermont, has looked carefully at the difficulties that go with the excessive diagnosis of diseases like breast cancer. He discovered that in women who die from other causes, an amazing 40 per cent have had microscopic changes in their breasts. These are common lesions that show up on mammograms and there is no way that any expert, no matter how skilled or highly experienced, is capable of knowing which of these will remain dormant and which will turn into cancer.

Neither, according to recent research, does a biopsy after a suspicious mammogram improve survival rates from breast cancer. A biopsy entails cutting through the suspected lump and invading the protective pocket that helps keep a tumour from spreading and, as a result, this very procedure which is designed to confirm the existence or non-existence of a cancerous lesion can actually encourage any cancer present to metastasize – to spread to other parts of the body. German researchers who looked at the survival rates of patients with breast cancer discovered that those who had had biopsies died earlier than those who did not. Even biopsies done with a needle rather than a scalpel do not appear to be safe – quite apart from what the worry over waiting for results and the pain involved in the procedure can do to undermine a woman's immune system. George Crile Jr, MD, a Surgeon Emeritus at the Cleveland Clinic in the United States, says, 'It gives credence to what our patients already think and tell us – that cutting into cancer spreads it and makes it grow.'

The point to consider from all of this is that it is time we stopped falling victim to the pronouncements and procedures of high technology medical procedures as well as to cancer itself as a disease. For the answers to its prevention lie mostly in our lifestyle. The answers depend upon things we can do ourselves to change the way we eat and live and think for the better and should not be left in the hands of abstract medical theorizing and the fear-mongering which too often accompanies it. As a recent editorial in *The Lancet* pointed out, 'Some readers may be startled to learn that the overall mortality rate from carcinoma of the breast remains static. If one were to believe all the media hype, the triumphalism of the profession in the published research, and the almost weekly miracle breakthrough trumpeted by the cancer charities, one might be surprised that women are dying at all from this cancer.'

Pre-cancerous Power

Another common procedure to which women are subjected is the Pap smear for diagnosing cervical abnormalities. Its name comes from a Dr George Papanicolaou who developed the procedure almost three-quarters of a century ago. It has since been refined and is now used as a way of identifying abnormal (often called *pre-cancerous*) cells as early as possible. Using a simple instrument inserted into the vagina, a doctor scrapes away a sampling of cells from the squamocolumnar junction of the cervix just inside the cervical opening at the bottom of the womb. These are then fixed on a slide with a chemical preservative and examined under the microscope by a technician or doctor used to reading them. Pap smears are frequently credited with the decline in the death rate for cervical cancer which has occurred in the past couple of decades. They, too, can be highly unreliable and produce a number of both false-positives and false-negatives, and there have been no controlled randomized trials that prove that they actually save lives. When a trial was carried out in British Columbia where mass screening by Pap smear had been done, deaths from cervical cancer did indeed drop. Not a lot could be deduced from this fact since they also dropped in the rest of Canada to just the same degree even when mass screening was not conducted. Meanwhile, in Britain, the death rate from cervical cancer has not dropped despite 40 million smears having been conducted. As Dr E. Robin points out in his fascinating book *Matters of Life and Death: Risks vs. Benefits of Medical Care*, the Pap smear is not only one of the most common and popular laboratory tests, it is also one of the most unreliable. He writes about one study where two Pap smears were taken from the same women at the same time. An amazing two-thirds of the women's two tests showed different results.

Cancer is not, as we have been led to believe, the inevitable curse visited upon innocent victims without warning. In the past five years a great deal of information has come to light about how the way you eat and live either protects or predisposes you to cancer. Forward-thinking researchers are awakening to hormonal links in the development of breast and womb cancer and finding ways of using natural hormones to protect against it. At the same time the evidence mounts that all those Pap smears and mammograms we have been putting ourselves through are not only pretty useless in protecting against cancer death, they may even be contributing to its development. Happily, the rest of the news about cancer which is emerging out of the bloodless revolution is all good – especially in terms of what it can do to protect your life and the lives of your daughters.

Cells Gone Wrong

Cancer is defined as a 'malignant neoplasm' – a powerful abnormal cellular growth which first invades and then eventually takes over normal tissue. Every cancer begins with an alteration to a single normal cell which causes an increase in cell division or reproduction as well as a loss of differentiation. Ordinary healthy human cells reproduce continually in a controlled manner as part of the body's normal growth and repair processes. This remains under the control of the body's normal patterning mechanisms which differentiate a cell from every other kind of cell in the body in line with the purpose this cell serves. Cancer cells are different. They multiply faster than normal and lose all definition so that newly replicated cancer cells become incapable of carrying out the tasks for which normal cells of a particular kind have been designed. Cancer cells revert to a more primitive form of cellular life, relying on glucose for their metabolism rather than oxygen, and avariciously reproducing, unchallenged by the body's normal control and regulating mechanisms. A woman's immune system, which is superbly designed to handle foreign invaders, finds it almost impossible to oust cancer cells because the membranes of cancer cells resemble closely enough the membranes of normal cells so that it does not recognize how dangerous they are.

No one knows for sure why cells become cancerous. There are two main theories. The oldest is known as the *genetic* theory. It says that a cancer cell is the result of damage to DNA (which holds the body's chromosomal codes for replication within it) which has been brought about by radiation, toxins or viruses. The genetic theory goes something like this. Damage is always occurring to the chromosomes of cells throughout the body and then being repaired by gene repair mechanisms. However, more damage can occur than a cell's repair processes can handle. When enough unrepaired damage accumulates, says the theory, cancer develops. A more recent theory about the origins of cancer – more likely according to a rapidly growing number of scientists as well as practitioners of natural medicine – is known as *epigenetics*. The epigenetic hypothesis insists that it is not time passing but

toxic elements within a cell's cytoplasm that trigger chromosomal changes which result in the cell's reverting to a more
primitive mode of behaviour. In effect, cells become cancerous in direct response to the toxic threat.

All this may sound like high-falutin' theorizing by abstract
scientists and of little relevance to any woman concerned
about the prevention and treatment of cancer of the breast,
cervix or womb, but it is actually great news. For where once a
woman was forced to see herself as a helpless victim of the
great demon cancer which struck without apparent warning,
we now know that there are specific lifestyle changes we can
make and actions we can take which not only help prevent
cancer but at the very least significantly prolong the life of a
woman who has it. These changes include cleaning up our
environment and following a diet that is low in fat, high in
fresh vegetables, rich in beta-carotene, and includes taking
supplements of the anti-oxidant nutrients such as vitamin C,
selenium and beta-carotene. Many studies also show that a
shift in attitude can both help prevent cancer and extend survival time in someone who already has it. So can the use of
certain natural hormones. All of this is particularly welcome
news since what has become blatantly obvious in recent years
is that the usual treatments for most types of female cancer –
surgery, radiation and chemotherapy, where toxic chemicals
are introduced into the body – have little success in treating
most kinds of cancer. For cancer cells can be hard to kill.
Preventing cancer is much easier than trying to cure it.

Hormone Links

Both breast cancer and endometrial cancer (cancer of the
womb) are related to a woman's hormonal balance. And
while endometrial cancer still remains relatively rare, in
recent years the incidence of breast cancer has increased
manyfold in industrialized countries. In the United States one
female in nine between the ages of one and 85 now gets
breast cancer and it is the leading cause of death among
women between the ages of 40 and 55. Only twenty years ago
the figure was one woman in 20. Now there are 180,000 new

breast cancer cases each year and 46,000 deaths while another 150,000 women submit to mutilating mastectomies. Worldwide, breast cancer is the most common cancer among women, accounting for 20 per cent of all malignancies. Britain has the highest breast cancer mortality rate in the world. In Britain, in 1992, there were 13,663 deaths from breast cancer and 53,000 total or partial breast excisions. Over 20,000 new cases are now discovered each year.

The relationship between the development of breast and endometrial cancer and sex hormones daily becomes more clear. Both breast tissue and endometrial tissue are sensitive to reproductive hormones. Oestrogens are well known to stimulate breast tumours in animals. Every published study on breast cancer turns up evidence that oestrogen – or, to be more exact, oestradiol and oestrone which are the most commonly prescribed oestrogens – is somehow related to breast cancer. The now-famous Swedish research carried out by L. Berkgvist and his colleagues at University Hospital in Uppsala, and reported in 1989, showed an increase in breast cancer after only seven years of oestrogen use. Several other studies have linked oestrogen replacement to increased risk of breast cancer, although not all studies as yet support this finding. Still many so-called medical experts continue to down-play the risk and insist that even women who have already had breast cancer are putting themselves under no special risk in taking oestrogen replacement or HRT, using both oestrogen and a progestogen.

When the dangers of oestrogen replacement first began to come to light, many doctors expressed the hope that they could minimize the risk of breast cancer by adding a synthetic progestin to the cocktail of hormones being given to women. This was a reasonable assumption since the progestins had been shown to offer some protection against endometrial cancer in women given oestrogen replacement. However, like many stopgap measures taken in medicine, this approach simply has not worked. This is perhaps not surprising when you know that the *Physician's Desk Reference* lists breast malignancies in beagle dogs as one of the side-effects of giving them Provera – one of the most commonly prescribed progestins in many countries of the industrialized world. The

Berkgvist study showed that taking an oestrogen/progestin combination (still commonly prescribed for HRT) quadrupled the breast-cancer risk compared with women who were not taking it.

Then in 1992, not long after the Berkgvist study was published, an important review of studies was carried out which examined the relationship between HRT and breast cancer, published in *Obstetrics and Gynecology*. It showed a 63 per cent increase in breast cancer risk for women on oestrogen/progestin-based HRT. Such findings have prompted many experts on breast cancer to set warning bells ringing. Dr Jonathan S. Berek, Director of Gynecologic Oncology at the UCLA School of Medicine, has said, it 'hits at the heart of our philosophy that patients should be on oestrogen and progestin. This questions the assumption that it is entirely safe, at least from the standpoint of the breast.' Meanwhile, evidence continues to mount that xenoestrogens and other environmental pollutants are also in part responsible for the rising incidence of breast cancer in the industrialized world. Yet more and more oestrogen/progestin HRT is doled out every year and our environment becomes more and more polluted by petrochemically derived oestrogen mimics.

Beware Oestrogen Dominance

Both breast cancer and endometrial cancer tend to develop during periods of oestrogen dominance in a woman's life. Breast cancer occurs most often in menstruating women with either normal oestrogen levels or high oestrogen levels but low progesterone – a set of circumstances most likely to present itself after the age of 35 when anovulatory menstruation becomes common in western women. Breast cancer also develops easily after menstrual periods have stopped when women are being given oestrogen replacement either on its own or together with a progestin but *without* natural progesterone.

A study carried out by Dr Linda Cowan which was reported in the *American Journal of Epidemiology* clearly showed the protective benefits of progesterone. Menstruating women with low progesterone levels were found to have almost five and a half times the risk of developing breast cancer. They also experienced ten times the number of deaths from malignant neoplasms compared with women whose progesterone levels were normal. Anyone willing to take the time to look in depth at what is known about the factors which predispose us to or protect us from breast cancer will find two things: first, oestrogen – particularly oestrogen unopposed by progesterone – lies behind the development of cancer; secondly, sufficient progesterone helps to protect from it.

There is a drug called tamoxifen now commonly given to women who have had breast surgery in an attempt to prevent cancer from recurring. The way tamoxifen works is simple: as a weak oestrogenic substance, it blocks the uptake of oestrone and oestradiol in breast tissue since it is taken up by oestrogen receptor sites on the breast, thereby protecting the breast tissue from the cancer-promoting oestrogens present in the body. Unfortunately the drug has some rather nasty side-effects. A growing number of doctors insist that the same results can be achieved by giving natural progesterone. The fact that tamoxifen works by protecting against oestrogen's effect on breast tissue is yet another thing which strongly supports the notion that oestrogen at levels that are too high is a major factor in the development of breast cancer. So is the fact that a woman's risk of developing breast cancer is much diminished by full-term pregnancies – particularly those that occur before the age of 18. (You will recall that the progesterone level in a woman soars during pregnancy, apparently conferring protection.) Women who have never had children have a much higher risk of getting breast cancer than mothers.

When men are given oestrogens as a treatment for prostatic cancer or after sex-change surgery, this too is accompanied by an increased risk of breast cancer. However, when a woman's ovaries have been removed before the age of 40, her oestrogen production decreases dramatically as does her risk of breast cancer. This protection is lost, of course, if she is given HRT. Recent research shows that strangely a woman's chance of survival after breast surgery is even influenced by whether or not her body is in a state of oestrogen dominance when it is performed. Menstruating women who have breast surgery carried out during the second half of their menstrual cycle – the luteal phase when progesterone is high to balance oestrogens – survive far longer than do women whose surgery is done early on in their cycle during the oestrogen-dominant follicular phase.

It may take 20 years before all of the measurements are in that will enable scientists to prove unequivocally that excess oestrogen in a woman's body allows both cancer of the breast and cancer of the womb to develop. From a commercial point of view it may be far longer. In the meantime we need to begin looking upon cancer not as some terrifying disease against which we are helpless but rather a result of biological and ecological imbalances which each of us is capable of taking action to rectify. For this is the truth of things. It is a truth much obscured by all the 'cancer drama' which surrounds us.

The Strong and the Weak

Even some of the weaker natural oestrogens themselves can have important roles to play in cancer prevention. You will recall that your body produces three main oestrogens or hormones with oestrus activity – oestrone (E1), oestradiol (E2) and oestriol (E3). In common parlance they are usually lumped together under the 'oestrogen' banner. Each of these oestrogens has unique characteristics. When you are not pregnant it is primarily oestrone (E1) and oestradiol (E2) which are secreted by the ovaries in relatively large quantities (measured in micrograms) while oestriol (E3) is only made in minute quantities as a by-product of E1 metabolism. During pregnancy, when the placenta becomes the prime site for oestrogen production, this pattern is completely reversed. Now oestriol becomes the dominant oestrogen and, at the same time, progesterone production by the placenta also soars. It is only oestrone (E1) and oestradiol (E2) which are highly stimulating to breast tissue that have been implicated in breast cancer, not oestriol. Studies carried out more than 20 years ago showed that oestradiol (and to a lesser degree oestrone) increase a woman's risk of breast cancer while oestriol is actually protective against it. For oestriol (E3) is a weak oestrogen. Like some of the phyto-oestrogens it appears to occupy receptor sites so that they are protected from the cancer-inducing properties of E1 and E2. So much weaker is E3 that the ratio of activity between oestradiol (E1) and oestriol (E3) is an amazing 1,000:1.

The Amazing Oestrogen Quotient

In animal experiments where both rats and mice were treated with cancer-causing chemicals and then one group was given oestriol (E3), researchers discovered that breast cancer was inhibited by this oestrogen. Much impressed by the protective effects of oestriol on animals, American researcher Dr Henry Lemon began to investigate how this oestrogen behaves in relation to human breast cancer. He developed a fascinating formula which he dubbed the *oestrogen quotient*, by which he meant the ratio of the cancer-inhibiting oestriol (E3) to the cancer-promoting oestrone (E1) and oestradiol (E2) in any woman. If a woman's oestrogen quotient is high then her body is producing a lot of the protective oestriol in relation to the other oestrogens. He theorized that in these women the risk of breast cancer would be reduced. If, on the other hand, a woman's oestrogen quotient was low then very little of the protective oestriol would be produced relative to the other two and she would be expected to have a higher risk of cancer.

To test all this out, Lemon measured the various kinds of oestrogen both in the urine of healthy women and those with breast cancer. In healthy women the average oestrogen quotient was 1.3 before menopause and 1.2 afterwards. Only 21 per cent of the healthy women had oestrogen quotients which were below normal. By contrast, in the women with breast cancer who had received no hormonal treatment of any kind, the average oestrogen quotients were between 0.5 and 0.8. A surprising 62 per cent of these women had values below normal. Lemon's work strongly suggests that women with breast cancer have low levels of oestriol relative to the other two oestrogens. It has also been confirmed by epidemiological studies. In countries where there is a low incidence of breast cancer, women tend to have high levels of urinary oestriol excretion and low levels in their blood compared with women in countries such as the United States where the incidence of breast cancer is high. Later on Lemon and his co-workers carried out another interesting study on women whose breast cancer had metastasized (spread to other areas of their body). One group was given oestriol in doses of between 2.5 and 15 mg a day. The other was not. By the end of the study an amazing 37 per cent of women who got the oestriol had either had their cancer arrested or experienced a complete remission.

In the light of what is generally expected in women with metastasized breast cancer such results are nothing short of astounding. Not only is there strong evidence that unopposed oestradiol and oestrone are cancer-causing in relation to breasts, both oestriol and progesterone – the two hormones which are produced in good quantity during pregnancy – help protect against it. Sadly the protective properties of natural progesterone remain largely unknown. Meanwhile to block the side-effects of oestrone and oestradiol on breast tissue it is not the safe natural oestriol (E3) with virtually no side-effects which is regularly used but rather the drug tamoxifen – known to increase the incidence of womb cancer when given to women. Why? There are probably several reasons. But without doubt one of the most important is that the protective powers of oestriol are little known by specialists let alone the average GP. Oestriol, the dose of which needs to be individualized for each woman, is a natural hormone derived from plant sources. As such, like natural proges- terone, it is a generic hormone of little interest to drug com- panies since there is no way it can be patented as a drug. It is worth noting that oestriol – by far and away the safest of the oestrogens – has all sorts of other useful properties. It has the ability to alleviate vaginal and urinary infections in post- menopausal women without causing breakthrough bleeding and eliminates vaginal dryness in the small number of women who need extra oestrogen after menopause. Yet oestriol (E3) is still rarely used. I suspect that only when women themselves demand it, will this change. (See p. 93 for more information about oestriol in relation to HRT)

Endometrial Help

Endometrial cancer (cancer of the womb) is not only relatively rare, it is much less dangerous than breast cancer. Because it tends to cause abnormal bleeding, it is not so difficult to diagnose early. It also tends to remain isolated for a long time before spreading to other parts of the body. The general treatment for endometrial cancer is hysterectomy. Once a woman who has had it has had her womb removed she is usually warned to stay away from HRT forever. When it comes to endometrial cancer, the relationship between excess oestrogen and its development is even clearer than in the case of breast cancer. As John Lee says, 'It is generally acknowledged that the only known cause of endometrial cancer is unopposed oestrogen. Here again oestradiol and oestrone are the culprits. When oestrogen supplements are given to postmenopausal women for five years the risk of endometrial cancer increases 6-fold, and longer term use increases it to 14-fold.' It is not only postmenopausal women who are at risk either. 'In premenopausal women, endometrial cancer is extremely rare except during the 5–10 years before menopause when oestrogen dominance is common,' Lee continues. 'The addition of natural progesterone during these years would significantly reduce the incidence of endometrial cancer as well as breast cancer.'

John Lee and other doctors working with natural menopause are not only suggesting the use of natural progesterone cream as a preventative measure against both endometrial cancer and breast cancer, but many of them also use progesterone as a way of helping to protect these women from progressive osteoporosis, and from urinary tract infections and vaginal atrophy which occurs in some women. In fact it was with these women – women who could not be given the oestrogens and progestins of ordinary HRT – that Lee first began his highly successful natural progesterone therapy. It was through his clinical work over many years that Lee discovered natural progesterone therapy would not only reverse osteoporosis and correct vaginal atrophy, it can also prevent the further development of all sorts of cancer in these women. None of the women Lee originally treated with progesterone who had had breast cancer have to his knowledge ever had any recurrence of the illness.

Fat Chance

Specific foods and nutrients can also play a vital role in protecting a woman from cancer of the breast or womb – in no small part because certain compounds in food actually help lower a woman's oestrogen levels. In a review of data from 12 case-controlled studies which appeared in *The Journal of the National Cancer Institute*, investigators concluded that 25 per cent of postmenopausal breast cancers can be prevented by changes in diet alone. Research shows that 60 per cent of breast, womb and ovarian cancers are associated with a diet high in fat for instance. In another study, where the dietary histories of 455 Italian women with ovarian cancer were compared with the histories of 1,385 normal women, a high-fat diet – especially from meat or butter – elevated the risk while a diet high in green vegetables, carrots, whole grains and fish provided the lowest risk.

High levels of most varieties of oestrogen are what you want to avoid to protect your body from breast cancer. Eating a high-fat diet rich in animal-based proteins such as meat and milk products increases a woman's concentration of these oestrogens dramatically. Oestrogens in your bloodstream are filtered through the liver where they become combined with elements that make them difficult to absorb. Then they are sent to the intestines to be eliminated from the body before any excess can cause damage to the body. But if you eat a lot of fat in your foods (and almost half the calories in the typical western diet come in the form of fats) then the intestinal environment becomes riddled with just the kind of bacteria that are able to break down oestrogen compounds so that the oestrogen is reabsorbed into the bloodstream. Not only does this increase the level of oestrogen-like compounds in the body it also tends to prolong what is known as a woman's 'menstrual life'. Menstrual life is how many years in a woman's life she actually menstruates. When it comes to assessing the risks of breast cancer women with a long menstrual life are twice as likely to get the illness as women with a short menstrual life. For example, American women who live on a high-fat diet rich in animal products on average begin to menstruate at around the age of 12 and do not go through menopause until the age of 50. This is considered a long menstrual life. Oriental women or young women on a vegetarian diet low in fat and only moderate in protein, on the other hand, begin menstruating later – around the age of 16 – and go through menopause earlier – at approximately 46 years old. They have a much smaller risk of ending up with breast cancer, although it is interesting to see that when Japanese women who have been raised on such a low-fat diet move to the United States and eat more of the high-fat western fare their risk of getting breast cancer rises significantly.

Alcohol drinking also increases your risk of breast cancer. All but three of the case-control and cohort studies reported recently in the *New England Journal of Medicine* which have investigated the association between alcohol intake and breast cancer incidence have shown a 40 per cent to 60 per cent increase in risk even with only moderate drinking. Sugar, too, is implicated in cancer development. An epidemiological survey of 21 countries showed that a high sugar intake is a major risk factor for the development of breast cancer in women over the age of 45.

A Passion for Healthy Foods

Just as certain kinds of diet predispose you to cancer so others can protect you from it. There are many anti-cancer constituents in common foods. They include methylated flavones, selenium salts, phenols, indoles, aromatic isothyiocyanates, protease inhibitors, and of course the important plant sterols. There are also certain foods which have proven anti-cancer properties. Many are soya based, such as tofu, miso, tempeh and tamari. Made from soya beans they contain plant sterols or phyto-oestrogens which have weak oestrogenic activity. Research shows that Oriental women who eat a lot of these foods have very little trouble with hot flushes around the time of menopause and afterwards. They also have very little trouble with any other menopausal symptoms, apparently because the weak oestrogens which the foods contain bind with oestrogen-receptor sites and protect them from the negative effects of circulating oestrogens in the body and from xenoestrogens from the environment. There are other foods which in their natural unprocessed state contain significant levels of plant sterols or phyto-hormones as well. They include corn, wheat, apples, almonds, cashews, oats and peanuts. Meanwhile the cruciferous vegetables, such as cabbage and cauliflower and broccoli, also boast anti-breast cancer elements such as indole-3-carbinol (I3C) which deactivates the oestrogen hormones that can encourage breast cancer. At the Foundation of Preventative Oncology in New York City researchers concluded a study examining the actions of these foods by saying that 'dietary I3C may provide the basis for a novel approach for preventing breast cancer . . .'

Natural fibre also offers protection against cancer. Fibre alters the metabolism of oestrogen in the bowel so that more is excreted and less reabsorbed. It has also been well established that optimal quantities of certain nutrients – most of them anti-oxidant vitamins and minerals such as vitamin A, C, beta-carotene and the mineral selenium have a great deal to contribute to cancer prevention. Researchers have discovered while examining 89,000 women nurses who were followed over an eight-year period that those who had an intake of less than 6,630 iu of vitamin A per day also had a 25 per cent higher incidence of cancer than women whose daily intake of the vitamin was above this level. The B vitamins too are important for immunity and may help prevent cancer. This group of vitamins is very much involved in the metabolism of oestrogen in the body as well as in good bowel function so that toxic wastes can be efficiently eliminated. Yet most of the B complex are destroyed or drastically reduced in the milling of flour and the preparation of convenience foods so that many women in the western world are deficient in them.

The best diet to follow for cancer prevention is low fat,

where less than 20 per cent of the total calories you consume come from fats – a primarily vegetarian way of eating that rejects highly processed convenience foods, eliminates processed oils, is high in complex carbohydrates and rich in fibre to help control the body's cycling oestrogen. Consider taking extra anti-oxidant nutrients to boost your levels of these important protectors and fortify your immune system to help protect against cancer as well. We are not powerless to deal with cancer. Banishing fear, losing our reverence for high-tech diagnostic procedures whose effectiveness needs to be questioned and taking back our responsibility for our own life and health hold the real promise for prevention. Knowing how is the first step, action is the next, action taken by we women ourselves with the help of our doctors and health practitioners. Once again, in the bloodless revolution, the power for change lies largely in our own hands.

Chapter Eight

Gremlins in the Architecture

Osteoporosis is a terrible disease. A progressive loss of minerals, bone mass and bone density, it affects men as well as women and can result in fractures of the hip, shoulder, ribs, vertebrae, forearm or wrist. Statistically, bone loss in women begins several years before menopause and then gets worse afterwards, creating an ever-increasing risk of debilitating breakages. In Britain, where the incidence of the illness has increased six times in the past 30 years, one in three women now develop it and one in eight men. In the United States, statistics are even worse. The illness currently costs the country more than eleven billion dollars a year. Twenty-five per cent of women whose hips fracture die within two years – not always directly from the fracture but from ending up in nursing homes where inactivity, alienation and loss of control over their lives defeat them. Today more women in the industrialized world die of fractures related to bone thinning than from cancers of the womb, cervix and breast put together.

Silent Killer

Osteoporosis is not a simple disorder. And it is most certainly not another so-called oestrogen deficiency disease, as some would still have us believe. Neither is it treatable by drinking masses of milk or stuffing yourself with calcium supplements. Surprisingly, both of these actions can actually make the condition worse. Like coronary heart disease which few people even know they have until a heart attack strikes, osteoporosis is an insidious illness. The *Harvard Medical School Newsletter* recently dubbed it the 'silent epidemic'. It develops secretly over the years until one day its presence in the body surfaces to devastate a life. It need not. The idea that is still taught in medical schools that bone mass decline is a normal consequence of ageing is quite simply false. There is nothing normal about bone thinning.

A few facts. Osteoporosis regularly occurs in men who are deficient in testosterone and in women who are deficient in progesterone. Black women have less bone loss than white women, big women less than small women and fat women less than their skinny sisters. Meat eaters are at far greater risk of the disease than vegetarians. A high calcium intake is often toted as essential in preventing bone thinning. Yet people in Third World countries whose daily intake of calcium is less than half our own have a very low incidence of the disease whereas in our culture its incidence is very high and continues to mount. Users of prescription drugs have more osteoporosis than people who do not take medication. And couch potatoes are far more prone to the condition than women who get regular exercise. To prevent osteoporosis you need to understand it. The earlier a woman learns about why it happens and the sooner she takes action to counter it, the better. Ideally this should be in her twenties and thirties. However, if those years are already long past, take heart. Despite all the fearmongering surrounding the disease, the truth is that there are actions you can take not only to halt bone loss if it has begun but even to *reverse* it – no matter what your age.

Living Bone

Bones may seem like tough inanimate objects but they are not. They are actually living support tissue which is constantly changing and growing. Bone is made up of a combination of a flexible non-cellular collagen matrix which has been embedded with hard and inflexible mineralized crystals. It is a kind of mineralized cartilage. Without the flexibility of collagen your bones would be so brittle they would easily shatter. Without the crystalline hardness of minerals they would resemble the soft cartilage of a shark. Unless you spent your entire life under water your skeleton would be unable to support the weight of your body. The combination of both this tensile strength from the minerals and compression strength from the collagen creates just about the finest structural resistance to breakage found anywhere in the living world.

Your bones are constantly being renewed, at a surprising rate. This is what makes it possible for breaks to mend and for a child's body to grow taller. There are two kinds of bone – *cortical* and *trabecular*. The heavy bones of your body such as the long bones of the legs and arms are cortical bones. Designed to give great directional strength, they are densely cast in spirals around tiny tubular channels through which cells can travel. Cortical bones renew themselves completely about every ten years. The other kind of bone (trabecular) is found in the vertebrae of your spine and at the ends of the long bones of the legs and arms – in places where you need compression strength. Trabecular bone is more web-like in its structure. And its turnover is even faster than cortical bone, completely renewing itself every two to three years.

When you are born, the growth hormone made by your body stimulates bones to grow at a rate that in general matches the rate at which the rest of your body is growing. Children start life at about 22–24 inches long, growing eventually to 64 inches, 69 inches, even 74 inches. The bones, muscles, tendons and ligaments all keep in touch via a mysterious and beautiful inner harmonic – of which bones are a part – that synchronizes growth rate. One day puberty arrives and the pineal gland switches on the reproductive hormones of the pituitary. The pituitary in turn activates the ovaries and the ovaries start making oestrogen and progesterone. When this happens women have a growth spurt for a year or so, after which they grow no more in height. Now the hormones of the ovaries take over. It becomes the job of oestrogen to slow up or moderate the rate at which old bone is being broken down. Meanwhile progesterone gets busy encouraging the manufacture of new bone. If the speed of these two processes are in complete harmony – working at the same rate – your skeleton will stay at that particular bone density. When new bone formation exceeds breakdown then your bones will grow more and more dense and stronger. But if breakdown begins to overtake new bone production then osteoporosis develops.

Bones can be thought of as similar to the fibres that make

a scarf or shawl – fibres that are knitted together with little spaces in between. When osteoporosis occurs not only have the fibres become finer, you actually have fewer of them. In effect you have lost a number of bone strands and each strand that is left has become thinner. Under the microscope, sometimes even with the naked eye, you can see there are spaces in such bone which make it look spongy and porous. That's where the word osteoporosis comes from. Whenever the resorption of bone is faster than the making of new bone you will have osteoporosis. In fact, osteoporosis can be described as the condition which happens when there is a relative deficiency of osteoblasts resulting in inadequate bone formation.

Personal Pacman

The ability of bones to break down and re-form depends on a process called *remodelling* which relies on two very special kinds of cells in the substrate out of which all bone develops. The first are called *osteoclasts*. If you have ever played the video game Pacman it is easy to understand how they work. It is the job of the oestrogen-modulated osteoclasts to travel through the spirals and web-like structures of your bone tissue like Pacman, seeking out old mineralized bone and then to gobble it up or dissolve it away (the proper name is *resorb* it) in order to make way for new bone. The minerals contained in the gobbled bone are released into general circulation and only empty spaces – called lacunae – are left behind. After the osteoclasts have done their Pacman work, along come the other kind of bone cells – the *osteoblasts*. These cells, whose activity is modulated by progesterone, are drawn to the same sites and make their way into these lacunae. There they get busy creating new bone.

When you are growing up your pituitary is pumping out growth hormone so the action of your osteoblasts dominates and more bone is created than is destroyed. Around puberty the activity of osteoclasts and osteoblasts becomes more balanced. Later on, however, the balance can shift in favour of the bone-eating osteoclasts while osteoblast activity declines. It is now that osteoporosis first takes hold. You get a shrinkage in bone mass since more bone is being resorbed than being built and more spaces are appearing than are being filled. If this goes on for a long time too many minerals can be lost and bone gets less hard and less dense until at last it becomes finely honeycombed and highly susceptible to breakage.

Stress Your Body

When any crystal structure, such as bone, is put under stress there are changes in the voltage of the electric fields around and through it. These electromagnetic changes draw the osteoclasts to the areas of your bones which need replacing as well as encouraging the production of new bone via the work of the osteoblasts which form the patterns of arcs and curves that create bone texture – a bit like weaving a scarf. When they are properly formed these patterns provide resistance to all the day-to-day stresses your bones are put under. In fact the more you stress your bones through exercise the better quality will be the electric fields that govern remodelling – provided, of course, you supply your body with all the nutrients it needs to create new bone tissue. All any woman needs to maintain good, strong, dense, well-mineralized bones is a good balance between the activity of her osteoblasts and her osteoclasts. A woman in the western world living a sedentary life and eating convenience foods will find this virtually impossible.

Secrets from the Grave

Once osteoporosis was considered a menopausal disease. If it occurred at all, and it was still pretty rare, then it would only happen at menopause or afterwards. A fascinating article appeared in the prestigious British medical journal *The Lancet* not long ago. During the restoration of Christ Church, Spitalfields in London, some skeletal material dating from between 1729 and 1852 was unearthed from the crypt. This gave medical researchers the chance to compare the rate of bone loss in the legs of these bone samples with those of present-day women of the same age. Using dual-energy X-ray absorptiometry (see p. 298), investigators discovered that there was significantly less bone loss in these women of 200 years ago compared to modern women despite our supposedly better diet. Equally surprising, when investigators calibrated bone density with age they could find no sign of a menopausal change in the unearthed bones. Now, however, unlike our ancestors, more and more women arrive at menopause having already lost between 20 and 30 per cent of their bone mass. And this loss begins much earlier than most woman realize.

It is during the five to eight years before menopause when, unknown to them, many women are experiencing anovulatory cycles that they are most vulnerable to bone loss. When a woman is not ovulating during a monthly cycle, no corpus luteum produces progesterone even though her periods may seem normal. Insufficient progesterone leads to insufficient osteoblast activity. For without enough progesterone the osteoblasts are unable to produce new bone properly so more bone is resorbed than built and osteoporosis sets in. Statistically bone mass in healthy women reaches a peak in their early thirties. After that osteoclast activity tends to increase while osteoblast activity decreases so that it declines gradually. At menopause the decline further increases for three to five years after which it tends to slow again to a rate of between 1 and 0.5 per cent a year. Most doctors still believe this is inevitable. It most certainly is not. To prevent it, to stop it and to reverse bone loss you need to do two things: change your lifestyle and get your hormone balance right. Let's look at hormones first.

Hormone Connections

Both oestrogen and progesterone help protect against osteoporosis. The average doctor knows that oestrogen replacement can slow down the rate of bone loss. This it does by regulating the 'gobbling' actions of the osteoclasts. What the doctor is probably not aware of, however, is the far more important role that progesterone plays both in protecting against osteoporosis as well as in reversing it. And where oestrogen's role is a minor one, progesterone's is a major one.

As far back as the early 1940s researchers noticed the relationship between the decline in female sex hormones and the development of osteoporosis. Not until the 1970s, however, did they discover that oestrogen replacement slightly decreased the rate of bone loss in women on HRT. Around the same time epidemiological studies indicated that there was a decrease in the number of fractures that occurred to women who had been put on HRT. With reports like this, backed by marketing and public relations money from pharmaceutical manufacturers eager to find new groups of women to sell their drugs to, it did not take long for statements to appear drawing the conclusion that, like menopause itself, osteoporosis is an 'oestrogen deficiency disease' and then spread the news far and wide that oestrogen replacement was the *treatment of choice* against the disease.

Unfortunately the news that was spread has turned out to be one of those dangerous 'half-truths' to which twentieth-century medicine is particularly prone. Yet it has continued to spread despite the fact that highly respected researchers and reviewers writing in prestigious medical journals, from the *Journal of the American Medical Association* and *The Lancet*, as well as every up-to-date standard medical text book, have long since refuted it.

The early studies on which the oestrogen-protection assumption were based had gross scientific defects. Some were carried out on too few participants to be significant. Others made use of imprecise methods for measuring bone density. Later scientific papers (post 1976) praising the value of oestrogen in managing osteoporosis failed to take into account that often either progesterone or a progestogen had also been included with the oestrogen supplementation. It could well have been that the minor benefits that were reported came not from the oestrogen itself but from the combination of the oestrogen and progesterone or oestrogen and a progestogen – or even from the progesterone or the progestogen itself. When medroxyprogesterone – a common progestogen – was used on its own without oestrogen in postmenopausal women, researchers reported that a small gain in bone mineral density of 5 per cent took place. It is not much but even this small gain is better than what can be achieved using oestrogen on its own. However oestrogen continues to be considered as the treatment of choice for osteoporosis.

A Touch of Evil

Unopposed oestrogen – that is oestrogen given on its own – carries with it serious long-term health dangers, both minor and major. They range from encouraging the laying down of fat stores in a woman's body and causing water retention to increasing her risk of endometrial cancer, liver disease and breast cancer. None the less, when hormone replacement began oestrogen was given on its own. These days, thankfully, most doctors are aware of the dangers of prescribing unopposed oestrogen and no longer do so. However, what they do prescribe – progestogen – is not safe either. Very few are yet aware that oestrogen's bone-protecting capacity is not all it is cracked up to be. Busy with their practices they often do not have time to examine the scientific literature closely.

Again it was Jerilynn Prior and her colleagues reporting in the *New England Journal of Medicine* who confirmed that oestrogen's role in osteoporosis prevention is only a minor one. In their studies of female athletes they found that osteoporosis occurs to the degree that they become *progesterone* deficient even though their oestrogen levels remain normal. Prior also made an extensive review of published scientific evidence in this area. It confirmed that it is not oestrogen but *progesterone* which is the *bone trophic* hormone – that is the bone builder. Prior and her team were even able to identify progesterone receptor sites on osteoblast cells. Nobody has even found osteoblast receptors for oestrogen. The only mechanism of action that oestrogen has on bone is that it helps inhibit osteoclast resorption, but it can do nothing to build new bone. The bottom line is that it is in women with *progesterone deficiency* where bone loss occurs.

Awakenings

It was pressure from hundreds of women with osteoporosis whose bone density tests only showed that they were getting worse that triggered Dr John Lee's experiments with progesterone. Many had already had one or two fractures and many were already on oestrogen replacement. Other patients he knew couldn't take oestrogen because of a past history of breast cancer. Some were already on a good diet and were trying to take enough exercise, yet still they all had progressive osteoporosis. Even in the core of women without a history of breast cancer, Lee, like so many conscientious doctors, had been deeply concerned about the possible long-term side-effects of giving oestrogen replacement. Since oestrogen is still produced by postmenopausal women, he asked himself, 'Could progesterone alone be enough to prevent and/or reverse osteoporosis?'

Tender Mercies

Lee began to test his hypothesis on women with postmenopausal osteoporosis using transdermal progesterone cream together with a programme of dietary changes, vitamin and mineral supplements, and modest exercise. Some of his patients were also given very small doses of oestrogen, particularly if they suffered from vaginal dryness. Lee carefully monitored his results, keeping records for more than ten years. When at last they were finally published his findings turned out to be nothing short of revolutionary. He had been able to accomplish the impossible. The natural progesterone cream had been able to halt bone loss whether or not the women taking it had been given oestrogen as well. More remarkable still, his patients showed an improvement of approximately 15 per cent in bone mineral density over a three-year period.

This had never been done – not with oestrogen, not with other drugs like calcitonin or the diphosphates nor with anything else. Patient after patient got better. Even more surprising, the women with the worst bones improved fastest. Some of them showed much greater than average improvement – a

30 to 40 per cent increase in bone over the three-year period was not uncommon. Those women whose bone density was fairly good when the experiment began improved more slowly until finally each woman (no matter what condition her bones had been in at the start of the study) had reached her optimum bone density and then kept it.

Witnessing the effect of progesterone on bone was one of the most dramatic things that Lee had ever seen in his long family practice. It has a similar impact on other doctors who gradually became aware of what Lee had been doing, including a number of orthopaedic surgeons who had been used to receiving referrals from Lee for his patients with broken bones. His patients stopped having fractures if they fell. Gradually, by word of mouth, the news spread. Before long Lee had treated hundreds of women successfully with a progesterone cream and simple lifestyle changes. Out of a group of 100 of his treated patients, selected at random, only three had experienced fractures. One fell down a flight of stairs carrying a television set and broke her humerus. She refused to have it set in plaster, put it in a sling instead and, to the amazement of her orthopaedist, found that it healed beautifully in under five weeks. Another was a woman in her seventies who had been involved in a serious car crash. Driving a little Volkswagen she had been crushed between two lorries. The accident demolished her Volkswagen and fractured both her knees. The orthopaedic surgeon who had screwed the broken pieces together and then watched them heal swiftly commented that it was the best bone that he had ever seen in a seventy-six-year-old. The third fracture, the result of a minor accident, was equally simple to heal. The other women treated with progesterone and a lifestyle change programme simply didn't have fractures any more.

An End to Osteoporosis

So there was Lee, a simple country doctor, with hundreds of patients who had been going through his office for some ten years, for whom he had records showing that their bones were greatly improved. He had women patients who had increased their bone mineral density even up to 50 per cent. Some of his patients were 45 years old, others were 75 years old when they started treatment. Age did not matter. Their bones were hungry for progesterone. The benefits his patients reported from progesterone and lifestyle change didn't end with osteoporosis prevention and the reversal of bone loss either. Women also reported a decrease in fibroids where they had been present, an increase in energy, a decline in aches and pains, and the disappearance of many other negative symptoms associated with PMS or menopause.

Hungry for Change

Although the successes of doctors, including Lee, who use topically applied natural progesterone are great news it might be tempting to think that all you need to do to prevent osteoporosis is to rub on progesterone cream every day and then sit back munching on junk food, certain that all will be well. The trouble is it just doesn't work that way. How you eat and live are equally important and need to be addressed if you are to have a future free of bone loss and avoidable fractures. A good treatment and prevention programme for osteoporosis needs to include carefully chosen vitamins and minerals which play an important part in osteoblast activity – vitamin D, vitamin C, beta-carotene, zinc and magnesium – as well as weight-bearing exercise for at least 15 minutes, preferably half an hour or more, at least three times a week. Without adequate exercise calcium cannot be incorporated into the bones since it is only when bones are put under physical stress that calcium is demanded. A good programme also emphasizes a way of eating which includes lots of calcium-rich leafy green vegetables and limits red meat to no more than a couple of times a week. It cuts down on alcohol and cuts out all 'sodas' and manufactured soft drinks for each of these in its own way affects the way calcium is used in the body. Many forms of purified protein such as casein, lactalbumin and egg whites – regularly used in slimmers' meal-replacement drinks – cause calcium loss too. In fact crash dieting of any kind is a common contributor to bone thinning in women.

Calcium Connections

In every case of osteoporosis calcium loss from the bones lies at the core of the problem. Calcium is the most abundant mineral in your body. It is vital for strong bones. So is phosphorus. After calcium, phosphorus is the next most prominent element in bone. The ratio of calcium to phosphorus is around 2.5:1. About 99 per cent of the calcium in your body is deposited in your bones and teeth although the remaining 1 per cent has some very important jobs to do. It helps regulate nerve and muscle contraction, for instance. It is related to the parathyroid function, and involved with blood-clotting and the metabolism of vitamin D. Calcium also enables your body to use iron properly and activate a number of important enzymes that help to regulate the passage of nutrients into and out of the cells. Finally, calcium is frequently called on – and called *forth* from bones – to balance the pH of your blood, rendering it more alkaline when it has become too acid from long-term stress, eating a lot of meat or drinking a lot of coffee.

If this makes you think you need to rush out and buy a bottle of calcium pills, think again. Despite all the vitamin manufacturers currently pushing calcium supplements, research shows that taking calcium supplements is of little help in preventing osteoporosis. It may even make the problem worse. Taking higher doses of calcium supplements can contribute to kidney stones and interfere with the metabolism of zinc and magnesium, both of which play central roles in building strong bones. The best way to get your calcium is to eat the right kind of foods, particularly green leafy foods and sea plants which are loaded with it in a form that is easy for the body to assimilate. The whole calcium issue is enormously complicated, yet it is very important to understand.

Metabolic Keys

For calcium to function properly in relation to bone building it has to be accompanied by phosphorus – but not too much phosphorus – as well as magnesium, vitamins A, B6, C, D, E and K. Zinc is also important since zinc is a co-factor in the intra-cellular conversion of beta-carotene to vitamin A which in turn helps manufacture the collagen matrix of bone. Zinc has to be present in sufficient quantities for the body's enzymes to make the conversion. Even the trace elements boron and silicon, needed only in the most minute quantities, play important roles in bone strength.

Forget the Milk

We have been led to believe that all you need for strong bones is to get lots of calcium either by popping pills or drinking masses of milk. Millions have been spent to propagate this fantasy. Yet, after three generations of milk promotion, osteoporosis has now reached epidemic proportions in the West while in countries where milk is not drunk it hardly exists. So negative an effect can milk and milk products, such as cheeses, exert on a woman's health that if you would care to experiment by leaving all milk products out of your diet for three weeks you are likely to find your looks and energy levels transformed for the better. This is not all that easy to do since milk in one form or another finds its way into most convenience foods. It is in breads and biscuits, and sauces. It is even in many nutritional supplements.

Milk is a food designed by nature for a very specific purpose – to feed young mammals until they can feed themselves. Cow's milk is made for cows and human milk for humans. As we grow up our bodies gradually lose the ability to produce *lactase*, the enzyme which digests the sugar in milk. This creates what is known as a lactose intolerance. Studies show that three out of every four adults in the United States have some degree of lactose intolerance. They are unable to digest milk properly. If they choose to include dairy foods in their diet they find their energy levels are lowered, their bodies can produce more mucus in an immune reaction, and that they experience food sensitivity reactions with symptoms that may include mood swings or depression as well as aches and pains, often with no sense of what may be causing it all. Milk is the most common food allergen in the western world. (Wheat follows close behind it.) Yet you find milk in one form or another just about everywhere – in cheese. cream, cream sauces, yogurt, ice-cream, breads and other commercially prepared food products. There is also mounting evidence that milk, the pure white food which we are continually told will give us good bones, strong hair and 'lots of bottle', may actually be toxic to adults. At Harvard Medical School, Dr Daniel Cramer discovered that using milk products increases the risk of ovarian cancer in lactose-intolerant women. After extensive analysis of lactose-intolerant women in 36 countries as well as meticulous examination of human and animal studies, researchers concluded that *galactose*, one of the sugars in lactose, is toxic to the ovaries and interferes with fertility. Some believe it may even trigger birth defects. Far from turning to milk as a source of calcium, most women who value wellbeing would be better off clearing out milk and milk products from their diet altogether. If you are going to cut milk out of your diet, you need to get rid of anything that might contain milk products such as milk solids, sodium caseinate, sodium lactate, milk fats, whey or lactose. So read labels carefully.

As for taking pills, a number of scientific reports have shown that calcium supplements do little to stop the loss of cortical bone tissue and have virtually no effect at all on trabecular bone in the spine and the hip where most osteoporotic fractures occur. Yet most people still believe that the best source of calcium is milk or milk products. The question which they rarely ask is where does the calcium in milk come from in the first place? Cows get calcium from eating green foods – grass, silage, herbs and plants. These are not the only plants which can take the calcium from the soil and turn it into a form available for absorption by animals. Beetroot tops, Chinese leaves, rocket, lettuce, seaweeds, herbs and broad-leafed green vegetables are all excellent sources of calcium. A cup of any of these vegetables supplies as much calcium as a cup of milk. And this kind of calcium is easily assimilated along with a collection of other important minerals and trace elements from such foods – all without having to deal with possible negative side-effects of using milk products. Include plenty of organic leafy green vegetables in your meals and you need never give calcium another thought. Incidentally, the reason why taking calcium supplements or drinking masses of milk has very little effect in halting – and none at all in reversing – osteoporosis is because it is usually not an *absence* of calcium in the body which is the problem so much as a *disorder in calcium metabolism.*

A Delicate Process

Calcium metabolism is a very complex process. The absorption of calcium from water or mineral salts in general tends to be highly inefficient. Only somewhere between 20 and 30 per cent of the calcium you take in through processed foods will actually be absorbed. Most of that then gets filtered through your kidneys and then excreted in urine and sweat or eliminated through the faeces. Many factors influence just how much calcium you will absorb at any time. When you are growing rapidly or when you place stress on your bones by doing weight-bearing exercise your absorption of calcium is increased. When your body is in great need of calcium it is also absorbed more effectively. In fact the smaller the supply of calcium available from your foods and the greater the need your body has for this mineral, the more efficient calcium absorption becomes. The opposite is also true. When large quantities of calcium are available – say if someone has been drinking a lot of milk or has taken masses of calcium supplements – then the absorption of calcium is markedly decreased. It is worth remembering that in the United States, where the consumption of calcium supplements and milk products is the highest in the world, so is the incidence of osteoporosis.

Acid Test

For proper assimilation, calcium needs an acid medium in the digestive tract. As people get older the hydrochloric acid content of the stomach tends to decrease. With this decrease comes a further decrease in your body's ability to assimilate calcium. Calcium absorption requires adequate vitamin D, too, which, together with parathyroid hormone, regulates the level of calcium in your blood. An adequate supply of the right kind of fat in the gut also facilitates the absorption of calcium. The mineral phosphorus is also essential to build bone. But if either calcium or phosphorus are taken in excess – as happens in the case of phosphorus in a typical western diet which includes processed meats, colas and diet drinks – then neither element can be used efficiently and bone loss increases.

Your body deals with any excess calcium that you take in by dumping it wherever it can in an attempt to restore a healthy balance between calcium and other minerals present. Chemical calcium supplements taken over a long period of time can bring about an increase in calcium plaque in the arteries as well as result in the calcification of soft tissues, but they won't make for stronger bones. Researchers at the University of Kentucky have found that calcium salt megadoses can actually decrease bone strength as well as induce internal bleeding. Studies show that animals fed calcium as salts at a dietary level of 2.7 per cent will die from profuse internal bleeding. Others report that pigs fed excess calcium have diminished bone mineral mass and lower bone-breaking strength. Taking drugs such as laxatives, diuretics, antacids and tetracyclines also impedes calcium absorption. So does coffee drinking. Like taking in too much protein, it causes calcium to be leached from your bone and carried out of your body. Once you begin to sense the enormous complexity and synergy involved with calcium absorption and use you begin to understand why it is probably best to get the calcium you need from a good diet. If you still feel you *must* take calcium supplements make sure they are low dose and in a form such as calcium EAP which is more readily absorbed than the usual calcium lactate or calcium carbonate which are cheap to make and form the basis of most calcium supplements. As far as oyster shell calcium or dolomite is concerned, avoid them like the plague. They can be filled with dangerous heavy metals.

The Magnesium Connection

What surprises most women – doctors too for that matter – is that it is taking extra magnesium that can make the greatest difference to good calcium metabolism. Magnesium is another element essential for the proper metabolism of calcium. Magnesium probably acts as a catalyst for more enzymes in the body than any other metal. Magnesium is plentiful in properly grown whole grains – brown rice, buckwheat, millet, whole wheat, whole rye and in legumes such as beans, lentils and peas, but low in highly processed foods. Adequate magnesium helps the body absorb calcium. Where there is a magnesium deficiency not only can osteoporosis develop easily but so can joint and soft tissue calcification. Low intra-cellular magnesium undermines immune functions too, making women susceptible to infection and such hard-to-handle conditions as ME, where women with low intra-cellular magnesium have been found to have unnaturally shaped bone mineral crystals.

Magnesium deficiency is common in women with or without osteoporosis. Milk is a relatively poor source of magnesium – another reason why it is a poor food for protection against osteoporosis. Magnesium deficiencies are particularly widespread in women over the age of 35 who have long been living on a western diet. PMS expert Dr Guy Abraham showed that giving women 600 mg of magnesium a day could bring about a significant increase in bone mass in nine months, although the women he treated were also given other vitamins and minerals as well as HRT so it is impossible to determine just how much of the improvement was due to the magnesium. In a recent Israeli study, however, where 31 post-menopausal women were given 250–750 mg of magnesium a day for two years, bone density increased 1–8 per cent in 75 per cent of the cases and remained unchanged in the remaining 25 per cent, while women who refused magnesium supplements altogether experienced losses in bone density of 1–3 per cent.

According to many recent studies, vegetarians have stronger bones and less osteoporosis than do meat eaters. A good, unrefined vegetarian diet which includes whole-grain breads and cereals, legumes and fresh vegetables is also moderate in protein and rich in magnesium, zinc, silicon and other bone-strengthening minerals. By contrast meat is high in protein. When you eat an *excess* of protein, calcium is drawn from your bones to help neutralize the acidic protein waste products. This creates a negative calcium balance. When forced to metabolize excess protein the body carries calcium away from bones and excretes it. Eskimos whose traditional diet was very high in protein (250–400 grams a day) with a high calcium intake of 1,500 to 2,500 mg a day were found to have the highest rate of osteoporosis of any group of people. By contrast, the Bantu in Africa who consume only 47 g of protein a day and get less than 400 mg of calcium – mostly from plant foods – remain free from osteoporosis. Of course, they also get plenty of exercise. Without adequate exercise calcium cannot be incorporated into the bones.

Kids' Teeth, Yes – Women's Bones, No!

For strong bones into your nineties, steer clear of a diet that is excessively high in protein, avoid diuretics (and if you are on them, ask your doctor to take you off them), steer clear of fluoride and don't drink fluorinated water. Fluoride is still wrongly recommended by some doctors as a substance that can help build bones. Although fluoride encourages the development of bone mass, at the same time it decreases bone strength. A large body of research links even low levels of fluoride in water with an increased incidence of fractures. In people undergoing fluoride therapy, non-vertebral fractures have been shown to increase by 300–600 per cent.

You should also avoid anything like an excess of alcohol or sugar which creates metabolic acidosis and leaches calcium from the skeleton.

Osteoporosis prevention is best started early, preferably in the teens, twenties and thirties while the density of bone is still increasing. It is easy to build good strong bones and establish lifestyle habits that can carry you through the second half of your life with no trouble. If osteoporosis has already begun, you will probably want to make use of topically applied progesterone to restore normal bone density and keep you permanently osteoporosis-free. Finally, just in case all this sounds like a tall order, take heart. The benefits an osteoporosis-protective lifestyle can bring to overall health are immense. Such a lifestyle also helps to keep your immune system functioning well, helping to protect you from illness, countering early ageing and enhancing your energy all round.

Chapter Nine

Phoenix in the Fire

One day, an ordinary day like any other, almost imperceptibly you sense something strange is happening in your body. A tiny flutter of heat begins to rise and sweep up your torso, neck and head. Then the strange feeling passes away again almost as quickly as it has come and you find now you are feeling just a bit chilled. Or maybe one night at 3 a.m. you awaken to find yourself drenched in sweat for no reason. 'Am I ill?' you ask, making a quick check through your body only to find that no, you do not feel ill. Then what on earth is happening?

The most common herald of menopause is the appearance of hot flushes. They are virtually synonymous with it in the experience of many women. An adjunct to hot flushes are night sweats where women awaken drenched in sweat, so much so that they not only need to change their night clothes but also the sheets on their beds. Both night sweats and hot flushes can be disconcerting particularly if a woman is fearful of them. Although a lot can be said about hot flushes, only two things are absolutely essential to know. First, they are *completely harmless*. Secondly, hot flushes are virtually the *only* symptoms among long lists of things usually attributed to menopause that genuinely belong to it. This was established by research carried out at Oxford and reported in the *British Medical Journal*. It compared mid-life women with mid-life men in an attempt to find out which of women's complaints were genuinely menopausal. Scientists reported that among those symptoms generally lumped together under the menstrual label – including aches in joints, migraine, depression and the rest – only hot flushes show a direct relationship to menopause itself. Another interesting study carried out in Canada by Pat Kaufert found that despite all the discussion over hot flushes, most women still look upon them as normal and believe that having them doesn't detract from seeing themselves as generally in good or excellent health.

Cross Currents

Menopausal women are not the only people who get hot flushes. They can also be common during pregnancy as well as just after giving birth. Men, too, will experience them after any kind of rapid withdrawal of sex hormones. Women of all ages get them especially strongly when their ovaries are removed surgically, and men when the testicles are taken out. So do people who for any reason have been given drugs antagonistic to gonadotrophin-releasing hormones. Such drugs cause testosterone levels in men and oestrogen levels in women to fall rapidly. At the time of menopause thinner women tend to experience more drastic alterations in their oestrogen – FSH/LH – levels and are therefore more likely that their bigger sisters to experience stronger hot flushes.

The standard medical treatment for hot flushes is oestrogen. And it is quite true that extra oestrogen will relieve the symptoms just like all the little leaflets tell you. What they don't tell you is that, if you decide to go on oestrogen for a few years 'to get you through the rough patch', when you come off it your hot flushes are very likely to return in force – whether getting off HRT turns out to be three or four years or as many as 15 or 20 years later. Extra oestrogen does not 'cure' hot flushes. It only masks them for a while. In any case, there is nothing to 'cure'. For hot flushes are not a symptom of disease. They are a *normal bodily change* associated with the transition between the menstrual years and menopause. Many physicians who work with natural methods of healing believe that, far from being a negative event, hot flushes can actually help cleanse the body. They can also be an indication of considerable vitality in the woman who has them. Most hot flushes happen without anybody ever knowing except the woman herself. Women always think they are more evident to the outside world than they are. And even if they are, so what? Why should a woman agree, even tacitly, to buy into the general consensus that menopause – like the swollen belly of pregnancy or the flow of menstrual blood – is something ugly to be hidden. To me all three seem proud badges of womanhood. If, as many women fear, men are troubled by the evidence of them, that is their problem. They are probably the kind of men who find it difficult to contact their own deep sexuality and who therefore feel uncomfortable with the birth-death-regenerative nature of life. Bless them and send a little prayer that one day they grow up.

No Great Matter

Back in the nineteenth century flushes were known as 'hot blooms'. Even then they were recognized as the most common symptom associated with menopause. The physiology of the hot flush is not yet fully understood. Medical dictionaries define flushes as 'vasomotor symptoms of the climacterium – sudden vasodilation with a sensation of heat, usually involving the face and neck, and upper part of the chest; sweats, often profuse, frequently following the flush.' During a hot flush blood rushes into the capillaries, the pulse rate rises and skin temperature goes up. Hot flushes do not appear to affect blood pressure, but they are often followed by a chilling phenomenon. Both oestrogen and progesterone play a role in internal temperature regulation. Hot flushes are triggered by the hypothalamus which among its many responsibilities holds overall control for body temperature as well as for directing the release of pituitary hormones. They can occur when a sudden lowering of the central hypothalamic thermostat takes place. The body trying to adjust its core temperature to this new setting produces heat loss by activating vasodilation (as blood flows through all the capillaries at the surface of the skin) and sweating.

At or near menopause the ovaries are programmed to decommission themselves. They no longer respond to the secretion of FSH from the pituitary as they used to by secreting oestrogen. The result is that the hypothalamus raises its production of GnRH – and its voltage. Finally the electric excitation spills over to affect an adjacent limbic nucleus involved in temperature control, causing a reaction which produces rapid temperature changes in the body. The capillaries are affected by consequent chemical or hormonal changes which take place in the tissues causing them to dilate and the nerves to be highly reactive.

Because hot flushes arise from neuroendocrine activity, heightened stress tends to make them worse. Similarly, placebos can often make them better through the complex interactive mechanisms of the immune, endocrine and central nervous system by which mind and body are linked. In most women hot flushes are at their most intense during the last year or so before menstruation ceases and during the first year or so afterwards. What do they feel like? This can differ just about as much as individual women do. Generally there is a flush of heat which sweeps your torso, neck and head. You feel the need to take off your sweater or jacket for a few minutes then will probably want to put it back on again since the body's reaction to vasodilation can leave you feeling a little chilled afterwards. Sometimes hot flushes can make your skin go red and even blotchy. Sometimes they are followed by perspiration which can either be no more than a little glow or as much as a torrent of water. Usually a hot flush lasts from a few seconds to a couple of minutes. Very rarely they can last as long as 15 minutes or more.

How often they come is another highly individual thing. A very few women seem to experience hot flushes – at least for a short period of their life – every hour or two. Others get them only at certain times of the day or night. Some women report up to 30 hot flushes a day while most experience only one or two. A few women don't get them at all. Most of the studies done on menopausal women are carried out in western countries where it is said that on average 75 per cent of women experience hot flushes. However, their prevalence in the whole world – bearing in mind the bias towards studies done in the West and the fact that in some primitive cultures women don't get them at all – appears to be that between the ages of 40 and 60 the number of women who get hot flushes ranges from 24 per cent upwards, depending upon the country of origin, diet and lifestyle of the women. Very few researchers have investigated at what age hot flushes begin but one study reports that in 60 per cent of the women who experience them they arrive on the scene some time between the ages of 40 and 50 while in 10 per cent of naturally menopausal women (that is those who have not undergone a hysterectomy) they began before the age of 41. The prevalence of hot flushes is virtually 100 per cent among women who have gone through an artificially induced menopause as a result of surgery. After surgery symptoms are much more intense and the flushes come much more frequently than they did before.

Factors that predispose women to hot flushes have also been little studied. What is known is that there is no correlation between hot flushes and socio-economic groups, employment status or medical status. The incidence of hot flushes is also not at all to be related to the age at which a woman began to menstruate nor to her age at menopause nor to the number of children that she has had. The one factor that does appear to correlate with hot flushes is that women that get them tend to have a lower body weight than women who do not.

Some of the most interesting work looking at the incidence of hot flushes has come from examining the effect of diet and cultural attitudes. In Indonesia and Japan women experience very few hot flushes, particularly compared to women in western societies. Mayan Indians in Mexico report no symptoms whatever at the approach of menopause other than the menstrual cycle becoming irregular. It would appear that there are significant dietary differences operating here. Japanese women eat lots of soya products which contain a high level of plant sterols. Urinalysis of Japanese women shows elevated levels of oestriol – the good-guy oestrogen – compared to western women and a diet high in natural phyto-sterols has the capacity to alleviate the symptoms of menopause. This could also explain the very low incidence of hot flushes amongst Mayan, Indonesian and Chinese women.

The Real Thing

Certain plants are high in oestrogen-like hormones – beetroots, potato root, parsley root and yeast, for instance, all of which contain around 70-80 picograms of these natural phytohormones per 100 grams. Natural unheated honey contains significant amounts while dry sage boasts 6,000 iu per kilogram. Clover is also high in phyto-hormones, as is alfalfa, fennel, celery, anise and liquorice. A diet which includes these foods should supply a much higher level of protective natural hormones to a woman's body and can help a great deal to alleviate hot flushes.

Research has also shown that oestrogen levels tend to be lower in premenopausal women with hot flushes than those without hot flushes. However, it is quite clear that low oestrogen levels, although they continually get the blame for hot flushes, are by no means all that is involved in their production. It is the sudden drop in oestrogen which is the issue. And once the hypothalamus and pituitary accustom themselves to lower levels of oestrogen most hot flushes gradually diminish. Sometimes low oestrogen is not involved in hot flushes at all. A small number of women go into menopause in their teens and twenties as a result of genetic abnormalities. These women seldom experience hot flushes. Hot flushes only happen to these women if they take supplementary oestrogen in HRT for a time and then stop. There are many postmenopausal women with low oestrogen levels who never have hot flushes while others continue to have them. Prior to puberty when oestrogen levels are very low, girls do not have hot flushes. On the other hand, hot flushes are reported by some women during pregnancy or immediately after giving birth when oestrogen levels are high. At John Bastyr College and the National College of Naturopathic Medicine in the United States a recent study of menopausal women showed that a formula of botanical substances rich in phyto-hormones was able to relieve the severity of menopausal symptoms including hot flushes in 100 per cent of the women studied, reducing the total number of symptoms by 71 per cent. Hot flushes were the most favourably affected of all symptoms despite the fact that oestrogen levels *decreased* in the treatment subjects during the period of the study.

Allergy Connections

There are certain things known to contribute to the incidence of hot flushes. If you are troubled by their intensity you might like to stay away from cigarette smoking, caffeine and hot spicy food. An overactive thyroid can cause hot flushes, too, as can untreated diabetes. Least recognized but in many cases also important, according to Dr Ellen Grant, author of the courageous book *Sexual Chemistry*, hot flushes may be the result of allergic reactions, particularly to foods or chemicals in the environment. The high levels of steroid hormones used in HRT tend to suppress certain vascular responses such as those which are connected with allergies and with the body's attempt to detoxify itself. When oestrogen decreases rapidly in a menopausal woman or in someone who has been taking extra hormones, then, according to Grant, the underlying allergy/toxicity or vascular reaction which was being masked by the hormones is exposed. Hot flushes can result. At the Charing Cross Hospital Migraine Clinic, Grant requested that her patients explore for themselves which foods gave them reactions such as migraine, headaches and rises in blood pressure as well as hot flushes. She found, as have many clinical ecologists and doctors well versed in the treatment of food sensitivities, that when an offending food such as milk, wheat, cheese, chocolate or oranges is removed from the diet hot flushes will either cease or diminish significantly.

The Power Rises

From an energetic viewpoint, according to eastern religions and traditional medicine, the experience of a hot flush is looked upon as a rapid release of *kundalini energy* – the cosmic creative energy which is said to rise up the spine refining the nervous system and activating the chakras or energy centres, each of which is associated with a different organ or system in the body as well as with different psychic or spiritual developments. The first chakra at the base of the spine is associated with survival energy, for instance, while the second chakra in the pelvis is connected with biological creativity, the fourth chakra in the centre of the chest is linked with the heart and with feelings of compassion, the sixth between the eyebrows governs clairvoyance and far-sightedness, while the seventh chakra is known as the thousand-petalled lotus. When activated it is believed to give the highest spiritual illumination. It is the seventh chakra which is responsible for the halo depicted around the heads of the saints, Jesus and the Buddha.

When the kundalini fire rises in the body it refines the nervous system so a woman becomes capable of carrying powerful healing energies, energies of wisdom and of peace-keeping, all of which throughout history have been viewed as the responsibility of the postmenopausal woman or crone. It can be useful to view hot flushes from this point of view. It is often helpful to see them as life energy. I have worked with many groups of menopausal women by approaching hot flushes in this way. We have looked at them not as something to be feared or concealed but rather as a sign that the creative fire of individual spirit, often long ignored, is demanding attention. Once you heed its call, not only can hot flushes cease to be a problem but the most phenomenal energy is often made available for whatever purpose a woman wants to use it.

I Lie Burning

The long tradition of European natural medicine views hot flushes as a means the body uses to detoxify itself as well as to enhance immunity. Recent research shows that even a slight rise in temperature in the body can be instrumental in doing both. A few months before she died, I interviewed Dr Dagmar Leichti von Brasch about menopause. A vital woman in her eighties and mother of five, Dr Leichti was director of the world-famous Bircher Benner clinic for 40 years and niece to Max Bircher Benner himself. When I asked her from the point of view of natural medicine what hot flushes are all about, she told me that, like night sweats, they have always been considered the means by which a woman's body deep-cleanses itself and refines itself for new physical and spiritual tasks. I also questioned Dr Leichti at some length about her own experience of menopause and about the experiences of the thousands of mid-life women patients she had cared for during the more than half a century she spent practising medicine. She told me that she believed from a spiritual point of view hot flushes and awakening in the night in sweat can be important events in a woman's life. 'They stop us from carrying on "as normal" which women are so apt to do – fulfilling their social roles. They demand that we pay attention to our bodies and to our lives,' said Dr Leichti. 'This is exactly what menopausal women are supposed to do.'

A vibrant and healthy woman, Dr Leichti ran the clinic in Zürich while fulfilling her role as wife and mother. She had the same experience during her menopause that so many perimenopausal and menopausal women have of awakening night after night in the wee hours of the morning for no apparent reason. When this happens it often occurs between 2 a.m. and 3 a.m. She told me she would find herself flooded by tears in the deepest sorrow. She would try to go back to sleep without success so she lay in bed night after night with tears streaming down the sides of her face. For a very long while Dr Leichti could not work out why she felt so sad – especially since every morning she would rise and go about her duties at the clinic feeling perfectly normal. Finally, after several months of this, she decided that instead of remaining in bed she would get up and go to her study to write down what she felt. 'Before long', she told me, 'I realized that I had begun to tap into new ideas which were exciting, to sense new possibilities and to see the world in new ways. It was during those early morning hours that I dreamed new dreams about my future.' Afterwards when Dr Leichti spoke to other women who had had similar experiences – waking in fear or grief, anger or frustration – she discovered that if they were able simply to allow themselves to feel whatever feelings arose from within, they discovered that hidden beneath these feelings lay wells of untapped creativity and bridges to the soul.

It is almost as though, from a spiritual point of view, hot flushes are like the Promethean fire of creation rising up within a woman demanding that she pay attention to who she is and find outlets for this fire.

I believe that Dr Leichti is right for I have observed that over and over again when a woman experiencing hot flushes overcomes her fear of them and begins to listen to the dictates of her soul, both the intensity and the frequency of hot flushes diminish. As one woman who had originally had severe flushes said to me when I asked her about them a few months after she had taken up dancing and drumming, 'Hot flushes? Oh, those. Yes, I guess I still have them. Most of the time I am so busy doing other things I love doing that I don't even notice.'

Living in Time

I, too, have had the experience of waking up night after night. I would awaken like clockwork at 3 a.m. to lie in bed in a state that can only be described as a mixture of terror and frustration. I could never go back to sleep for another couple of hours – some nights not at all. I kept feeling that I wanted to get up and *do* something. I had a strange desire to leave my house and walk barefoot down the path through the woods to the sea. Then the fear would arise, a fear of doing something so unconventional – something different from what I was used to doing. Perhaps it was a fear of madness, I don't know. At that time I had no idea that what I was feeling had to do with my coming menopause. I was menstruating normally and had only begun to have the odd hot flush which did not worry me or seem particularly strange since it felt very much like I feel during vigorous exercise. Later on, just at the point of my periods stopping, I began to brave getting up at night. I would go into my studio, turn on the lights and work. At that time I was finishing my first novel. Then after two or three hours I would climb back into bed again and sleep for an hour before getting up to send my youngest son off to school. I relished that hour. Such a deep and blissful sleep came then – a sleep full of dreams and new visions. Later I was to discover, as Dr Leichti had, that the work I did during my night vigils was the most creative work I had ever done.

Since then, having spoken to dozens of women who report similar experiences, I have come to believe that hot flushes, night sweats, night awakenings and many of the other events associated with menopause often bring to the surface parts of ourselves which we are not living out fully. In Leichti's case it was old sorrow, in my own it was profound frustration about my work and a great deal of fear, in other women it can be resentment or grief, sadness or even wonder and a new kind of joy. Don't try to batten down the hatches and carry on 'as normal'. All of this is not to say that if you have severe hot flushes you should not do something to alleviate them, however. It is worth consulting wise-woman lore. Recent research into the effects of a number of so-called old wives' treatments for hot flushes and other menopausal conditions strongly support their effectiveness. Still, much of how you experience something depends on your point of view.

The mythologist Joseph Campbell used to tell a story about a conversation he once had with Alan Watts, the writer on Zen Buddhism. He had told Watts about a problem he was having with his wife. She was always late. Campbell said invariably he would make an appointment to meet her somewhere, then he would have to sit and wait for half an hour or more before she arrived. After a while Campbell assumed that this was the normal thing for men to do because, after all, it takes women a long time to get out of the house. The problem was, he told Watts, that he always became irritated by having to wait. He would get so aggravated that when she finally did arrive he had a tendency to be unpleasant. Watts told Campbell, 'Well, your problem is that you want her to be there and you're wishing for a situation which is not the one you're in. Just realize that you are ruining the experience that you could be having while waiting by thinking it should be otherwise.' After that, Campbell transformed waiting for his wife into a spiritual exercise. 'The place where I was became so goddamn interesting I wasn't bored at all. Often times it made me hope that Jean would make me wait a little longer,' said Campbell. 'That would have been impossible until Alan suggested shutting out any thoughts that my situation should have been otherwise.'

Within each woman lies a similar ability to transmute that which seems frightening into a source of power. The phoenix is a mythological bird who, when consumed by fire, is born anew and rises from the flames to soar to greater heights than before. But the secret of the phoenix is always hidden, waiting for a woman bold enough and persistent enough to uncover it.

Chapter Ten

Double Indemnity

Plants hold powerful medicine for women. Even to state such an obvious truth seems absurd since every culture in the world from the beginning of human history has turned to herbs and foods as medicine. Yet as women in the post-industrial world we find ourselves in the absurd position of having to rediscover our medicinal and health-promoting heritage, not only by unearthing long-neglected local practices passed on verbally from woman to woman but also by investigating herbal traditions from other parts of the world – Tibet, China, India, Japan and Native America. The benefits of making medicinal plants a part of your day-to-day life become more obvious when you realize that the origins of most drugs lie in plants.

Quinine (the core anti-malarial drug) is derived from cinchona also called Peruvian Bark, for instance. It is the white willow that first supplied the analgesic acetyl salicylic acid which has now been replaced by its chemical analogue aspirin. The lovely foxglove yields digitalis for ailing hearts. Morphine, ephedrine, codeine and atropine all have plant origins. And when it comes to preventing or treating women's symptoms – from PMS to hot flushes – little works better or is more long lasting than the gentle art of plant power. It is an art with two branches. First is the use of botanicals either singly or in a combination *medicinally* as treatment for specific problems. Second, less well known but equally important, is the health-promoting benefits of incorporating plants rich in minerals, enzymes, fibre and phyto-hormones (plant-derived) and other beneficial phyto-chemicals, as *foods* in your normal daily diet.

Secrets of the Yam

When it comes to using a plant to benefit women, the Trobriand Islanders from Papua New Guinea have a few secrets well worth knowing. The Trobriands are a little group of flat coral islands not far from Northern Australia. The author Paul Theroux visited them and then reported on his visit for *National Geographic* in 1992. In these islands a form of wild yam grows in abundance. It is central to the island's social activities and forms the basis of the islanders' diet. Trobrianders, as it happens, have an almost perfect diet. It is low in fat with no fried foods and just about everything they eat is fresh. Their yams are grown in fields then carried to the villages and stored in beautiful wooden houses built in the centre of each village which look a bit like small cathedrals. In most of these yam houses a four-foot giant specimen is suspended in a frame of lashed poles. The yam represents not only food to them but also prosperity and the powers of life – in much the same way that corn was revered in Native American cultures. So sacred is the yam considered to be in this matrilineal society that men are not allowed to harvest the vegetable. If a man even accidentally comes upon a procession of women bringing yams from the fields, he is attacked and sexually ridiculed. His clothes are confiscated by the women and he is sent back to the village stark naked – a laughing stock.

Masters of self-reliance, the Trobrianders have little interest in the outside world. They greatly value the preservation of their own culture, however. They also value sexuality which is treated in a natural matter-of-fact way and around which there is no guilt. They encourage teenage sex and boys and girls aged 14 or 15 share *bukumatula* (bachelor houses) in which they are given complete privacy. Each year, at harvest time, a month-long yam festival is held during which all marriage is suspended and yams are eaten prepared in a myriad of ways from creamy porridge drenched in coconut milk, to boiled, steamed and baked dishes. 'For a reason that no one can explain,' reports Theroux, 'the birthrate is lower than might be expected.' After the Theroux article appeared in *National Geographic* the editor received a number of letters from readers. One was interesting. It came from a physician in Caracas, Venezuela, Mely Lechtich de Révai MD, who wrote: 'Yam of *Dioscorea* was long known by certain Mexican Indians to have a contraceptive effect. In 1939 Dr Russell

Marker, an American chemist, determined the molecular structure of diosgenin, a steroid substance with progesteronic effect derived from the yam root. Based on this information, Organon, a leading producer of contraceptive pills, uses the diosgenin from the Mexican yam roots as the raw material for some of its products.'

Diosgenin, you will remember, is the stuff from which the natural progesterone used in progesterone cream is derived, as are any number of other patented hormones sold as drugs by pharmaceutical manufacturers. Not only is the progesterone derived from wild yam a cornerstone of the bloodless revolution but, like the Trobriand Islanders' sacred vegetable, certain yams such as *Dioscorea villosa* and *Dioscorea Mexicana* are also useful as food supplements or natural medicines in the treatment of PMS and menopausal problems. Rich in phyto-hormones or their precursors, they can help protect against cancer and against the oestrogen dominance which underlies female ailments. In the future wild yam may turn out to be the best method of natural birth control available. It appears to work well for most women who have tried it and, unlike contraceptive drugs, it has no negative side-effects. Indeed, it boasts a long list of positive benefits.

Contraception au Naturel

Willa Shaffer is a remarkable woman, a Texas midwife who has dedicated her life to serving women's health and who trained in nutrition, midwifery and reflexology. She has for decades used plants to enhance the health of women of all ages. Shaffer first experimented with wild yam some 15 years ago as a means of staving off threatened miscarriages and eliminating PMS and menopausal miseries and found she got excellent results with it. Wild yam could be taken daily month after month, year after year so long as it was needed to counter a woman's negative symptoms. Shaffer reports, as have others who use this plant regularly, that in addition to banishing the symptoms for which it is being taken, wild yam can improve a woman's energy levels, enhance digestion, eliminate aches and pains normally associated with ageing or rheumatic conditions and balance emotions. It also appears to be a perfect antidote to lost libido, helping to restore a woman's capacity for sexual pleasure when it has been lost. But most interesting of all, and potentially revolutionary if controlled studies are ever carried out on it, is Shaffer's rediscovery of the secrets of wild yam used for birth control.

Shaffer had been continually faced with recurrent symptoms and serious health problems caused by birth control pills in the women whom she looked after. Then in 1976 she came upon an article in a small American magazine called *The Herbalist*. The article talked about the healing properties traditionally associated with the wild yam and about its use as a contraceptive. Excited by the possibility of a benign alternative to the Pill, Shaffer passed the article around among her patients. They were keen to try the plant. After some initial difficulty she was able to locate a source of dried wild yam in capsule form. She began to test it on scores of women. Then in 1986 she wrote a little booklet about her experience with the yam, *Wild Yam, Birth Control Without Fear*. It makes fascinating reading.

The ages of the women whom Shaffer tested ranged from 17 to 47. They came from many different backgrounds – some were black, some Caucasians, others were Latin Americans or had Native American blood. During her four-year test period no negative side-effects to the plant were reported by any of the women. There was no evidence, for instance, of weight gain, or cramps, hormonal changes, swelling, or any of the other unpleasant symptoms associated with prescription birth control. Out of the first 75 women who tried it, 56 were still using it as their sole source of contraception four years later. Of the 19 who did not continue, three decided to get pregnant, stopped taking the yam and had babies, six forgot to take it or did not take it as directed (i.e. they took too little or did not continue steadily), and ten dropped out of the experiment or were lost track of. Only one woman became pregnant despite the fact that she *religiously* took the wild yam – possibly, Shaffer believes, because her own specific requirement for the plant for use as a contraceptive was much higher than average so she should have been taking more. She was a woman who had always said of herself, 'Every time my husband just hangs his pants on the bedpost, I get pregnant!'

Dosage Decisions

In the beginning, Shaffer had no idea how much wild yam to use for birth control. Working together with a doctor who was familiar with the plant, she settled on three capsules in the morning and three at night which would supply a total of 3,000 mg or 3 g a day of the powdered dried root. Shaffer discovered that it is important to take the wild yam for eight weeks before relying on it as a sole source of contraception. Should a woman forget to take the herb for one day or more she needs to use an alternative method of birth control such as a condom or diaphragm as well as the yam for a couple of weeks before relying entirely on the wild yam again. In the course of experiments with the yam Shaffer also found out that all sorts of menstrual and menopausal problems are resolved by its use including painful menstruation, irregular menstruation, mood swings, depression and hot flushes, together with scores of other supposedly hard-to-treat conditions. Almost by chance Shaffer had rediscovered what the Trobriand Islanders, the Central and South American Indians and many other primitive cultures have known well since ancient times, that in several species of the wild yam is to be found an inexpensive, totally beneficial plant capable of giving a high degree of protection against unwanted pregnancy while enhancing women's health. It is quite a discovery – one which needs serious scientific investigation – yet the average doctor remains totally ignorant about the wild yam.

The women I know who use wild yam for birth control take 3 to 3.5 g of powdered root a day – either *Dioscorea villosa* or *Dioscorea Mexicana* – in other words 1.5 to 1.75 grams in the morning and in the evening. Just how many capsules this amounts to if you choose to take it in capsule form depends upon the weight of the capsules. They report, so far without exception, that the wild yam they are using for birth control has also eliminated PMS, made heavy periods lighter, enhanced their energy and helped to balance their emotions.

Whether proper scientifically controlled studies will ever be carried out to validate Shaffer's anecdotal evidence depends more than anything else upon ordinary women becoming vocal enough to demand them. And if trials did validate wild yam as a reliable method of birth control it could not only literally save governments millions that might be used in others ways (for contraceptive drugs are pricey and plants very cheap and widely available), it could also protect hundreds of thousands of women from the potential side-effects of pharmaceutical contraceptives.

For two generations feminists have quite rightly insisted that women's bodies belong to women themselves and that each woman must have the right to choose whether or not she becomes pregnant. As women determined to exert control over our own lives we have, perhaps, been too ready to back drug-based contraception complete with all of its negative side-effects because there seemed to be no alternative. Our doing so has too often wreaked havoc in women's lives. Drug-based contraception still continues to disrupt the biology, long-term health and emotions of millions of women in the world. Now seems an appropriate time to re-evaluate our position. As Shaffer herself says, 'Can you imagine the change it would cause if wild yam would be used on a large scale? So many severe problems caused by the controversial birth control pills would be extinct. Let's all pray that people become more aware of the safe herbal remedies and preventatives that are available.' She then goes on to muse, 'John Heineman states in his book that recent clinical evidence has shown that when the extract of mallow flower was administered to dogs (which have male reproductive organs that are anatomically similar to men) it causes substantial infertility by inhibiting the production of sperm in the testicles.' Finally she adds, 'Now if I could only get my hands on some mallow flower . . .'

Like wild yam, many of the plants and botanical products most useful to women are rich in phyto-sterols – compounds whose molecular structure is akin to the body's own hormones. Vegetables and herbs which fall into this category include celery, fennel, ginseng, alfalfa, liquorice and red clover. Hops (*Humulus lupulus*) are so rich in plant sterols that exposure to them can affect the onset of menarche in girls. 'It was girls and women picking hops who first drew attention to the fact that hops have an effect on the genital organs,' says Rudolf Fritz Weiss, author of *Herbal Medicine*. 'Before machines were introduced, hop pickers used to spend several weeks at this work and it had always been known that menstrual periods would come early in young girls while they were there.' The fresh hop plant contains significant quantities of plant hormones similar to a woman's own oestrogens. They not only affect the menstrual cycles of women but can also suppress libido in men. This is the cause of *brewer's droop* familiar to beer-drinking men and what has given beer its reputation for raising expectations while inhibiting performance. It is also why the *British Herbal Pharmacopoeia* suggests hops as a treatment for persistent erection.

Mission Impossible

All sorts of supposedly impossible healing tasks can be accomplished when phyto-sterol rich herbs are used medicinally. But, sadly, few women know much about how to use them since so many of the old herbal protocols have been all but forgotten in the last 50 years. When I began to research the use of herbs for menstrual and menopausal problems I was surprised to find that when you examine the scientific literature on phyto-sterol-rich plants, surprisingly few of the known benefits are listed. Most of the information we as women need to take control of our health and future life still has to come from other women by word of mouth. Occasionally, however, I came upon a book which is genuinely useful. Susun Weed's *Menopausal Years* is a real gem. Weed spent three years talking to more than 10,000 women about their menopause and then produced a handbook replete with practical advice and simple wisdom. She has, in effect, gathered many wise-woman practices and made them readily available to women. So has Willa Shaffer, whose knowledge not only of wild yam but many other useful plants comes from half a century of working with women and finding ways of helping them through every kind of health challenge.

Author of *Midwifery and Herbs*, *Wild Yam*, *Birth Control Without Fear*, as well as *Diary of a Country Midwife*, Shaffer learned her skills in childhood when plant treatments were the order of the day in dealing with almost any kind of illness. As a child she had suffered from bronchial disorders and pneumonia and she was usually given lobelia along with other plants. But then in her teens, in the early 1930s, she found she could no longer locate supplies of common plants for medicinal purpose for pharmacies were by then busy converting their stocks of natural products into drugs. (It was then, by the way, that in North America pharmacies began to be known as 'drug stores'.) From then on Shaffer spent some 30 years in poor health until in desperation she turned back to plants to help and was at last able to heal herself. This prompted her to learn everything she could about medicinal plants, nutrition and reflexology and to use what she had learned in her practice as a midwife. Shaffer now has women from as far afield as Central America and Europe consulting her for help. Like every wise woman worth her salt she gives of her knowledge freely to any woman who needs it. Both Shaffer and Weed draw heavily on plants rich in phyto-sterols for the herbal treatments they recommend.

Green Afternoons

'Usually,' says Susun Weed, 'phyto-sterols are most concentrated in perennial roots (such as dandelion and ginseng), leaf buds (such as briar rose and blackcurrant) and hard berries (such as vitix and saw palmetto).' Unlike highly concentrated chemical hormones and drugs, plants such as these work gently and holistically in their effect on the body – many of the non-steroid components of a particular herb supporting the actions of the active phyto-sterols. 'Your body's access to phyto-sterols,' Weed insists, 'is increased when glycosides, saponins, minerals and flavonoids are also present in a plant. Renowned hormone-balancing herbs such as Dong Quai/Tang Kuei, black cohosh and sarsaparilla contain a dozen or more of these constituents, each of which offers slightly different hormonal building blocks.' Among the most widely used phyto-sterol-rich foods and herbs are sage, red clover, sarsaparilla and sassafras, liquorice root, alfalfa, hops, wild yam and yarrow. Phyto-sterol-rich rhubarb root and hops have been used for generations by doctors and herbalists in the treatment of menopausal symptoms including hot flushes, vaginitis and secondary amenorrhoea. Now, in Britain and Europe, these two botanicals are sometimes given in the form of a product called Phytoestrol. Made by Pharmazeutische Fabrik Goeppingen Carl Mueller in Germany this botanical consists of 90 mg of extract of hops and 4 mg of rhubarb-root extract. Doctors who use the product insist that, unlike drug treatments, it carries no negative side-effects. One enthusiastic advocate of Phytoestrol is British naturopath and homeopath Dr Harald Gaier who uses the product regularly with women patients. Says Gaier, 'It is not as fast acting as conventional hormones, but Phytoesterol brings lasting improvement to many women and they have no drug interaction dangers or incompatibilities or side-effects that accompany them.'

A three-month double-blind placebo-controlled pilot study was carried out in the United States and reported in the *Newsletter of the Office of Alternative Medicine of the National Institute of Health* in 1993. It looked at the hormonal and symptom-relieving properties of a combination of traditional botanical medicines on perimenopausal women including *Glycyrrhiza glabra* root (liquorice), *Arctium lappa* root (burdock), *Dioscorea villosa* root (wild yam), *Angelica sinensis* root (angelica) and *Leonurus cardiaca* (motherwort). These botanicals were given in capsule form in equal parts. After three months all participants in the test groups showed a reduction in the severity of menopausal symptoms compared with only 6 per cent of women in the placebo group. Seventy-one per cent of the test group reported fewer symptoms – of which hot flushes, vaginal dryness, insomnia and mood changes were the most common – as opposed to 17 per cent in the placebo group.

Plant sterols are also known to act either indirectly or directly on the cells of connective tissue including bone cells. This may be one of the reasons why postmenopausal women living on processed foods – which are very low in sterol hormones – have a significantly higher level of arthritis and osteoporosis than other women. Dr Joseph E. Pizzorno Jr and Dr Michael T. Murray of John Bastyr College in Seattle are enthusiastic about the use of plant-based sterols as opposed to conventional drug oestrogens in the treatment of female ailments, including osteoporosis. 'Menopausal women commonly receive oestrogens to help allay the hot flushes, nausea, bone loss and other symptoms of this decrease in the body's own natural hormone level,' they write. 'While generally effective, both synthetic and natural oestrogens may pose significant health risks including the risk of cancer, gallbladder disease, and thromboembolic disease. Phyto-oestrogens have not been associated with these side-effects.'

The general consensus among doctors aware of plant power and familiar with the use of botanical substances and foods rich in phyto-hormones is that the right plant foods and treatments can help balance oestrogen dominance and maintain health while at the same time preventing premature ageing, degenerative diseases and the hormonal disruptions which manifest as women's ailments.

Hormones Good and Bad

Phyto-hormones act upon the body in very different ways from synthetic drugs and the xenoestrogens that pollute our environment as well as our bodies. Hormone drugs and oestrogen mimics in our environment are very strong. Typically when they bind with the body's receptor sites they interfere with metabolic processes since – unlike natural hormones and their precursors – they are incapable of being changed by the body's own enzymes into other useful compounds. Nor can they be easily eliminated to restore hormonal balance where necessary. On the other hand, phyto-sterols or plant hormones are weak in their actions. They usually come to us through our foods in the form of precursors which the body can then make use of to synthesize whatever hormones it needs. As John Lee says, 'Phyto-hormones are very different from the xenoestrogens which have an excessive oestrogenic effect on a woman's follicles and are responsible for the widespread oestrogen dominance now developing in women. They are gentle compounds which can be substituted for the body's oestrogens. They occupy the same receptor sites but with less and less effect. As such they tend to protect a woman from the xenoestrogens doing damage. These phyto-sterols "fit in" to a woman's metabolism. Her body recognizes them and knows how to use them. I consider them a very benign and helpful source of hormones.' At the Dunn Nutrition Unit at Cambridge, the work of Adene Cassidy and her team confirms Lee's assertions. Phyto-oestrogens do indeed compete with human oestrogen, blocking the stronger oestrogens from stimulating cells. This is why a diet high in soy bean products such as tofu plays such an important part in protecting Japanese women from hormone-mediated diseases.

When weak oestrogens from plants bind with receptor sites, they also help *protect* the body from both negative hormone and hormone-like influences by encouraging the elimination of these 'bad' sterols and allowing the body to readjust its own hormonal balance naturally. The vitamins, minerals and phyto-sterols in fresh foods eaten as close as possible to the state in which they come out of the ground – or carefully and naturally fermented as the Japanese do – can bring to a woman's diet a supply of phyto-hormones sufficient to mitigate most of the female symptoms that plague us in industrialized countries. Professor of Clinical Gerontology at the University of Cambridge, Kay-Tee Khaw is another expert who voices enthusiasm about natural phyto-hormones from plants and stresses the importance of a wholesome diet of natural foods in preserving and enhancing a woman's health. Khaw believes such a diet may help lower the risk of osteoporosis, breast cancer and heart disease. Quoted by Gail Vines in an article 'The Challenge to HRT' in *The New Scientist* Khaw says, 'We have become so obsessed with looking for magic potions . . . that we are not asking the real questions about lifestyle that can have profound effects.' She continues, 'Clinical medicine is the end of the line. Everyone asks, how could this have been prevented? We need to understand what causes some people to be healthy, and others not. If people today had the same fracture rate as existed in the 1950s in Britain, one in two hip fractures would not happen. We need to understand what is going on.'

The Wilder Shores

When it comes to eating, the best protection from menstrual and menopausal problems is a 'primitive' diet of fresh foods which is low in fat, high in raw fruits and vegetables, and whole grains and legumes in their unprocessed form, plus a few fresh seeds and nuts. It is important also to include plenty of foods rich in phyto-sterols such as soya products, sprouted seeds and grains. Such dietary change is not some wishful action to carry out in the hope that it just might make a little difference to your life. In a study carried out in Britain where women were switched to a diet rich in phyto-hormones derived from soya flour, red clover sprouts and flaxseed oil, researchers reported that the menopausal symptoms of 25 women were significantly reduced by such alterations alone. In another study carried out in Scandinavia and reported in *The Lancet* three years ago, researchers discovered that Japanese women who eat large quantities of phyto-sterol-rich foods including soya products (who, you will recall, also have a very low incidence of breast and uterine cancer and experience very few menopausal or menstrual problems) eliminate an astounding 1,000 times as many phyto-oestrogens in their urine as do Finnish women. In effect their bodies have become saturated with phyto-hormones which both trigger the elimination of the bad sterols and also spill over themselves as waste. With this kind of phyto-oestrogen intake researchers reported the risk of breast cancer is only a fifth what it is among American women on a typical western diet. In the United States, studies of Seventh Day Adventist women on vegetarian diets show that they not only have a very low incidence of breast cancer, they are recognized as the healthiest people in the western world. Studies also show that they have low levels of oestrogens in the blood and they excrete much higher levels of oestrogens in their urine than do meateating women.

The Emulators

A high-raw way of eating, such as that outlined in *The New Raw Energy* which my daughter Susannah and I researched and wrote, has long been used by doctors and health practitioners trained in natural methods of healing both to protect from and to counteract menstrual and menopausal symptoms which have resulted from hormonal imbalances. In part this is because such a diet – in which 50 to 75 per cent of your foods are taken fresh and raw – supplies a very high level of essential nutrients and enzymes which encourage optimal metabolism and help detoxify the body of whatever might be interfering with metabolic processes. But a raw energy way of eating is also high in phyto-hormones from raw seeds, nuts, vegetables and fruits to help the endocrine system rebalance itself. And because these foods are mostly eaten fresh the beneficial plant substances they contain are easily assimilated when you eat them.

But foods do need to be fresh. You can lose 50 per cent of the vitamin C in a fresh cabbage within the first 24 hours after picking. After 48 to 72 hours you can end up with a mere 5 per cent of what was originally present. Just as vitamin levels decrease when foods lose their freshness, so too are the levels of phyto-sterols in natural foods diminished when a food we buy has been grown in a far-away country, harvested before it is ripe, and shipped thousands of miles before it ends up on our table. After picking, the synthesis of phyto-sterols within a plant ceases while oxidation processes which destroy vitamins and hormones speed up.

Green Magic

Some of the best hormone-rich foods to add to your diet both as a protection against trouble and for the sake of overall vitality are the green foods: spirulina, chlorella, the seaweeds, sprouted alfalfa and green barley. Eating some of the green foods every day can slowly over a period of several months help replenish what may have been lost for many years. It is something that is very difficult to do any other way for in order for minerals to be well assimilated they have to be highly bio-available – your body needs easily to be able to make use of them. Most vitamin mineral supplements are not bio-available. Seaweeds, chlorella, spirulina and green barley are also wonderful cleansing foods to help detoxify the body of excess oestrogens as well as other pollutants such as heavy metals like lead, mercury and aluminium, which may be interfering with metabolic processes, and they are excellent energy enhancers. Try ten days on green foods coupled with other high-raw phyto-sterol foods such as those included in Miso Detox and Buildup (see Resurrection, p. 365) and you may be delighted that so much benefit can come to you so quickly. The body is always attempting to strengthen and heal itself and is hungry for those elements from foods that can help it do so. Green foods have much to offer.

Age of Treason

Orthodox medicine's almost total disregard for the use of phyto-sterol-rich plants in the treatment of women's ailments is of recent origin. It is as though with the coming of patentable drugs centuries of traditional methods were dismissed with the wave of a hand. 'Uterine tonics' made from sterol-rich herbs and plants were used for centuries to treat all different kinds of female complaints. They still work. Once you get to know the actions of various herbs, you begin to develop a feel for the character of each botanical and a skill that enables you to call on the plant or plants you need just when you need them. But it is important to remember that plants are slower acting than drugs so you need to be patient. It is often necessary to use a herb for a few weeks or even longer before you will experience its full benefits. Having said that, I have frequently found that a herb will bring almost immediate relief.

One big advantage of using botanicals is that many, when taken over a period of time, will do the job for which they were being taken so well that you no longer need to use them. (See Field and Forest, pp. 346–364.) Another important thing to remember when using herbs is that they often work well in combination, and there are some good combinations on the market. (See Resources for what is available.)

It is essential that the supply of herbs you are using is clean – preferably organically grown. Some herbs on the market today have been grown in countries where pesticides and herbicides are sprayed heavily. Others are not fresh or have been irradiated or are contaminated with chemicals. Often suppliers themselves are not even aware of how the dried plants have been handled. Once you have your herbs it is a good idea to keep them in airtight jars in the refrigerator so they stay potent for as long as possible. Having worked and played with plants, herbs and tinctures for many years I have developed the deepest respect for their beauty and their power. Each plant has its own unique personality which you can turn to for health or strength when you need it. I keep herbs in my garden, cut them fresh in summer and use them dried in winter for everything from cooking a soup and making a salad to healing a cough, banishing a headache or clearing a room of negative energies. I also keep a whole row of litre and half-litre bottles of plant tinctures just behind my desk in the room in which I work and call on them frequently when help is needed – for energy, to calm stress or to ward off an impending infection. The support which plants can give a woman going through her passage to power is nothing short of miraculous.

Chapter Eleven

Order Out of Chaos

Life feeds upon life. Modern practices destroy food's *wholesomeness*. Wholesomeness is a property very hard to measure except in terms of the degenerative effects that eating foods without it has on our bodies. Destroy a food's wholesomeness and you destroy its integrity as well as its ability to support health at the highest levels. And once the health-giving integrity of any food has gone it has gone for good. It can never be compensated for by vitamin and mineral supplements or by eating cereals to which extra fibre and vitamins have been added. You can analyse every bit of information available about an apple, break it down into its chemical constituents and quantify the level of each one. You can then gather all its constituents together again but you still won't be able to make an apple. Only *life* can do that.

The secret to eating for high-level health is making use of wholesome foods radiant with life energy that increase mental and physical energy and protect from premature ageing while restoring hormonal order. The theory is simple, the practice gets more complicated. The first step is forsaking once and for all convenience foods with all their fragmentation and hidden fat and sugar for a life-generating way of eating based on simple wholesome foods grown on healthy soils, fresh, and eaten as close as possible to the state in which they come out of the ground. Next comes incorporating foods rich in phytosterols. They include raw foods, concentrated green foods, and naturally fermented high-chi foods from the Orient such as miso. You also need to be savvy about body energy – what enhances it and what depletes it – and about food allergies, how they can undermine health and vitality and about how to avoid them. It is important to become streetwise about fats, too, since nothing can foul up a woman's hormonal system like processed fats in foods, and *junk fats* are just about everywhere these days. Finally, you need to address the question of nutritional supplements. The decisions you make about how and what you eat from the age of 35 onwards largely determines the kind of menopause you will have and how protected you are from osteoporosis. These same decisions are responsible for how slowly or rapidly your body ages and how much energy you have to do whatever you want to do with your life. Much of what follows I have investigated in previous books – *Lean Revolution* for example – but it is so central to understanding how our bodies function, that it is worth restating here. Let's tackle energy first.

Witness to the Fire

Carbohydrates are your body's main source of energy for all its functions. However, just any old carbohydrate won't do. Only *complex* carbohydrates – fruits and vegetables, unrefined grains, sea plants and legumes – provide steady lasting energy throughout the day. They also protect you from blood-sugar problems, mood swings and the chronic fatigue that is prevalent in the lives of many women over the age of 35, which leads them to binge on sugar or coffee or pep-up pills just to keep going. Sugar cravings are common with PMS and indulging them can be dangerous to a woman's long-term hormonal health. Women with PMS eat three times as much refined sugar as those without. Eating sugar causes your body to excrete magnesium and interferes with the liver's ability to deactivate harmful oestrogens. Adequate magnesium is essential in preventing PMS and menopausal symptoms as well as in keeping immunity high. It helps the body to inactivate excess oestrogen, clear painful menstruation and reduce lower abdominal and back pain. Many of the ill-effects of dairy products also appear to involve magnesium. Dairy products are nine times higher in calcium than magnesium. Eating them regularly can upset the calcium/magnesium balance, interfering with the metabolism of important B complex vitamins and making PMS symptoms worse.

One of the major energy problems caused by eating processed foods full of *simple* carbohydrates like white flour and sugar is that it brings about a progressive decline in your body's ability to metabolize sugar. Unlike natural foods full of protective fibre, refined and processed foods are highly concentrated foods. Fibre is no longer present to dilute their concentration and to slow down the rate at which the simple starches and sugars they contain are absorbed into your bloodstream. Such foods are far more *calorie dense*. When you eat them year after year they begin to overwhelm the body – especially the pancreas – causing blood-sugar problems and mood and energy swings that wreak havoc with your health.

Refined and highly concentrated convenience foods devoid of their natural fibre make your blood-sugar curve rise steeply as a lot of sugar is pumped quickly into your system then force it to drop off quickly so that after a couple of hours you get an energy slump and feel hungry again. It is little wonder. Believe it or not each teaspoon of sugar in the jam you ate was refined out of 6 to 12 feet of sugar cane and in the processing all the protective fibre and other nutrients, such as chromium, which your body needs for its proper assimilation, were lost. So a couple of hours after breakfast you have to reach for a bar of chocolate to keep going. If the snack you choose is, say, a couple of biscuits or a sweet roll you take in another 4 spoons of sugar – the sweetness of 9.6 metres or 32 feet of sugar cane – which you get in one big bang with no protective fibre to slow down its release into your blood. This jolts the pancreas forcing it to respond quickly by producing more and more insulin to keep your blood sugar from going too high.

The Dark is Rising

Continue to eat concentrated foods full of simple carbohydrates year after year and your blood glucose levels will tend to get higher and higher as the pancreas is continually forced to release more and more insulin in an attempt to control it all. Even though insulin is still being produced in high concentrations your body will have become insulin resistant – that is your cells no longer respond normally to insulin and the body's ability to control blood sugar is lost. When this happens the calories from your foods are more and more easily converted into fats, or triglycerides, which are then laid down as fat stores on your belly, hips, thighs and bottom and you have also increased your likelihood of getting heart disease and other degenerative conditions.

Simple carbohydrates such as white sugar, white flour, cornflakes and white bread are *high* on what is known as the *glycaemic index*. This means that they cause the blood-sugar level to rise quickly, contribute to insulin resistance, can disturb appetite and make energy maintenance difficult. Foods high on the glycaemic index are foods to avoid. They include glucose, most packaged breakfast cereals such as cornflakes, instant mashed potatoes, maltose, white rice, white pasta, white bread, sweet biscuits, potato crisps and most processed packaged foods. For lasting energy and good health it is important to choose natural foods which are lower on the glycaemic index – fresh vegetables, apples and non-tropical fruit, oats, brown rice, sea plants, wholewheat spaghetti, soybeans, lentils, sweet potatoes, lima beans and kidney beans as well as fruit sugar from apples and oranges. These are foods that you can feel comfortable in eating a lot of. Don't get misled by the nonsense that is written on the packaging of foods you buy either. Read the ingredients carefully and watch for hidden sugars which could interfere with the fat-burning process in your own body – glucose, sorbitol, invert sugar, corn syrup, maltodextrin, dextrose, barley syrup, malt sugar. Even many products which claim to be sugar-free contain one or more of these, all of which are just another name for sugar.

Caffeine Freedom

What place do coffee, tea and soft drinks have in a healthy way of eating for women with menstrual problems or passing through menopause? Very little. Certainly they should not be drunk every day. Quite apart from the negative effects of caffeine – an ingredient in coffee, tea and many soft drinks – drinking coffee messes up blood sugar. Caffeine, technically known as trimethyl xanthine, is a habit-forming drug. It has been shown to be responsible for headaches, insomnia, nervousness, anxiety, and that familiar wired mental state which keeps you buzzing for a time intellectually but tends to disconnect you from your instincts and, in some women, even from having a good grip on reality. Caffeine gives you a quick lift and the illusion of energy only to let you crash down a couple of hours later when you are inclined to reach for more.

Caffeine has mutagenic effect too – that is it is capable of crossing the placenta to cause permanent damage to an unborn child as well as breaking apart the chromosomes in your own cells and interfering with the repair of DNA. Drinking coffee stimulates the secretion of acid in your stomach disturbing natural appetite control mechanisms and making you far more likely to end up with an ulcer than your non-coffee-drinking cousin. Actually, caffeine acts as a stimulant to the central nervous system in a rather curious way. It makes you *feel* more mentally alert. But tests show that in reality it creates more confusion and nervousness. In animal experiments very high doses of caffeine have been shown to create psychotic behaviour. Coffee also tends to raise blood pressure and to increase the risk of coronary thrombosis. Drink five cups each day and your heart attack risk goes up by 60 per cent. Coffee also makes the blood more acid which in turn draws calcium from your bones to try to re-establish a healthy acid/alkaline balance. Drinking more than 2 cups of coffee a day is one of the things you should not do if you want to prevent osteoporosis.

And tea? It too contains caffeine – 100 mg to coffee's 120 mg in a regular-sized cup. Tea also contains tannic acid which is an irritant to the digestive system. There is also evidence that drinking tea in quantity interferes with iron absorption from foods. Even if you have always been a committed 6 to 8 cups a day tea or coffee drinker, after a couple of weeks on good water you will find you don't miss it. Then when you have an occasional cup it becomes a simple pleasure rather than an addiction.

Cut the Soft Drinks

The average intake of soft drinks in the West has risen to 8 to 12 cans a week in some countries – between 400 and 600 a year. Women and children are the biggest users. Many colas, squashes and soft drinks also contain caffeine. And they are far too high in sugar. They bring nutritionally empty calories into your body which you can ill afford. A 330 ml (12 oz) tin of cola contains 7 teaspoons of sugar – about 40 grams. Colas are full of chemicals to pollute your body and preoccupy your liver's elimination processes. As for the 'diet' varieties, quite apart from the proven fact that drinking them will do absolutely nothing to help you lose weight, they are an even more chemically unpleasant cocktail full of excess phosphorus and additives which only pollute your body and further contribute to calcium loss from bones. Stay away from them. They are also full of phosphoric acid (the chemical used to etch glass) which, when your body tries to eliminate it via the kidneys, combines with calcium, leaching this vital mineral from bones, teeth, nails and hair. Fizzy colas are major contributors to osteoporosis in women.

All Fats Not Equal

Now let's look at the issue of fats. For the kind of fats you eat determines greatly the hormonal health of your body. Each of us in the West consume about 175 grams of fat a day. That makes 63 kilograms a year. Between 40 and 50 per cent of our food calories come from fat. The biscuits you buy in your local supermarket are well over 40 per cent fat and the munchy-crunchy snacks which masquerade as health bars seldom contain less than 50 per cent. For good long-term health you need to reduce your fat intake down to between 15 and 25 per cent of the calories you eat. You also need to take great care to make sure that these fat calories are the right kind. This is not always easy to do.

All fats and oils in our foods are made out of fatty acids. A fatty acid is a molecule that contains an acid part and a fat part. Chemically it consists of a chain of carbon and hydrogen atoms to which one oxygen atom is attached. A molecule of fat differs from a molecule of carbohydrate (which is also made out of carbon, hydrogen and oxygen) by the fact that the fat contains a lot less oxygen. This makes it highly concentrated and is why there are nine calories to each gram of fat while only four calories in each gram of carbohydrate or protein.

Fats can be roughly divided into two groups – saturated and unsaturated. A saturated fat is a fatty acid with a molecule where each carbon atom is connected to a hydrogen atom so that there are no empty *spaces* to allow one or more of the carbons to reach up and join together with molecules of other substances in your body. Because of this, saturated fats (found in meat, dairy products like cheese, ice-cream, milk, and the tropical oils like palm kernel oil and coconut) are stable, inactive and virtually inert in your body. Their major *raison d'être* is to provide calories in a concentrated form which can later be burned as energy. Eat too many foods full of saturated fats and they do their best to lay themselves down as fat stores. You will get as much saturated fat as you need from your food without ever giving it a second thought.

Unsaturated fats are different. They are made up of fatty-acid chains which *do* have empty spaces – carbon atoms with open arms which are not connected directly to hydrogen atoms. Unsaturates come in two forms: *mono*-unsaturates, like olive oil, and *poly*-unsaturates, found in corn, sunflower seeds, peanuts and many other foods from which they are extracted. Thanks to their free spaces, mono-unsaturates and poly-unsaturates are much more biologically active, more able to easily take part in important biochemical changes in your body that produce energy, create hormones, and help burn stored body fats. The right unsaturated fats are essential to a woman's hormonal health all through her reproductive life and beyond. That is the right *kind* of unsaturated fat. But there is a lot of hokum spread about unsaturated fats by sellers of margarine and producers of processed junk foods. Just because a label says 'unsaturated' it doesn't mean the food in the packet is good for you. Ninety-eight per cent of them are not. You have to be shrewd about what you buy and really know the ropes. This means going a bit deeper into the whole fat issue. Bear with me. An understanding of good and bad fats can revolutionize your health.

Bare Essentials

Your body can make all the fat it needs for daily metabolic processes except for two essential fatty acids, linoleic and linolenic. These are found naturally in fresh foods, in seeds and nuts, in vegetables and fish, even in wild meat such as game. For optimum health you need no more than 2 to 4 tablespoons of these essential fatty acids a day yet despite our high fat intake in the West, they can be as hard to find in modern convenience foods as the proverbial hen's teeth. These two unsaturates help you burn body fat and build energy; they also help your body manufacture important hormones. Linoleic and linolenic are called essential fatty acids because that is exactly what they are – essential to human life and health.

The moment you remove an unsaturated fat from the food in which it comes you produce what is known as a *free-fat*. A free-fat is any fat which has been separated out from the food in which it occurs in nature – corn oil for instance, peanut or groundnut oil, sunflower oil, safflower oil, as well as any margarines or biscuits or other foods containing them. Free-fats are something women should avoid like the plague. Through complex operations involving the use of heat and unpleasant chemical solvents, food manufacturers turn our natural fatty acids contained in wholesome fresh foods into highly artificial fat products which damage health. It takes an amazing 12–15 ears of corn to produce a mere dessertspoon full of the golden oil. All the protective 'packaging' of fibre, vitamins and minerals gets thrown out in the process or fed to pigs. Advertisers are continually promoting products full of 'poly-unsaturates' as though they were healthy. It is a lot of rubbish. Most poly-unsaturated fats are not at all healthy. Let me give you an example of what I mean. In addition to the common process 'hydrogenation' which turns an unsaturated fat into a saturated one, making an oil into a solid fat like margarine by adding extra hydrogen atoms to spaces on the fatty-acid chain, there are other processes commonly used in food processing which degrade or completely destroy the health-giving properties of whatever essential fatty acids a poly-unsaturated fat may contain.

The Good Guys and the Bad Guys

Natural, unadulterated, unsaturated fats for health come in a chemical configuration known as a *cis* form. This is the *only* form a woman's body can use for anything except pumping up her fat stores. Cis fatty acids are destroyed by modern processing procedures such as bleaching, hydrogenation, heating and deodorizing, which turn out the golden oils that shimmer from the shelves of our supermarkets and with which the mass-produced foods we eat today are riddled. These procedures alter our healthy cis fatty acids into unhealthy *trans*-fatty acids by rotating the hydrogen atoms on the fat molecules so that they change sides. Cis fatty acids – the good guys – are rather like 'gloves'. Like natural hormones which key into hormone receptor sites, they fit perfectly on to the 'hands' of the molecular fat receptors in your body. Trans-fatty acids are bad guys. Like the drug-based hormones and xenoestrogens they don't properly fit into your body's metabolic machinery. Their presence can even block fat receptor sites, interfering in your body's ability to produce important hormones involved in reproduction, causing PMS and menopausal miseries.

Since trans-fatty acids don't occur in nature, like many hormone drugs, your body has never developed any mechanisms for making use of them. It treats them as foreign invaders rather like toxic wastes and does its best to try to protect you from any detrimental effects they can have on your body (such as furring up your arteries) by laying them down in fat tissues. A first principle of trouble-free menstruation and menopause is to *eliminate free oils, hydrogenated fats and processed foods from your diet.* Every processed fat contains unhealthy trans-fatty acids. Not one mass-produced margarine on the market is genuinely health-promoting despite all the advertising designed to convince us to the contrary. Nor are all those golden oils, salad dressings and biscuits, breads or ready-made meals containing them healthy. So don't be misled by the words 'contains poly-unsaturates'. Margarines and cooking oils are *junk fats.* Your body cannot use them for health and, because their presence actually blocks the uptake of cis fatty acids, eating them can lead to fatty-acid deficiencies and hormone chaos. The ordinary saturated fat that you find in steak or chicken is healthier than such artificially produced, hydrogenated, unnatural fatty acids. It is important to read every label, and anything that says it contains hydrogenated vegetable oil or partially hydrogenated vegetable oil, leave on the shelf.

Don't assume you can believe everything you read on food labels either. Look on any packet that lists the protein, carbohydrate and fat content, and the calories per serving, and make some quick calculations to tell you what percentage of the calories in the food are fat calories. Here's how to work it out quickly.

Say a particular packet of biscuits contains 145 calories per 100 gram serving, made up of 4 grams of protein, 19 grams of carbohydrate and 7 grams of fat. Multiply the amount of fat by ten (rounded up from fat being nine calories per gram); i.e. add a zero to the number of grams of fat per serving to give you how many of the calories per serving are in the form of fat. Then compare this figure with the total calories. In this case it would be $7 \times 10 = 70$ calories of fat in each 145 calories. Now divide 70 by 145 and you get 0.48 – the fraction of those calories per serving which come from fat. This tells you the biscuit calories are about 48 per cent fat calories. As this is way above the limit of 25 per cent for optimal health, reject the packet.

As far as the golden vegetable oils that you find on supermarket shelves are concerned, don't use them. On your salads, instead of using salad oils, use *cold pressed extra virgin* olive oil. This oil is not a poly-unsaturate with many free spaces on its molecules, but a mono-unsaturate with only one free space which makes it highly stable. It is the best overall oil for salads. You can also use it in tiny quantities for wok-frying vegetables.

So just where do you get the important unadulterated essential fatty acids you need and how do they work? The answer to the first question is simple.

Essential fatty acids are found in abundance in nuts, beans, grains and seeds, and soya products, as well as in olives and other plant foods. Soy beans are an excellent source, so are grains like wheat and barley, oats and maize. What happens in your body when you eat these foods is that the linoleic and alpha-linolenic acid they contain are converted into other fatty acids that are needed for various purposes, provided, of course, that your diet is not full of junk fats that prevent these conversions from taking place. It is important to buy your foods really fresh. Reject any grain or seed or nut which does not taste and smell absolutely clean and keep your nuts and seeds in the fridge. With the exception of avocados, nuts and olives, most of these whole plant foods have a low fat content. Animal foods, however, have a much higher fat content. Even the leanest steak boasts 50 per cent of its calories from fat while the more delicious fat-marbled variety can be as high as 80 per cent. Butter and cream go even higher, offering 100 per cent of calories from saturated fats, none of which you need for health.

Clever Conversions

In your body the essential fatty acid linoleic acid is converted by an enzyme called the delta-6-desaturase enzyme into gamma linolenic acid, or GLA. These days it has become well known as a way of improving the skin and as a treatment for female problems including PMS. GLA is in turn changed into prostaglandins and different fatty acids such as arachidonic via other metabolic steps. Linolenic, the other essential fatty acid, is present in pumpkin seeds, flaxseeds, soy beans and walnuts, as well as in oily fish such as wild salmon, mackerel, sardines and wild trout. Because of the way they are fed these days, farmed fish such as trout and salmon contain more and more saturated fat and less and less linolenic acid. Linolenic is similarly converted through the action of an enzyme called delta-5-desaturase into eicosapentanoic (EPA) and then on to docosahexanoic acid (DHA).

A major reason why GLA from evening primrose oil, borage oil or starflower oil has such a positive effect on the body is that, because our western diet is high in junk fats or trans-fatty acids, we often have difficulty making the conversion from linoleic to gamma-linolenic. Similarly in recent years, fish oils containing EPA and DHA have been prescribed –

particularly for athletes, slimmers and people at risk from heart disease – because as we get older there appears to be a decline in the enzymes that are necessary to make these conversions. One of the best ways of getting extra quantities of essential fatty acids is to buy vacuum-packed flaxseeds, pulverize them and sprinkle a dessertspoonful or two on your cereals or salads every day.

Cry Wild

More than fifty years ago Hans Eppinger, chief doctor at the First Medical Clinic of the University of Vienna, discovered that a high-raw way of eating leads to increased cellular respiration. This it does in a number of ways by creating a kind of positive feedback loop where one thing in turn stimulates another until cell metabolism is heightened. It eliminates accumulated wastes and toxins from cells and tissues. It supplies the level of nutrients essential for optimal cell function. And, perhaps most important of all, it heightens the micro-electrical tensions associated with cell vitality so that even cells in a particularly sluggish and neglected system are revitalized. They become better able to burn calories in the presence of oxygen and to produce energy efficiently both for overall vitality and for carrying out the housekeeping on which the health of your body depends.

Capillaries are minute blood vessels which form the vast network of microcirculation throughout your body. It is their responsibility to deliver oxygen-rich blood for it to be used by the cells. So important are these fine vessels that nature has supplied you with incredible lengths of them. If you were to attach all the capillaries in your body end to end they would measure some 60,000 miles in length – more than twice around the world. On the state of your capillaries depends to a great extent the condition of your body as a whole. For they are the arbitrators of cell nutrition, respiration and elimination. It is through these capillaries that nutrients and oxygen are carried. Each of them has tiny 'pores' which allow plasma but not red blood cells to seep through and pass into the body fluid. This is how nutrients are delivered and wastes eliminated from tissues. Without a good microcirculation, metabolism cannot take place efficiently. That is why the capillaries play a vital part in the successful elimination of excess fat deposits with all their stored toxins.

Unfortunately, over the years, the capillaries of women living on the average western diet become twisted, distended and highly porous. When they do, proteins seep through and deposit themselves between the tissues and the capillary walls, where they interfere with proper oxygen exchange and impede nutrient delivery and waste elimination. This can gradually starve cells, tissues and organs of all they need to function properly and can also lower cellular metabolic activity. Such changes in microcirculation lower overall vitality, since none of your body's parts are receiving the oxygen and nutrients they need for healthy metabolic functions. They also predispose you to degenerative illness and to rapid ageing. A high-raw way of eating helps restore normal microcirculation and thereby not only heightens metabolism, which is necessary for rebalancing hormones and for maintaining good energy as well as maintaining normal weight, but in a very real way it also rejuvenates your body.

Life Generating Diet: Low-fat, Low or No Dairy, High-Fibre Natural Foods	Western Diet: High-fat, High-protein, Convenience Foods
Normalizes weight	Promotes overweight
Stabilizes emotions	Promotes emotional instability
Alleviates breast tenderness	Exacerbates breast tenderness
Reduces breast cysts	Increases breast cysts
Relieves PMS	Exacerbates PMS
Lowers risk of osteoporosis	Increases risk of osteoporosis

Lowers risk of cancer of
    breast, ovaries and womb
	Increases risk of cancer of
	    breast, ovaries and womb

Protects from diverticulosis	Encourages diverticulosis
Reduces risk of heart disease	Increases risk of heart disease
Alleviates heavy periods	Exacerbates heavy periods
Relieves endometriosis	Exacerbates endometriosis

Protects skin and body from premature ageing	Encourages premature ageing of skin and body
Reduces risk of varicose veins	Increases risk of varicose veins
Lowers risk of gallstones	Increases risk of gallstones
Eliminates constipation	Encourages constipation
Relieves chronic fatigue	Exacerbates chronic fatigue
Reduces risk of bowel cancer	Increases risk of bowel cancer

Sacred Hunger

Ideally the foods you eat on a high-raw diet should be chosen from fresh, organically grown vegetables and fruits, for these foods offer the highest complement of substances of nutritional value to an organism. But for me, as for most people, this is just not possible. I grow my own herbs and a few fruits and vegetables in my garden in the country but half of the time I live in a flat in the city and there I have little access to anything which has been organically composted. Making at least one meal a day a big raw salad made out of sprouted seeds and grains and all sorts of raw vegetables – from raw beetroot to raw herbs, carrots, cauliflower or what-have-you – solves, at least in part, the dilemma about organically grown foods. Since you've grown the sprouts yourself, you *know* that they haven't been subjected to any chemical treatments and, because you have used (or should have used) spring water for them, you know that they do not contain any undesirable minerals or other chemicals. And your salad is an excellent source of top-quality protein, essential fatty acids and natural sugars. When seeds are sprouted the starch in them begins to be broken down and turned into natural sugars which are easy to assimilate and provide energy to heighten your mood. Finally, and probably most important of all, remember that home-grown sprouts are brimming with life energy. This life energy is as yet little understood: it is only beginning to be measured by sensitive instruments. There are no better raw foods than sprouted seeds and grains. Clive McCay, Professor of Nutrition at Cornell University, once researched the sprouted soy bean and declared that he had discovered an almost perfect food: 'a vegetable which will grow in any climate, will rival meat in nutritive value, will mature in three to five days, may be planted any day of the year, will require neither soil nor sunshine, will rival tomatoes in vitamin C, will be free of waste in preparation and can be cooked with little fuel . . .'

Red Dragon

The Japanese are without question the healthiest of any industrialized nation. Sadly this is now changing thanks to the invasion of western convenience foods and eating habits into their culture. However, there is still much we can learn from them. Unlike twentieth-century western medicine and nutrition, which are both limited by their linear chemical thinking, the Oriental approach to health and nutrition takes into account the importance of manipulating life energy or chi in order to create the balance and harmony in the body on which good health depends. Their whole approach to food selection is traditionally energetic in character. It is a balancing of yin and yang energy in food selection and of the various tastes – sweet, bitter, sour, burnt, and so forth – which are said to influence the energy flows that regulate the secretion of hormones and the function of the various organs and systems. Whole grains, legumes, and vegetable foods are good foods for *centring* energy (the body's chi) while sugar and meat and dairy products are very far from the perfect balance of yin and yang and so tend to render its energy off-centre and unbalanced. Meat and dairy products are very *yang* (dense and contracted in nature) while sugar and sweet things are *yin* (very expansive and cooling to the body). When you eat sweets, the body, needing balance, begins to crave meat and vice versa. For optimal health choose *centring* foods – the same wholesome grains, vegetables, local fruits and pulses which contemporary researchers and clinicians from Pritikin to Ornish have discovered help heal the body even of long-standing chronic conditions.

According to traditional Japanese nutrition the major

cause of women's health problems in the West is our consumption of dairy foods, excessive sugar and meat. The Japanese and Chinese have never included milk products in their diet. They have always insisted that the human body was not designed to consume cow's milk and that eating milk products year after year causes the body to degenerate. Increasingly, western nutritionists are beginning to side with the Oriental view. The two most common foods to which people tend to be sensitive are milk and wheat. This is not surprising since convenience foods are replete with these two foods. There is much we can learn from the Oriental approach to food and health.

In Japan there is as yet little awareness of a high-raw way of eating for healing and enhancing health, but this is compensated for by the tradition of slow natural food processing and preservation they use to create their staple foods – miso, kuzu, umeboshi and brown rice vinegar. Unlike our high-tech food technology, the Japanese traditional methods of handling foods for preservation and the creation of dishes such as miso actually improves a food's health-giving quality by enhancing its chi. Traditional miso is made by combining *kogi* (cultured grains or soy beans which have been fermented) with soy beans, salt and water and then letting it ferment naturally from between three months to two years. Many naturally processed foods such as these play an important part in the modern system of macrobiotics which (like the high-raw approach to health) has been credited with an almost infinite ability to support the body's healing of itself.

Nutritional Supplements

One of the most common questions women ask is, provided my diet is good, do I need to take nutritional supplements. Ideally no. The best sources of vitamins and minerals are organically grown foods. No supplements can or ever will compete with them in health-promoting properties. Certainly no amount of nutritional supplements, no matter how wisely chosen, will ever replace a good diet. Many large-scale studies show that women in the western world are deficient in nutrients such as zinc, some of the B vitamins, magnesium and others. For women who have been exposed to high levels of xenoestrogens and who for years have eaten the standard supermarket fare while living stressful lives, specifically chosen vitamins, minerals, trace elements and certain essential fatty acids can greatly enhance health.

The best nutritional supplements are the superfoods like spirulina, seaweeds, chlorella, green barley and wheat grass. They contain complexes of important vitamins, minerals and trace elements in a form that is balanced and easily assimilated by the body. Anti-oxidant nutrients and metabolites such as vitamin C, vitamin E, beta-carotene, coenzyme Q10 and selenium can be helpful too. They improve the immune system's function and are helpful in warding off illness and degeneration. Magnesium is vital for good immune function and hard to come by in processed foods while zinc strengthens the immune response. Women who are athletes or who do a lot of physical activity need greater quantities of magnesium than others and almost certainly more zinc as well and these can only be supplied by nutritional supplements. So do older women.

Every woman is a complete biochemical individual so only the roughest guidelines about nutritional supplements can be given. Specific nutritional programmes are best devised with the help of a skilled nutritional adviser since most doctors receive virtually no nutritional guidance in relation to their medical training. (See The Professionals, p. 404, for guidelines and suggestions.)

Finally, although to my knowledge nobody has done any hard research into the subject, from the experience of women themselves it seems obvious that many women's dietary needs and desires change after menopause. Most women find they feel better on a mostly or completely vegetarian diet which eliminates dairy products, caffeine and meat. There are exceptions, however, so it is important to experiment. A few women actually need meat and do far better if they eat it during and after menopause. Certainly if you decide to eat meat it needs to be from healthy animals (see Seeds of Change, p. 378) and low in fat.

Chapter Twelve
Body Heat

For a few women exercise is such a normal part of their lives that they do it regularly without thinking. It makes them feel good so they run or swim, play tennis, do yoga, row or attend dance classes. For most of us, however, heavier exercise is something that can seem rather daunting – especially if you haven't done any for 30 years. From our earliest introduction to physical activity in schools our perception of exercise gets coloured by the confusion that exists between sports skills and fitness. Being skilful at a particular sport does not necessarily have much to do with being fit. Many women who discovered in school that they were not natural athletes are still put off the idea of taking up some form of regular activity because they feel they lack physical prowess, that they will simply be 'no good at it.' Being good at something is completely irrelevant. What matters is simply that you use your body by setting it in motion and letting it experience the kind of movement for which it was made. It can be useful to look at whatever your own unconscious assumptions may be regarding exercise so you can clear away any cobwebs. For exploring the possibilities of what exercise can do to change you for the better is a life-expanding experience. It can be one of the most exciting journeys a woman can take at any time but especially in the middle of her life. And this is particularly true if, like me, your natural tendency is to curl up into a ball and flop on to the sofa.

Dr Walter Bortz of the Department of Medicine at the Palo Alto Medical Clinic in California published a fascinating paper in which he reviewed more than 100 studies showing that the sedentary lifestyle which has developed in the past 50 years in the West causes bodily damage. Disuse through inactivity increases levels of cholesterol and triglycerides for instance. It also reduces *vital capacity*, that is your ability to take up and use oxygen. Bortz found that the average sedentary 45-year-old has lost half of the ability to take up and use oxygen. With that loss comes all sorts of degenerative changes to the body that even most doctors still think are a part of normal ageing. What is so wonderful is that when a sedentary person gets into regular exercise for a year, he or she can restore the ability to take up and use oxygen to that of a 25-year-old. The benefits of restoring vital capacity are superior to any drug or medical treatment in existence. This is particularly true for women in mid-life and beyond. As one of the world's foremost authorities on exercise, nutrition and good health, Dr Michael Colgan says, 'There is no longer any doubt: exercise can save your life, while couch potatoism creates an existence that is nasty, sick and short . . . *exercise directly prevents disease.*' (The italics are mine.)

Numerous studies show that most bodily changes associated with age have little to do with years passing. They are instead the result of negative shifts in what is known as our Lean Body Mass (LBM)-to-fat ratio – that is decreased muscle mass in relation to fat – which occur as a result of simple disuse. There is a widespread belief that as women get older their body metabolism naturally slows down and therefore it is normal that we grow steadily fatter. Yet here, too, inactivity is the culprit.

Your Lean Body Mass is always shifting. Being inactive makes it shrink. So does going off and on slimming diets. Crash dieting causes you to shed muscle tissue. Yet when lost weight is regained it is regained in fat, forever decreasing the weight of your LBM. This is why the more you diet the flabbier your body becomes. And because crash dieting shrinks LBM, it also shrinks your metabolism so it becomes harder and harder to stay thin until finally you need to starve yourself (and often ruin your health) to keep the scales right. It is little wonder that when your muscle tissue is as good as it is in a wild animal or a healthy child, your own brand of radiance shines through.

What I didn't know until recently, however, is the more you strengthen your LBM, the easier it is to get rid of psychological hang-ups, fears and all those other niggling things that hold you back. When it comes to using exercise as a bridge to freedom for women in mid-life it is muscle you need to work with. To do so brings about a fascinating metamorphosis and a highly individual one. It will not change you in any intrinsic way, nor will it turn you into someone else's idea of who you should be or what you should look like. It will only help make you more what you are. As you work week after week with the right kind of exercise, even a body which may have been distorted over the years through stress, poor eating and lack of movement, metamorphoses into the true form that is hidden within it. That is where resistance exercise comes in and the best form of resistance exercise is weight training.

Catalogue of Rewards

Working with weights does not mean that you will end up with a killer body. Quite the contrary. Exercise to build muscle, using light weights and many repetitions, is the most effective way of enhancing LBM. It chisels and defines arms, legs, torso, hips and bottom, even if they have been neglected for many years and have lost their natural tone and shape. So good is this kind of body-building at improving LBM that until recently no one considered that it might be an excellent form of protecting against degenerative illnesses such as coronary heart disease as well.

There was a time when aerobic exercise was considered king for health, fitness and longevity. Now, thanks to new research into the effects of weight training at prestigious centres such as McMasters University in Ontario, we know that aerobic exercise combined with weight training is the very best you can get for health, fitness and longevity as well as good looks, stamina and energy. As a result, the much-respected American College of Sports Medicine have recently revised their long-standing assertion that aerobic exercise held the key. Their new programme advises a minimum of two sessions of weight training a week using ten different exercises to enhance the large muscles of the chest, back and legs as well as three sessions of aerobic exercise. Ideally, I think three sessions a week are needed, each between 30 minutes to 1 hour in which you combine resistance movement with some aerobic activity to warm up and cool down (see p. 420–421). Then you get the best of both worlds. Be sure too to walk as much as you can in the open air.

The right exercise also helps prevent degenerative diseases such as cancer and heart disease. An eight-year study which followed more than 10,000 men and 3,000 women and was reported in the *Journal of the American Medical Association* looked at the long-term effects of physical fitness. It found that sedentary women have a 460 per cent higher mortality rate than those that took exercise more regularly. Men in the low fitness category had a 340 per cent higher rate.

Exercise Brings Benefits	Disuse Brings Trouble
Builds strong bones	Renders bones porous and fragile
Increases life-expectancy – on average by seven years	Precipitates deterioration of arteries
Clears anxiety and depression	Lowers noradrenaline levels and makes you more subject to depression
Enhances mental clarity	Induces fuzzy-mindedness
Enhances immune functions – increasing the levels of lymphocytes, interleukin 2, neutrophils and other disease-fighting components of the immune system; also lowers cancer rates in women	Encourages aches and pains to develop as the cells accumulate lactic acid after even the mildest exertion and suppresses immune function
Encourages more restful sleep and greater relaxation	Fosters emotional instability
Improves both mental and physical flexibility	Makes ligaments and tendons lose strength and flexibility so you are more easily injured
Increases mental and physical energy	Causes muscle and brain cells to lose the enzyme capacity for maintaining energy

Increases insulin sensitivity, helps to maintain energy levels and protect against diabetes	Undermines energy and encourages blood sugar disturbances and disorders in glucose metabolism
Improves the elimination of wastes	Contributes to the development of constipation, haemorrhoids and varicose veins, and can lead to disturbances in bowel function
Alleviates symptoms of PMS	Exacerbates symptoms of PMS
Lowers cholesterol – especially the 'bad' low-density lipoprotein (LDL), one of the best predictors of cardiovascular disease	Increases levels of cholesterol, LDL, and triglycerides
Encourages good Lean Body Mass-to-fat ratio	Encourages flabbiness and the laying down of fat stores in the body
Normalizes blood pressure	Fosters rising blood pressure as the years pass
Keeps sex hormones at optimum levels	Causes sex hormones to decline which affects skin, psyche and libido

Caterpillars into Butterflies

I have always been fascinated by the idea of transformation, you know the kind of thing, frogs into princes, Cinderella becomes the belle of the ball. Most people believe that in *real* life transformation is not possible. They have obviously never worked with muscle. Quite apart from all the mind-boggling new research into how the *right kind* of exercise can rejuvenate your body, in the past year I have discovered for myself that exercise is a great deal more than something you do to counteract ageing or protect yourself from heart disease. It can foster personal metamorphosis of the deepest order – physical, emotional and spiritual. Not only is such transformation possible, it is virtually guaranteed – provided you are patient and provided you are willing to put real *muscle* behind it.

A year ago I made a decision to explore just what kind of transformation was possible for me by working intensively with muscle. I had just finished writing a book, *Lean Revolution*, which examines in depth a way of regulating normal weight in the body. In the course of my research I had come to understand the enormous importance of enhancing Lean Body Mass (LBM). I knew that *skilful* weight training (not the slap-about kind you see carried out in most gyms) is the fastest and most efficient way to do this. So I searched out someone who could work intensively with me as a trainer to shift the LBM-to-fat ratio in my own body. I found a Welsh champion weight lifter, Rhodri Thomas, who said he would take me on. When we began to work together I was scared to death that after the first two hours I would collapse in a heap. After all, I am no athlete. However, I was keen to find out for myself just how change happens through muscle so we trained for six days a week. Every day we would work with weights backed up by aerobic exercise such as running, swimming and cycling, interspersed with other activities like squash and tennis – just for relaxation. I found to my amazement that I did not collapse. Instead I watched as all sorts of deep changes began to take place. Muscles I didn't know existed slowly and quietly began to surface through my flesh. I discovered that the psycho-physiologists are right – feelings, thoughts and past experience are indeed held within our own flesh. All sorts of old memories, feelings and fears seemed to be encoded in some mysterious way in my muscles. As you work muscle intensively sometimes these rise to the surface to be lifted off, much as the body is detoxified of physical toxins on a fast. Frequently I found myself pushed to my absolute limits. Then the gym floor would be covered equally with my sweat and my tears. Still, thanks to Rhod's presence and a will that came out of somewhere deep inside me I kept working.

Now, a year on, I am glad that I have. I have discovered that not only does working with muscle in this way transform the body in an outer way by changing LBM-to-fat ratio and reshaping your body, which has all sorts of wonderful rewards but, in many ways even more wonderful, it helps develop from within a slow but steadily growing sense of self-confidence, clarity and independence. For many, myself included, this is a deep change which would have been virtually impossible to come by any other way. It now seems to me that working with muscle slowly and steadily day after day builds a powerful bridge between one's inner and outer world. So now when I think back to all those fairy tales about transformation, about frogs and princes, for the first time in my life I feel I am beginning to understand them and to understand what real transformation through the body is about. It is not all glitzy like they say in the movies. It is slow and inexorable. Yet it brings in its wake gifts far beyond our wildest dreams.

Chapter Thirteen
The Alchemy of Energy

Many years ago the brilliant Nobel laureate Albert Szent-Györgyi, who isolated vitamin C, was prone to asking a peculiar question at dinner parties: 'What is the difference between a living rat and a dead one?' According to the laws of classical chemistry and Newtonian physics there should be no fundamental difference. Szent-Györgyi's reply to his own question was simple yet revolutionary: 'Some kind of electricity.' Living systems are first and foremost energy systems. And the 'electricity' of which Szent-Györgyi speaks is the mysterious life energy which distinguishes us from inanimate things in the universe. The alchemy of energy deals with the means of enhancing it.

The biochemical approach to natural menopause which we have been looking at so far involves things like the manipulation of hormones, changes in diet, and the use of selected botanicals which aim to bring about changes in the body's functioning through *physical* or *chemical* means. And they are terribly important. There is no substitute for supplementing a natural hormone like progesterone where it is needed, or for using botanical products to shift hot flushes, restore emotional balance and banish insomnia, just as there is no effective way of improving bone strength and density unless, in addition to any hormonal support needed, you exercise and follow a wholesome diet ensuring that the vitamins, minerals and trace elements your body needs are optimally supplied. But there is another equally essential dimension to health, emotional wellbeing and spiritual development which such approaches only address obliquely if at all. In the linear, drug-based thinking of the late twentieth century this dimension of health and healing is too often neglected: the *energy* dimension.

The Order of Energy

Your body is not just a collection of physical and chemical events. Like all living systems it is a unified collection of energy fields. Take action to alter the quality of these fields and you can change the way your body functions for ill or good. You can even change how you think and feel. In a living organism it is energy, not chemistry or physical form, which is *primary*. Shift it and the organism will in turn alter itself chemically and physically. This is how acupuncture works and why practising certain martial arts can so affect health and personal power. And this is what lies at the core of energy medicine.

A great deal of the most advanced diagnostic equipment used today in orthodox medicine – from ECGs (electrocardiograms) for looking at heart function and EEGs (electroencephalograms) for examining brain function as well as MRI (magnetic resonance imaging) and EMGs (electromyelograms) – already make use of the principles of energy medicine. Rather like Dr McCoy's approach to healing on *Star Trek*, the new energy medicine goes way beyond mere diagnostic techniques such as these. It looks set to become the medicine of the twenty-first century. Sometimes an energy approach to health and healing employs mind-shifting techniques such as meditation and body movement like Tai Chi to improve the way the body feels and functions. At other times it makes use of external energy carriers such as homeopathic remedies or space-age equipment which subject the body to external fields of some sort (magnetic, sonic, acoustic, electrical, light waves). Whatever its source, the aim of all forms of energy treatments – from the use of something as simple as the Bach Flower Remedies to actions of the advanced light beam generators – is to enhance life energy by restoring energetic *order*. Energetic order is the key to high-level wellbeing. It lifts vitality and intensifies mental clarity, enhances spiritual awareness and triggers self-healing while at the same time improving the specific function of the body's various organs and systems. After an energy treatment the liver works better and can metabolize hormones well, the adrenals are strengthened so a woman is better able to handle stress. Re-establishing energetic order improves the function of the pituitary and hypothalamus, which are responsible for the control of hormones, and makes the assimilation of nutrients and micronutrients from the foods we eat more available to us. But to understand a little of how the energy dimension works we need to leave behind for the moment the biochemical world we have been exploring and move into the realm of high-level physics – the interface between consciousness and physical reality.

Negative Entropy

Two of the most important laws of physics are the laws of thermodynamics. Simply put they are an attempt to understand events in the universe by studying the kind of energy changes which accompany them. The First Law of Thermodynamics states that the quantity of energy in the world remains constant. Energy is neither created nor destroyed it is simply transmuted from one form to another. The Second Law of Thermodynamics is central to an understanding of why energetic order lies at the core of physical and spiritual wellbeing and how energy medicine can be used to enhance health. It is best formulated in terms of *entropy*. Entropy is a measure of *disorder*. This Second Law is known as the *law of entropy*. It describes the way that, left to their own devices, all things in the world become disordered: iron rusts, buildings crumble, dead flowers decay, and so forth. In short, everything tends towards *maximum* entropy, a state of maximum disorder in which all useful energy has been decreased. But what is remarkable about living organisms, including our own bodies, and what still puzzles the world's finest scientific minds, is that, despite the law of entropy, so long as we are alive our bodies maintain themselves in a state of fantastic improbability. In the words of Albert Szent-Györgyi, who spent most of his life trying to penetrate this mystery: 'Life is a paradox . . . the most basic rule of inanimate nature is that it tends toward equilibrium which is at the maximum of entropy and the minimum of free energy. The main characteristic of life is that it tends to decrease its entropy. It also tends to increase its free energy. Maximum entropy means complete randomness, disorder. Life is made possible by order, structure, a pattern which is the opposite of entropy. This pattern is our chief possession, it was developed over billions of years. The main aim of our existence is its conservation and transmission. Life is a revolt against the statistical rules of physics. Death means that the revolt subsided and statistical laws resumed their sway.'

Of the Highest Order

In a way which no one has ever been able to explain, living organisms, unlike things in the inorganic world, are superbly equipped to maintain energetic order. This in turn supports physical and biochemical wellbeing. It is something which makes virtually no sense within the paradigms of chemistry and Newtonian physics. Where by rights there should be little difference in the chemical and physical processes taking place within a living body and those that occur in a corpse, in reality there is every difference in the world. Living systems create for themselves a high degree of *negative entropy* – despite the fact that events in the universe as a whole are running wild to destroy it.

For despite the innumerable destructive processes continually going on in and around us, we have the power to resist entropy and to maintain energetic order. Indeed, there is every indication that so long as we live we are continually involved in the process of creating even more order. This we do both individually in the repair functions of our cells and enzymic systems and also from an evolutionary point of view since living organisms appear to continue to differentiate into ever more complex and highly structured organisms as time passes. And the better the quality of order in our bodies the healthier and more vital we remain, regardless of age.

Negative Entropy means Menopausal Freedom

From an energetic point of view, ageing is the process which transports a woman's body from a highly ordered internal state towards maximum entropy, i.e. death. There are two ways in which this can happen. Either energetic order and the biochemical harmony which depends on it is steadily eroded so that the body and mind slowly but surely degenerate (as they do in most people these days) or we can take informed action to support energetic order and maintain negative entropy to the highest degree. By taking the second route we are able in effect to *die young late in life*. But such a goal can never be accomplished entirely by manipulating chemistry alone. One of the first scientists to recognize this was another Nobel laureate, the physicist Erwin Schrödinger. He took a close look at the scientific contradictions implicit in the living state and concluded that so long as the human body is alive it resists entropy and avoids decaying into an inert state of equilibrium through metabolism – by eating, drinking and assimilating various kinds of information from the environment. As far back as 1944 Schrödinger wrote: 'Every process, event, happening – call it what you will; in a word, everything that is going on in Nature means an increase of the entropy of the part of the world where it is going on. Thus a living organism continually increases its entropy – or as you may say, produces positive entropy – and thus tends to approach the dangerous state of maximum entropy, which is death. It can only keep aloof from it, i.e. alive, by continually drawing from its environment negative entropy . . . What an organism feeds upon is negative entropy . . . which is in itself a measure of order. Thus the device by which an organism maintains itself stationary at a fairly high level of orderliness really consists in continually sucking orderliness from its environment.'

From an energetic point of view a woman's body is an *open living system*. As such it is constantly processing energetic and chemical *information* which comes to us not only through the kinds and combinations of foods we eat and the way we prepare and process them but also from the air we breathe, the ideas on which we allow our minds to play and the electromagnetic environment in which we live. In effect, as Schrödinger believed and, as a long tradition of natural medicine both in Europe and the Orient has taught, to ensure a high degree of vitality and to protect ourselves from degener-ation, we need to 'suck order' from our environment. To maintain the kind of energetic order that best fosters health and spiritual development during menopause and afterwards, we need a constant supply of the right information from the outside world. Energy medicine can supply some of the best available. Treatments such as soft laser therapy, microcurrent therapy, scalar wave therapy, magnetic field therapy and light-beam therapy can all be used to help restore order to a body in which it has been degraded. The level at which these kinds of treatments work is profound as are the effects they are able to bring about both mentally and physically.

One of the most knowledgeable people in the English-speaking world about energy medicine and its practical applications is Dr Robert Jacobs. A naturopath, homeopath and inventor, Jacobs has spent the last 25 years developing and using leading-edge equipment such as the lightbeam generator, which radiates photons of light to help restore energetic balance at a cellular level, and crystal magnetic beds designed to relieve stress in the body and re-establish order on a molecular level. Jacobs is a true visionary. He is the direc-tor of two charities: The Society for Complementary Medicine in London and the Society for Human Development in the United States. They are dedicated both to advancing the sci-ence of preventative medicine and immune enhancement and to providing leading-edge holistic clinical treatment to those fighting critical illness as well as to ordinary people striv-ing for optimal health. Both charities are funded by private individuals and organizations and much of their work is devoted to bringing help to people suffering from critical ill-nesses, such as AIDS, who are unable to afford treatment. But Jacobs is just as interested in helping otherwise well people develop their mental, physical and spiritual potentials to optimal levels. To this end he uses the latest generation of homeopathic medicines plus advanced nutritional approaches as well as state-of-the-art energy-based treatments, all of which can be particularly useful to women whose hormones are in flux and who want to regenerate and rejuvenate their systems.

Soft Laser Therapy

Not long ago researchers discovered that coherent light – laser light – can exert as strong an effect on biologically active points on the body as can acupuncture needles. Since then laser therapy has emerged as a potent force for human health. In the right hands it can aid the healing of internal structures. Soft lasers have been used to treat the body ever since it was discovered that by stimulating the body's energy centres, including acupuncture points, on the skin's surface you can bring about important energy shifts to enhance organ and system functions. A soft laser looks like a long-armed robot with a big gold head at the end of each arm. These are positioned over clusters of biologically active points to the liver, adrenals, thymus, pancreas and various areas of the brain to enhance the function of these organs and glands. Laser light also impacts cellular mechanisms in the local area on to which it has been directed by raising the body's own healing capacity in that area manyfold. Several interesting hospital studies have been carried out using lasers on burns, diabetic ulcers, bed sores and skin problems from acne and eczema to ageing skin.

Lightbeam Therapy

Another important instrument in energy medicine is the lightbeam generator. It relies on a high-frequency static electric field along with a specific spectrum of emitted light. This piece of equipment looks like a black box from which a long cord emerges. At the end of that is a small electrode that emits an electric spark. The lightbeam can be used to re-polarize cells using electrostatic energy to enhance cellular functions and repair. The static electric fields created by it significantly alter intracellular enzyme activity. By increasing ion potential they facilitate enzymic functions. The same fields also enhance nerve impulses to a given area by exerting a positive electrochemical effect on the nervous system so there is less resistance to electrical energy flows. Lightbeam therapy also acts on the cell's potassium-sodium ion pump to improve the assimilation of nutrients and bring a better elimination of wastes. Used over whichever areas of the body is appropriate – internal organs such as the pancreas, kidneys, adrenals or anywhere there is nerve impairment – it can help break down blockages in the lymphatic system while exerting a separate direct healing effect on skin, bathing it in ozone and in the static fields to improve skin metabolism. The light-beam generator is an excellent instrument for treating skin lesions of all sorts including acne, eczema, rashes, and infections. It can also help to rejuvenate skin by increasing the flow of ions and enhancing the enzyme activity in cells.

Magnetic Field Therapy

Every living organism, including the human body, is made up of atoms consisting of a nucleus which carries a positive charge circled by negatively charged spinning electrons. It is the spinning of electrons that create the magnetic fields of an atom. The magnetic fields of the atoms can be influenced from outside the body and it is this mechanism which forms the basis of electromagnetic treatments. As well as influencing the state of the body by acting upon it at an atomic level, electromagnetic applications in energy medicine induce changes in tissue voltage, improve the activities of the body's enzymes, enhance ion transport at a cellular level and affect membrane potentials. This in turn results in heightened tissue repair and wound healing, improved immune functions, the reduction of inflammation, and can bring about the elimination of allergic sensitivities and the re-establishment of energetic harmony in the body as a whole.

On a physical level stress shows up as a loss of order in the body and a disruption in homeostasis. Magnetic field therapy lifts off stress by inducing a state of deep relaxation, stimulates circulation and enhances the use of oxygen and the assimilation of nutrients at a cellular level while improving the elimination of wastes. Throughout the ages exposing living organisms to magnetic fields has been known to have bacteriostatic properties and to bring about wound healing – effects which have now been confirmed by twentieth-century science. Modern magnetic field therapy is an extension of all this. It can take a number of different forms. Pulsed magnetic field treatment is one which is well known. It is often used in the treatment of athletic injuries for enhancing the healing of soft tissue and bone by orthopaedic specialists such as Robert Becker MD, who has been nominated for a Nobel prize three times. Solid state magnetism is another form where large high-power magnets are placed near the body to create a negative magnetic field. American physician William Phillpot reports remarkable results with this form not only in the treatment of physical conditions but also in mental states. There are also a number of magnetic beds and magnetic devices on the market, most of which sadly are not very good since their manufacturers often wrongly use mixed fields – both positive and negative – and only the negative fields can bring long-term benefit to the body. The best form of whole body magnetic field therapy I have come across is the kind Jacobs uses. It comes from lying on a specially constructed bed or table in which not only high-powered solid state magnets emitting a negative field have been embedded but also optical grade quartz crystals. Quartz crystals create a piezoelectric field (an electrical charge) which intensifies the biological activity of the magnets and creates resonance in the body, opening up areas of blocked energy. Each crystal acts rather like a tuning fork – or a small resonator. By creating beneficial resonance the body is able to maintain its own natural state of resonance which is order and balance. Lying on such a bed is in itself a wonderful treatment.

Scalar Wave Generator

This is the most esoteric of all the instruments currently used in energy medicine. A scalar wave device emits a form of pure information that is carried into the body via opposing electrogenetic frequencies which canal themselves out leaving only the scalar. Scalar waves themselves are non-electromagnetic in character. They are capable of acting on living organisms at a sub-atomic level. Certain frequencies of scalar have been shown to destroy viruses and bacteria. Other frequencies have been developed for military purposes because they have destructive powers. But by far the most interesting and beneficial use of scalar waves to the body and psyche is when a sweeping range of beneficial frequencies are used to which the body can be exposed en masse, thereby enhancing its own healthy resonances and efficiently helping to restore energetic order. A scalar wave generator is an instrument which can be used either in a doctor's office or at home as a tool for helping to keep the body in top form. It is something that I would never want to be without. I carry a scalar instrument all over the world with me to enable me to maintain a high level of energy even when I am crossing time zones. I also use it day and night when I am working long hours so I don't overtax my body. You place the head of the instrument over whatever area of the body appears to need attention – the adrenals, the liver, the spleen, the head. But the benefits of the instrument can, in effect, be carried to the whole of the body, enhancing its natural resonances.

The Energy of Beauty

Ironically, probably because many of the techniques involved in twenty-first-century energy medicine are so far away in their approach from twentieth-century drug-based medicine, one area in which energy medicine is already being put to practical use is that of beauty treatments both for the face and for the whole body. Few beauty therapists using energy instruments come close to the results of body therapist Beth Jacobs. This is perhaps not surprising when you consider that she also happens to be Robert Jacobs' wife. Beth Jacobs, who originated the Gagnon System of total beauty, works in a unique way by combining a broad base of training in body therapy – encompassing movement, muscular manipulation and structural reorganization – with the use of specialized energy equipment such as the soft light laser, lightbeam generator, microcurrent and magnetic fields. The usual beauty therapy takes an approach that might be described as trying to stick things back together with safety pins and chewing gum to give the illusion of restoring lost youth. Beth Jacobs' energy approach to beauty, however, is genuinely holistic. It aims not at illusion or cover up but at maximizing a woman's natural radiance from the deepest levels, no matter what her age, and at the same time helping to bring energetic balance to her mind and body.

Each year the skin's biochemical processes slow down a little as a result of free-radical damage, internal and external pollution and ageing. When skin cells are stimulated by certain electric currents, lightbeam photons or magnetic fields, this opens up the flow of energy, improving both the skin's biochemical functions and the look of the skin. Such stimulation also improves cell metabolism so that skin cells are able to absorb more nutrients effectively and to eliminate waste products. This kind of bio-electrical or magnetic cell-tuning enables tissues to regain integrity. In the right hands, a dozen or so of such energy treatments spaced over a few weeks can bring about a non-surgical facelift, eliminating all sorts of energy blockages in the rest of the body at the same time as improving lymphatic drainage which, when it is poor, causes a woman to retain wastes and water and produces aches and pains in her muscles and joints. The power of energy medicine used to enhance good looks lies in a marriage between the energy-enhancing equipment being used and the skills and wisdom of the therapist using it. Sadly, many of the new electronic approaches to beauty have become more like the latest fads. As a result, various machines now grace the rooms of salons yet they are being used by therapists who can be incompletely trained and have little grasp of the potential for overall rejuvenation and regeneration of skin and body which lies in their hands. In such circumstances, much of the power of energy therapy is lost. It is important to choose a therapist carefully. You can spend a lot of money and get very little in the way of results. Just because someone uses an electronic gadget of one kind or another doesn't mean they are practising good energy medicine. For that you need leading-edge scientific equipment and fine practitioners of the art. It is a rare combination.

Bodymind

By no means does all energy medicine come in the form of space-age equipment, however. Practitioners of ayurvedic medicine, qigong, yoga and meditation have throughout the ages insisted that consciousness plays the central role in governing physical and psychological health. For generations the power of the subtle energies of consciousness or the mind to influence the body have been preached. Only recently, however, have researchers begun to draw scientific maps of how this occurs. Much of their new knowledge comes out of a fascinating medical and biochemical discipline with an absurdly long name – *psychoneuroimmunology* – or PNI for short. Far from being two separate entities, mind and body are more like opposite ends of a *bodymind* continuum – two aspects of a living being – and PNI is the scientific study of bodymind. Western scientists working with mind/body medicine such as Dr Joan Borysenko and and Dr Candice Pert, former Chief of Brain Biochemistry at the Clinical Neuroscience Branch of the National Institute on Mental Health in the United States, have been charting in measurable physical terms some of the pathways by which mind influences energetic order for better or worse. They have also been exploring ways and means of empowering people by discovering mental and physical techniques which can enhance that order.

PNI first rose to prominence in the late 1970s, then broadened its base to include high-level physics and psychology, out of which a new science of consciousness is being forged – another way of looking at life and health from the point of view of energetic order which creates the underlying patterns of the universe. It sees human beings as part of a universal energy field, interconnected with all of life, and recognizes that the action of hormones in your body plays a central role in bodymind functions and the way in which thought is directed in turn affects hormonal balance.

Leading researchers in the field of PNI have discovered that the human mind, which includes our conscious thoughts and unconscious impulses as well as what could be called our superconscious or transcendent mind and our emotions, are all elaborately interwoven with every function of the body via nerve pathways and chemical messengers, such as the endorphins, neuropeptides and hormones. A powerful hormonal/nerve relationship exists between your sex steroids like the oestrogens and progesterone via the pituitary, the adrenals and the hypothalamus. Known as the *hypothalamic pituitary adrenal axis*, it links thoughts and emotions with physical responses. New evidence even suggests that a few of the body's chemical messengers may be made of a single molecule whose configuration can actually be altered by a person's mental, emotional and spiritual state, to create new forms.

With each passing month more scientific maps of bodymind are being drawn. They show how what you think and feel powerfully influences the level of vitality you have as well as how slowly or rapidly you age and the shifts of hormones in your body. It is because of these connections that so many hormonal disturbances in a woman's body have psychological or emotional components – from endometriosis (where the lining of the womb proliferates out of control) to PMS, to dysmenorrhoea (painful periods) and amenorrhoea (the absence of a menstrual period). A woman's hormonal symphony, which is an important element of her bodymind, is such an important piece of music that it ideally should not be tampered with. The introduction of an artificial hormone or drug to a woman's body can be like trying to add an African rhythm to a baroque fugue. When the various receptors of hypothalamic and pituitary hormones are faced with having to cope with synthetically altered hormones, this can distort the balance in the endocrine system and disturb energetic order in the body as whole. Via the hypothalamic pituitary adrenal axis it may also lead to a disturbance in a woman's thinking functions and to her emotional balance. So, by the way, can the mental and spiritual stress of her feeling trapped in a job or a relationship which she hates or which offers her soul no nourishment. By contrast, the regular use of a meditation technique, of an energy-based exercise practice such as the Chinese Tai Chi, of biofeedback through which one learns to exert conscious control over bodily processes or of regular prayer is a way of bringing energetic order back to the body – not only through the mechanisms of PNI but in other ways so far only partly understood by doctors and scientists working in the fields of PNI. This, too, is an important branch of energy medicine.

Homeopathic Energetics

Products can also be used to help restore energetic order. Take homeopathic medicines. The latest research into the ways in which homeopathic remedies work shows that their actions belong not to the realm of chemistry but to the domain of quantum physics and the field of energy medicine which is taking shape out of it. In using ordinary chemical medicines and drugs, generally speaking, the higher the dose the greater will be the effect. Just the opposite is the case with homeopathy. In homeopathy the more a medicine is diluted, the higher its energetic potency becomes. Homeopathics are made by a process which entails diluting a substance or compound again and again in alcohol or water and then succussing it – shaking is vigorously. Lower doses of homeopathic remedies still contain traces of the substance from which they have been made even though their primary actions lie in the way the particular remedy's energy resonates with the energetic order of the person or animal being treated. But, once any homeopathic is diluted one-in-a-hundred 24 times or more, no trace remains of the compound or substance from which it was made. Examining such remedies, using nuclear magnetic resonance (NMR) imaging, researchers are able to do readings of their sub-atomic activity. One researcher who has looked closely at the mechanisms by which they act is German biophysicist Dr Wolfgang Ludwig. Ludwig has demonstrated in other ways that homeopathic remedies emit measurable electromagnetic signals and that the nature of dominant frequencies in these signals are specific to certain remedies. So are the Bach Flower remedies. These inexpensive and effective products for restoring harmony to mental or emotional balance can be very useful to women in their menstrual and menopausal years.

The homeopathic remedies most commonly used in menopause and hormonal complaints tend to be *Lachisis, Sepia, Pulsatilla, Apis, Aconite, Calcarea Carbonica, Cimicifuga racemosa, Sulphur* and *Phosphorus.* But in the hands of a good homeopath, a remedy prescribed is always determined by a total picture of a woman's constitution and symptoms. This is one of the reasons that research validating the actions of homeopathic remedies can be hard to carry out. Unlike drugs which are constantly given to any patient with a particular complaint, in homeopathy the same condition may call for completely different remedies according to the constitution of the person being treated. That being said, there was an interesting open study published in 1992 which investigated a German homeopathic combination remedy for menopause and PMS known as Mulimen. Made from *Agnus castus*, black cohosh, sepia and St John's wort, it was given to women over a three-month period. Out of 82 women treated, around 49 experienced significant relief from their symptoms from this alone. Half of the women who had been experiencing hot flushes became completely free of them.

Energetic Soul Alignment

If I could choose only one health-enhancing product for use year in and year out it would be Vita Fons II (see Resources, p. 502). Vita Fons II is a second-generation version of something known as *Vita Florum*, developed by Elizabeth Bellhouse as a vehicle to carry what might be described as the energy of perfect balance and order. According to Bellhouse, each human being consists of seven different and interdependent levels of being: *body, soul, brain, emotions* and *mind* – all of which are meant to communicate freely with the *divine core* via the *spirit.* When, for any number of reasons, the human spirit does not resonate in harmony with its divine core a person's energetic order becomes distorted, energetic order is undermined and optimal wellbeing becomes degraded. This can manifest in many ways – physical illness, emotional disturbances or spiritual pain. When used on the body, Vita Fons II products are designed to help restore resonance with the divine core of an individual – the only element within each of us which is said to be totally perfect. This in turn strengthens a person's psychic and spiritual bodies and heightens an organism's natural abilities to maintain order, which in turn helps create physical health or restores it where it has been lost. It also encourages each individual spirit to create conditions which allow the perfection of his or her divine core to influence all aspects of a person's life.

Since the power of Vita Fons II is entirely non-chemical, its energy can be carried to the body in a number of different mediums – in water, in a tablet, in an ointment, lotion, massage oil, salve or talcum powder. It is used over any areas of the body where there is discomfort as well as over energy centres at the navel, heart region, solar plexus and forehead. Because it is the energy in Vita Fons II and not the material substance from which it is made that does the work, it is not the amount of any Vita Fons II product which you use that is important but rather the frequency with which you use it. When well, a woman of, say, 50 years old might use the water six times a day to maintain order. If she were ill she would increase the frequency of use depending upon the severity of the illness.

The company which produces Vita Fons II is controlled by a non-profit charitable trust whose purpose is to make available this high order of energy product to all who want it. The products are available throughout the world either by mail order or through appointed importers. Reports of the positive transformation and physical healing from users are by now legion. Bellhouse has written an interesting book, *Life's Flowering*, which delves into the subtle nature of Vita Fons II, how it works, and what the value of this very special energy is in the modern world.

Energy medicine will unquestionably become the medicine of the future for no other reason than that, once we gain an understanding of how to use it most effectively, it is capable of accomplishing with a minimum of effort what chemical and physical treatments can only do very clumsily. Used skilfully, it is without the dangerous side-effects that are implicit in the use of drugs. 'Chemical medicine is likely to become a subset of medicine as a whole,' says Robert Jacobs. 'Perhaps 80 percent of medicine in the coming century will be energy medicine and 20 percent chemical medicine.' What is already clear is that health in menopause, as in every other part of a woman's life, depends upon supporting energetic order of the highest quality. It may be 30 years before we have a firm grasp of just how much these remarkable treatments and products have to offer in restoring and enhancing order in the body. In the meantime, there is a lot each one of us can do using what is already available to make this a possibility in our own lives.

Chapter Fourteen

Distant Thunder

Since the Industrial Revolution we have been steeped in paradigms or models about health and medicine which are frequently in opposition to the basic principles of natural law –
principles which have been affirmed throughout history by all
the great religions of the world and recently validated by scientific discoveries in high-level physics. They include an
awareness of *wholeness* which implies the interrelatedness of
all things, an acknowledgement of the *energetic nature of life*,
and an appreciation that health and illness are not two separate states (the former to be preserved at all costs and the latter to be wiped out as quickly as possible), but rather opposite
ends of the life continuum. What each of us experience at any
moment in relation to health and illness is nothing more
than a particular degree within a multiplicity of degrees at
some point along that continuum, an expression of the birth-
death-regeneration cyclical nature of life.

Our western health/medical paradigm or model looks
upon the phenomenon of the universe, at life itself, as an
accidental occurrence, nothing more than a complex but ultimately explainable series of chemical and physical reactions
to be studied, classified and manipulated to our advantage.
Such a paradigm or model, unconscious though it is in most
of us, has led to our considering both doctor and ailing
patient as separate from the health/disease process. It has
also led us to ignore any relationship between mind or spirit
and an organism's state of health. Finally, it has created a tendency towards treating disease as a measurable, quantifiable,
pathological state affecting specific tissues, organs or systems
which has little relationship to the thoughts, feelings and
lifestyle of the sick person – that illness arises entirely as a
result of outside events such as trauma, infection or simply
bad luck.

Science of Fragmentation

Such a model has had value. It has provided us with an elaborate science of diagnosis enabling us to identify innumerable disease conditions. It has also made possible the study of specific effects of a myriad of chemicals and drugs, which may be used to 'fix things' – to kill the microbe or wipe out the symptoms. Unfortunately, it has also resulted in our losing sight of the woods by confronting only the trees. By listening only to the tumour or the infective agent present in a disease state without reference to the overall condition of the person who is sick, we have become deaf to whatever possible 'messages' may be being spoken from the unconscious or superconscious mind. We have eliminated the possibility, through listening to these messages, of learning more of the 'language' of illness and health, and of how to work with the body's own processes to help transform the former into the latter. Instead, our modern way of operating with illness has become to eradicate a symptom, to replace a defective part or to suppress a pathological process. It is an approach described by theologian Paul Tillich as 'unhealthy health.'

Such is the thinking behind most conventional treatment offered women for menstrual and menopausal problems. In an attempt to alleviate symptoms regardless of long-term costs to the physical and spiritual health of the woman being treated, there has as yet been little attempt to identify the reasons why female complaints have taken on epidemic proportions in the twentieth century. Nor, too, are questions much asked about the relationship between the health of the individual and the health of the planet. Until, as women, we demand that they be asked, until we come to the point where, instead of looking at disease from a linear, masculine point of view as an entity to be suppressed or destroyed at all cost, we begin to see it in a female way as an expression of the cyclical nature of life fully connected with a human being's feelings, dreams, disappointments and the environment in which we live, we will have to content ourselves with makeshift half-solutions to complex female problems.

Growing Market

During the first half of the twentieth century menopause was viewed as a natural physiological occurrence which rarely required medical intervention. Only after synthetic hormones (the oestrogens and progestogens) were developed did it come to be described as a hormone deficiency disease. The medical profession has gradually extended its scope of action way beyond that of the diagnosis and treatment of disease which used to be its purpose – to encompass the 'control' and 'management' of what was considered a perfectly normal event in a woman's life. One doesn't even need to fall into the paranoid trap of suspecting conspiracy to wonder about the coincidence between the demographic emergence of the post-war baby-boomer market – more than 100 million women in the United States and Europe alone coming of menopausal age – at the same time that menopause has been labelled a deficiency disease. The potential market for hormone drugs is the largest in history. Pharmaceutical manufacturers have only begun to tap it.

Once you define menopause as a disease then you need to find a 'cure' for it. In making use of the cure (HRT drugs) you are putting the body at risk of cancer and numerous other side-effects, no matter how infrequently they occur. If, instead, you choose to define menopause as a natural change in a woman's life, a passage from one stage of her life to another physically, emotionally and spiritually, then you are faced with an altogether different challenge. You are not trying to *cure* anything. You are instead in the business of affirming this change as natural, and looking out for information and techniques that can not only make it as easy as possible (as we already have with natural childbirth) but also of helping each woman use her symptoms whether they be emotional or physical as roads to further empowerment. There is no money in such an approach, and most of the men and women who are the trailblazers in the natural menopause revolution are neither wealthy nor selling anything other than the truth.

A Complex Web

The practice of medicine and the training that any doctor receives has to be constantly updated because things change so rapidly. Every doctor is faced with choices about whether to go for further education after leaving medical school. In organized medicine, both in Europe and the United States, most information and continuing medical education offered to doctors comes from pharmaceutical corporations. Doctors' lives are very busy. They are filled with the demands of their patients. It is not all that easy for them to keep up with the constantly evolving scientific research that can enable them to make shifts and alterations in the treatment methods employed.

Most of the post-graduate education which our doctors receive after they leave medical school (even our specialists, such as endocrinologists and gynaecologists) comes not from the experience of other doctors nor even from reading scientific journals but straight from the medical-industrial complex. This is a close-knit association of pharmaceutical manufacturers, organized medicine and medical regulatory agencies at government level. But the medical-industrial complex has its limitations. It does not have to be corrupt to be vulnerable to the same weaknesses and human prejudices that the rest of us suffer from. The manufacture and distribution of drugs to the public is a multinational business on which medical research itself is dependent for some of the billions of pounds of grants offered to doctors, biochemists, university scientists and other organizations throughout the industrialized world to enable them to carry out their research. This creates a complex web in which the medical establishment, pharmaceutical manufacturers and government regulatory bodies are closely connected to one another, so much so that many people at the top of their profession in one group will shift, often more than once during their career, to another group.

The goal of a pharmaceutical company, just like the goal of any business, is to make a profit. In this case profit comes from the sale of drugs which carry a patent, that is drugs which are chemically unique. When a patent belongs to a particular company, the company is protected against any of its competitors selling the same product. Such a company is quite naturally not interested in carrying out research on non-patentable medicines such as widely available herbs or natural progesterone, regardless of how great their health benefits may be. Neither are they going to inform doctors about the potential such natural compounds might have for improving human health. To do so would undermine their own sales. Instead, the flow of research money out of pharmaceutical manufacturers tends to be directed towards establishing the efficacy of patented drugs. As a result, scientists working in research, as well as doctors whose largest source of information after leaving medical school comes from the medical-industrial complex, tend only to have experience with the use of patented drugs. They remain largely unaware of natural products or techniques which can be used but are non-patentable. This is the main reason why it is not surprising when a government official, industry-supported consultant or academic expert speaks out against some natural form of treatment. Be it hydrotherapy, acupuncture or the use of a compound like natural progesterone, he is likely to dismiss its value. Such people often have very little, if any, personal knowledge of the subject.

In many ways it is little wonder that doctors are so ill informed about differences between the actions of natural progesterone and those of the progestogens with which it is so often confused, especially when even the medical references to studies inaccurately refer to various synthetic progestogens as 'progesterone' in discussing their actions and side-effects. What does seem particularly sad is that occasionally even some of the most conscientious researchers – professionals who have spent much of their career informing the public about the long-term dangers of using hormone drugs – can fall prey to the same error.

What are the arguments against the use of natural progesterone and who has come out strongly against it? Surprisingly, very few doctors, even very few gynaecologists, who prescribe HRT regularly to their patients have even voiced an opinion – probably because they are still not aware of it as an alternative and because, like much of the medical literature on the subject, they wrestle to clarify the confusion between a synthetic progestogen and progesterone itself – the same molecule that is found in a woman's body.

So far Britain's most vocal opponent of natural progesterone use has been the writer Dr Ellen Grant – a researcher and expert in the use of a nutritional approach to female problems, from PMS to menopausal troubles. I have always had enormous respect for Dr Grant's work. Almost single-handedly she has gathered material together and made public the long-term dangers of the use of contraceptive pills. Over the years I have learned much from her. However, when it comes to the progesterone issue, Dr Grant is vehemently opposed to it. In fact she opposes strongly the use of *any* steroid hormones – natural or artificial.

A few months ago in response to an interview with John Lee about natural progesterone which appeared in the newsletter *What Doctors Don't Tell You*, Grant wrote an article called 'Hormonal Mayhem' in which she expressed her opinion that natural progesterone supplementation, like the use of synthetic progestogens, is riddled with dangers. She claimed John Lee had made three fundamental mistakes – asserting that progesterone supplementation is safe, regarding natural progesterone as any different to the synthetic progestogens, and claiming that osteoporosis is in some way related to progesterone. Grant writes that 'even small amounts of extra progesterone, estrogen or testosterone at key times during pregnancy can interfere profoundly with physical and mental development and sexual orientation', citing animal studies by Dr Gina Schoental to support her statement.

Out of respect for Ellen Grant's opinion, and because it was important to me before incorporating the information on the use of natural progesterone into this book, I carefully examined the references on which she was relying to back up her assertions, including Gina Schoental's work. I was surprised to learn that, when contacted, Dr Schoental confirmed that her work had never involved progesterone.

In the same article Dr Grant also warns of the dangers of progesterone use, claiming that progesterone suppresses immunity, that together with viruses and chemicals it acts as a co-carcinogen (cancer causer) and has a number of other negative actions. When I later examined in depth the papers cited by Dr Grant to support her assertions, I, and a doctor colleague of mine who went over them with me, were forced to disagree with many of the conclusions which she drew from them.

There are three ways in which the natural progesterone molecule which is chemically identical to the progesterone produced in a woman's body is a unique hormone. First, it is the main precursor of other important steroids such as the corticosteroids. Unlike the progestogens, it is not an end-product molecule. Second, it provides many important intrinsic functions in the body. Third, it is remarkably free of side-effects such as those listed so extensively for the synthetic progestins. So far the lack of distinction between natural progesterone and their synthetic analogues appears largely a semantic problem wrought by the use of the word 'progesterone' as a generic term for progestogens as a whole. It is little wonder that the average GP or gynaecologist is likely to be ill informed on the subject of natural progesterone and its use.

It is my belief however, that in time – given the mounting numbers of women whose wellbeing is restored in part at least through the use of natural progesterone – even those who know little or nothing about it will come to see how much it has to offer. The people who are going to be most instrumental in bringing this about are the key players in the bloodless revolution – women themselves who report to each other, to the press and to their doctors their experience of its use. After all, it was only through public awareness of the existence of food allergies and the profound effects they can exert on health that the medical profession slowly came round to looking at the issue and finally to taking it into account. So, I suspect, will it be with natural progesterone.

At the moment many doctors – ignorant of xenoestrogens and unaware of the oestrogen dominance to which they contribute – still insist that women need to take oestrogen either together with a progestogen or on its own as menopause approaches. They tell you that the risk of cancer is minute in comparison with all of the protection that HRT provides and that it will automatically relieve the anguish of hot flushes and numerous other troublesome symptoms which are supposed to result from menopause. What they don't tell you is that there are other, safer, easier and less expensive ways – both in terms of money and in terms of potential strain on the body and psyche. These include natural herbs, natural progesterone products, dietary change, homeopathy and lifestyle change. And the reason they don't tell you is because, by and large, they do not know. In the face of the elaborate network which disseminates information about drugs, there is so far no economic or political pressure group who could even begin to compete in public relations terms to give the other side of the story.

Beware of Watchdogs

In the western world it is the United States Food and Drug Administration (the FDA) which takes the lead in the approval of a food or drug for distribution. What the FDA decides today becomes a blueprint for action in other countries tomorrow. When, a few years ago, a poisonous batch of the amino acid tryptophan was discovered in America the FDA took this amino acid entirely off the market. Country after country followed suit and it has never returned. In 1962 the FDA was given broad powers to regulate 'articles intended for use in the diagnosis, cure, mitigation, treatment, or prevention of disease in man or other animals' as well as 'articles (other than food) intended to affect the structure of any function of the body of man or other animals'. There is a popular misconception that the FDA is an effective and efficient watchdog constantly looking out for the interests of people by testing the safety and efficacy of various drugs, nutritional products and remedies. This is simply not the case. It is the pharmaceutical manufacturers not the FDA who test the products they have developed. They then submit their results to the FDA for its approval. The average cost of testing a single new drug today is phenomenal – £112 million. Even if a product or drug receives FDA approval this does not mean it is safe. There are instances where pharmaceutical manufacturers have withheld information about side-effects, and many more when serious side-effects have been discovered only after years of a drug's use by hundreds and thousands of patients. Manufacturers of simple natural remedies are unable to afford the huge expense of applying for FDA approval. The safety and effectiveness of various botanical products and natural progesterone creams is well supported by clinical experience over decades. But these remedies are not publicized widely and few doctors therefore know about them. There is also virtually no money available to carry out the tests necessary to receive FDA approval on a generic product which cannot be patented. So natural remedies and approaches to health often remain well-kept secrets – publicized, if at all, only by practitioners who have used them and know they work and women whose lives have been changed by them.

Drug or Cosmetic

Remedies such as natural progesterone creams, pellets and oils are effective and safe. However, companies which manufacture them not only in the United States but in other countries are in the absurd position of being unable to say anything publicly about their efficacy. With the exception of natural remedies already widely in use in the United States, when the major amendments to the Food, Drug and Cosmetic Act were made in 1962 that demanded lengthy and expensive testing to prove a drug's efficacy, natural generic remedies could not be sold as such. In fact, manufacturers of natural treatment products and nutritional supplements are not even allowed to give their products names which suggest how they are to be used. This means that natural products need to keep a low profile. You will find that natural progesterone creams will not even say 'progesterone' on the label, they must speak in veiled language about 'wild yam extract' instead. And they will be referred to as 'cosmetics' simply because if they were correctly labelled they would have to be categorized as drugs and could not be sold without a licence. One of the unfortunate things about the position in which the FDA has placed manufacturers of these products is that there is no way of establishing the quality of one product as compared to another by being able to inform customers about a product's manufacture and what standards it maintains. So, together with the two or three best natural progesterone products, you can find some copycat second-cousin versions manufactured by companies without the best technology and without the real knowledge to produce a high-quality product. Meanwhile the women who may have heard about natural progesterone cream and want to try it find it very difficult to know which is the best product to buy.

In 1994 a British company called Higher Nature began importing a good range of natural progesterone products into Britain. They were responsible and intelligent in the way this was done. The company provided seminars for doctors and other health practitioners as well as talks for the general public and the press, inviting doctors of the calibre of John Lee to present their clinical findings, background information on progesterone and protocols for use. Higher Nature set up a panel of trained nutritionists whom professionals and non-professionals alike could contact by telephone for further information and advice. They also made available research papers as well as independently produced reports and books to anyone wishing to buy them. The reception for the new products turned out to be excellent, particularly since a growing number of far-sighted British doctors soon became highly enthusiastic about the results their patients were getting from their use.

Within a few months, the company was forced to stop selling the products except by prescription. This is how things have remained since. As it stands now, any woman in Britain wanting to make use of a good natural progesterone product has two options. Either she goes to a doctor who she knows works with them and hopes that, after examining her, s/he will prescribe them, or she can order the products – quite legally – from abroad for her personal use only. Yet the protocols for the use of these valuable products remain hard to come by for a woman who needs them. Meanwhile the biggest irony is this: what few doctors are aware of is that the routinely prescribed combinations of oestrogen/progesterone now used as HRT have in fact *never* been approved by the FDA for use as hormone replacement therapy for postmenopausal women. As Gail Sheehy says, 'I also found that Provera has never been approved for treatment of menopause by the US Food and Drug Administration. Notwithstanding, the FDA's Advisory Committee on Fertility and Maternal Health Drugs stated in 1991 that this combination of hormones [i.e. oestrogen progestogen combinations] may be used indefinitely by a woman with a uterus. Asked what proportion of the female population over age fifty would be suitable candidates for long-term consumption of oestrogen alone or combined with synthetic progesterone [sic], the committee replied, "Virtually all". A blank cheque.'

As Ellen Hodgson Brown who wrote the introduction to *Breezing Through The Change* says, 'The FDA has never approved the oestrogen/progestin combination as hormone replacement therapy for postmenopausal women, so its long-term risks are unknown. What research does show is that progestins may reverse the cardiovascular benefits of oestrogen; and they do *not* reverse its increased risk of breast cancer and may increase it. Synthetic progestins also come with a long list of side effects many women are unable or unwilling to endure.'

In recent decades women have taken greater and greater control over their own lives. We have exercised choice about whether and when to have children, about the kind of relationships we have with our men or with other women. Yet what I see happening is that our assertion of choice and independence is being used and fed into the HRT mania which interferes with the very freedom of body, mind and spirit which natural menopause can offer a healthy woman. For the process which Noam Chomsky has named 'manufacturing consent' is most certainly taking place in the continued insistence that women at menopause are fundamentally in need of medical management. Meanwhile, the revolution in natural menopause now seeded continues to expand, its primary thrust coming from women themselves. After all it is we who fought for our right to choose to bear children or to remain childless. It is we who demanded that our men be allowed into the delivery room and that we have the choice of a drug-free childbirth at home. And it is my belief that women will ultimately decide how to handle menopause or indeed just how much handling of it is needed.

As it once was with natural childbirth, the knowledge about how to use many of the best natural products and treatments for women can only come from individual scientists and, ultimately far more important, by word of mouth from women themselves – women who, having struggled to find their own way through menopause and out the other side with what information they could glean, pass on their knowledge to other women who need guidance and help. One day I hope there will be a self-supporting organization rather like La Leche League to give practical advice to women who need it. That kind of information is the best you can find anywhere because it is information based not on theoretical ideas but on practical experience and bonds of respect not only for the female body and psyche but for the magnificence of life itself. It also has nothing to sell except the truth.

THE SCIENCE OF MYTH

Chapter Fifteen

Moonstruck

It is not easy to be female at the millennium. In the past half century a woman's place as defined by society has undergone drastic shifts and revisions, many of which have offered us greater freedom of choice. Women have demanded, and to some degree achieved, equal opportunities at work with men. We have refused to spend all of our lives in supportive roles. We have sought out new ways of relating to our families, work colleagues and friends – as well as to ourselves. We have also gone a long way towards eroding long-standing negative assumptions about the female, the idea that as women we are too emotional, too unfocused, too fickle, to accomplish anything significant. We have proved that women have good minds and are capable of high achievement academically, in business and in the arts. Yet being a woman in today's world demands that we be willing to live the life of a juggler. Each of us has become involved in a never-ending task of trying to keep the balls of our life's roles in the air – professional woman, mother, worker, lover, wife, achiever – while we get through each day, and week and year.

Daughters of the Father

Many women have chosen to walk away from the limited self-sacrificing lives they watched their mothers lead – lives which too often produced grief and bitterness as the menopause years approached. Instead of following in the footsteps of the traditional female whose primary role was concerned with nurturing, they have looked towards the male world for their mentors and role models as a means of giving credence to their need for a sense of purpose, for their ambition, intellect, direction and definition of success. They have opted for achievement in the world by becoming *daughters of the father* – women who identify with the traditionally male focus on power, independence, prestige, money and glamour, and for whom anything less than carrying out 'important work in the world' is simply not enough.

Other women have simultaneously tried to live out the male ambition inherited from the world of their fathers and also to redefine their fostering female energies in the hope that they will be successful in the world yet still be able to raise their children and fulfil their sexual and emotional needs. They try to make lives for themselves which they hope will not end in sorrow as the lives of countless generations of previous western women have.

Still others have decided to reaffirm traditional values as *daughters of the mother*. They have chosen to create lives for themselves dedicated primarily to nurturing the ambitions of lovers or husbands and devoting themselves to the development of their children so long as they remain within the family.

These are only a few of the possible choices now open to women in a world where shifting economic, social and personal values have undermined the established social order and made choice possible. Whatever path we choose, somewhere deep within each of us searches for meaning and longs for freedom – whenever we have time to think about it between caring for children, paying the bills and trying to look like we have just walked off the cover of *Vogue*. Such are the warp and woof from which our lives are woven during our thirties and early forties – lives which often include a career as well as further education, motherhood, loverhood and a myriad of other things. Such is the ordinary world of today's woman.

So great are the demands on women now – many of them self-imposed – that we are often in danger of losing track of our own souls and of burning ourselves out. There is no place for the old female rituals in our lives. In other cultures, among the Native Americans for instance, women would leave the tribe for a few days each month to enter the soul realms and experience the Moon Lodge during menstruation. There, in the presence of other women, they gave themselves permission to enter altered states of consciousness, to restore their energies and to express the wildness of their own creativity – a creativity which at the dark moon time of menstruation has nothing to do with nurturing or relating to men or to children.

We have no such opportunity. Instead, many women, unaware of the value of venturing into the soul realms, choose to 'control' their moods and cycles by taking hormones – not only to avoid unwanted pregnancies but even to regulate events so that a business meeting doesn't come up in the middle of a menstrual period when they might not be as rational or as socially acceptable as at other times. Then, sooner or later, every woman gets moonstruck. When it happens the ordinary world in which she has been living is rent asunder. She is being initiated into the mysteries of the dark blood. Menopause has arrived.

'Isn't it wonderful,' the editor of the woman's page of a national newspaper said to me one day, 'science has finally conquered women's biology.' 'What are you talking about?' I replied. 'Oh, you know,' she went on, 'it's great. We don't have to menstruate any more and we don't have to have babies thanks to the Pill. We don't even have to go through menopause or get old now that we have HRT. At last women are set free from their biology. I'd like you to write a piece on it.' It took me a few seconds to recover from the shock of hearing an intelligent woman voice an opinion so far away from my own sense of what being female is about. I knew there was no point in even discussing the issue. I said that the idea didn't grab me and walked out of the office literally stunned by how carelessly this poor frazzled daughter of the father could dismiss a million years of inherited woman power, wisdom and blood. She had done it with the wave of a hand and the swallow of a pill. Then, almost as an obituary, she had proposed a 750-word article on modern women's new-found 'freedom'. At the door I turned to look at her. There sat a haggard 35-year-old, who looked 50, hunched over her computer, smoking cigarettes. Three years later someone told me she had just had her womb removed.

Wasteland Echoes

The editor's sense of freedom, like much of the so-called 'freedom' we hear about, is certainly of a very limited kind. Since all freedom is won at a price, I cannot help wondering how high a price we are paying and if it is real freedom at all. I know too many dynamic, successful women who appear to have everything. Yet, when you sit down with them alone, away from the glitter of their busy lives, they describe feeling out of sync with themselves. A sense of sterility and stagnation permeates their lives, and they carry a feeling of emptiness and even of betrayal, yet from what and by whom they rarely know. Many have aimed for the top and arrived. So now what? Where is the next challenge, the next battle to be won, the next social occasion? They tend to pack their days with duties and appointments, always uneasy that if they stop for a moment they might let somebody down or their lives might fall apart.

Just as our mothers and their mothers before them embraced the expectations of their culture – that fulfilment would come through being a good wife, a good mother or a good servant – women have now taken on another cultural stereotype. We have learned to do things logically. We have largely bought into a male stereotype based on the attainment of academic, financial or artistic success. We have thrown ourselves headlong into the male world and many of us have 'made it' within that world's terms. Yet, in the wake of our success, we often find ourselves pursued by a confusing sense of barrenness and despair that further achievement in the world, new love affairs or the prospect of a facelift can do nothing to cure. It is at this point that many women, myself included, first hear the call to adventure. It comes as a powerful challenge to leave the ordinary world in which we have lived decades of our lives and set out in search of answers. Why did this happen? What was wrong? What secrets have we forgotten and what connections have we lost in our obsession with *doing* things and our tendency to opt for chemical control of our body's cycles? And what are we missing out on?

When I began the research for this book these were some of the questions I set out to find answers to. The search led me down two paths which at first seemed so separate that I did not see how they could possibly meet – science and myth. First I explored the biochemistry and physiology of a woman's body, entering the fascinating world of shifting hormones and trying to make sense of it. When I discovered the phenomenon of oestrogen dominance and realized that most of the physical and emotional agonies of menstruating and menopausal women in the West have resulted from the same male-orientated, blinkered, linear view of reality that has poisoned our planet, it overwhelmed me. How could we as women continue to buy into values and ways of living which not only did not serve the coming to fruition of our own talents and our capacities for joy but were inexorably destroying the earth? Where had all our real freedom gone and our power – not power in the male sense of *power over*, but in the female sense of *power to*? I also delved deep into the past in search of archaeological findings and archetypal connections that might give clues to just what as women we had lost and how any of these lost treasures might be rediscovered. This led me into the realm of myth and ritual. I discovered that the two worlds – the world of science, with all its shifting biochemistry and rising and falling hormones, and the world of myth, peopled with archetypes, symbols, goddesses and rituals – not only meet, they are blended within a woman's body and psyche. And where they meet is a cauldron of blood.

Blood Mysteries

According to written records, since the beginning of human history, the power of creation was believed to reside in the blood that pours forth from a woman's body. It ebbs and flows with the waxing and waning of the moon. Blood has always been credited with magical power and with containing the essence of a person's soul – 'one's life blood'. Medieval physicians believed that a young woman's menstrual blood could cure leprosy and act as an aphrodisiac. For centuries, rituals for taking in spiritual powers involved ingesting menstrual blood; it was mixed with red wine and taken as an alchemical drink. Ancient Egyptians, Celts, Persians and

Taoists in China all held similar beliefs about menstrual blood and carried out similar rituals. In Ancient Greece during planting festivals women mixed their menstrual blood with corn seeds then spread them upon the earth for fertility. In the seventeenth century when William Harvey wrote his famous scientific treatise on the circulation, he referred to the flow of blood through the body as the *coursing of spiritual power*. Even our word 'blessing' is derived from the Old English *bloedsed* which means bleeding. Menstrual blood and the blood of childbirth are the only blood given freely, that is shed without wounding. Not only metaphorically but speaking strictly from a scientific point of view, human life cannot be created without the blood in a woman's womb. So profoundly did an awareness of the power of a woman's blood touch the lives of primitive people that native words for menstruation carry connotations of spirit, divinity and magic – of the supernatural and of the sacred. Ancient Hindus taught that all life is created out of the congealing of Great Mother's menstrual substance which had been worked and thickened to form curds or clots from which the crust of solid matter emerges. Their goddess of creation Kali-Ma 'invited the gods to bathe in the bloody flow of her womb and to drink of it; and the gods, in holy communion, drank of the fountain of life and bathed in it, and rose blessed to the heavens'.

Moon Goddess

A woman's average menstrual cycle is 29½ days – exactly the length of the moon's passage from new to full and back to new again. In primitive cultures, where women live in close physical proximity to each other, and their natural menstrual cycles are not disrupted by such things as exposure to natural light, electromagnetic fields, drugs and hormones, not only do they menstruate at the same time, ovulation tends to occur when light is brightest at the full moon and menstruation begins during the moon's dark phase – at new moon. There is by no means anything pathological in any woman in the modern world not cycling in this particular natural rhythm, but it has been demonstrated that the menstrual cycle can be regulated according to the exposure to varying degrees of light which mimic the waxing and waning of the moon's phases. Under such circumstances the three phases of the moon – waxing, full and waning – correlate exactly with the monthly cycle of ebb and flow of female hormones – the oestrogen-dominated proliferative phase, ovulation, the secretory luteal phase and menstruation itself.

In the realm of myth and symbols these three phases are superbly mirrored in the three phases of every woman's life: childhood, before the sex hormones begin to flow, the childbearing years which begin at the menarche, and the postmenopausal years of the goddess in her crone guise. In ancient cultures the moon was considered the source of fertility and birth. She ruled destiny and time, the secrets of the unseen world, transformation, death and regeneration. It was the moon's power that quickened all of life. Sowing and harvesting were done in harmony with her ebbs and flows. It was the moon growing bright then darkening and disappearing altogether each month that taught people that nothing in life is constant. The only thing on which you could rely was change. The moon became a symbol of the cycle of transformation that makes its home in a woman's body while woman came to rule all things that involved change.

Archaeologist Marija Gimbutas, the late Professor Emerita at UCLA, is the acknowledged world expert on neolithic goddess-centred cultures in prepatriarchal Europe. Author of more than twenty books, she paints a richly detailed picture of their social structure, agriculture, customs, rituals, religion and art. Much has been learned in recent years about the nature of the goddess-centred cultures which existed for literally tens of thousands of years in Europe and Asia. The miniature sculptures that have been unearthed in the past twenty years give insight into the great variety of female manifestation of the divine which appeared as long ago as 27,000 to 25,000 years BC. Three thousand of these have been found in Siberia alone. In *The Civilization of the Goddess*, a monumental encyclopaedic book which has already changed history, Gimbutas writes, 'According to myriad images that have survived from the great span of human prehistory on the Eurasian continents, it was the sovereign mystery and creative power of the female as the source of life that developed into the earliest religious experiences. The Great Mother Goddess who gives birth to all creation out of the holy darkness of her womb became a metaphor for Nature herself, the cosmic giver and taker of life, ever able to renew Herself within the eternal cycle of life, death and rebirth.'

We learn from ancient sources that, like woman herself, the Moon Goddess has many faces. At the new moon she is the Virgin Goddess wrapped in enthusiasm for new beginnings as seeds sprout and first shoots appear. When her second phase begins so does puberty. Buds turn into flowers and flowers to fruits as virgin becomes transformed into Divine Mother in charge of procreation and sexuality. She is the pregnant goddess, mistress of animals, bringer of life, the madonna. As the moon begins to wane, woman passes through her next initiation to a time of harvest and a time of death during which all that is old becomes compost for new life. It is the Dark Goddess who rules the darkness of the moon, death and rebirth. Ancient statues of the Dark Goddess carved in bone, marble, alabaster or clay are often white – for white is the colour of death. Bones are turned white by the elements. The big breasts and hips you find on statues of the Divine Mother are replaced by stiff nudes. The Dark Goddess is often shown without breasts, her hands either on her chest or extended along her sides. She is shown with an enlarged pubic triangle, for the Dark Goddess of the waning moon is not only goddess of death but of regeneration. She rules the time in a woman's life when all that has run its course, all that is outmoded or no longer meaningful must be destroyed to make way for a more authentic life. She rules menopause.

Dark Goddess

Menopause is the initiation of the Dark Goddess. It is the passage during which a woman is asked to confront the possibility of her own death and probe the mysteries of decay, dismemberment and regeneration. As menopause approaches often a woman wants to spend more time in nature and to feel her spirit fed by the earth. The fear of menopause and the fear of the crone, so widespread in our society, are nothing more than a reflection of a fear of death itself. For in our modern world we have forgotten the great cyclical flow of birth, flowering, death and regeneration that is hidden within the circle of the moon, as it is within all life, and reflected in the circle of our own souls. Our patriarchal culture denies cyclical time and views events as linear. In linear time the end is not connected with the beginning and birth and death are not two events in a continuing cycle of life but opposites – the one to be celebrated the other to be resisted at all costs until the bitter end. It is no wonder our society wants to blank out menopause and to reject the older female. It is the only way in the fearful fragmented world we live in that human beings can deny for a time their own mortality. And so the Dark Goddess remains a focus of fear and loathing in stereotypical male-dominated linear thinking. Any woman who does not break through the limitations of such thinking and move beyond it risks becoming so paralysed by fear that she will look upon the crone as an enemy to be resisted. In truth she is the archetype and medium by which the internal split that took place thousands of years ago between woman and her feminine nature can be healed.

The Dark Goddess is death's priestess. It is she that wipes out old patterns and then, acting the role of the midwife, gives birth to new forms of living. She can seem a terrifying figure to women approaching menopause. She has so long been repressed within our psyches that when at last her energy rises and she makes her presence known, it can sometimes arrive on the scene like an earthquake or a volcano – some eruption of nature that occurs when pressures held too long within the earth are released. Yet she has always been present in our lives, she has appeared each month as the moon grows dark and menstrual blood flows. Now, at menopause, the Dark Goddess comes at last to rest within a woman's being. For instead of being released each month, the dark blood of creative power is retained within a woman's body and made available for her use.

Spokeswoman for the Dark Goddess is the crone. Her presence in a woman's life is usually easy to spot. She appears whenever we experience any drastic and dramatic changes – the death of a loved one, loss of a job, disfiguration. She is the teacher who guides us through the transformation that is demanded of us. She is there in our deepest despair and at times when we connect most powerfully with our own creative fire. She is the handmaiden that nurtures us through dark nights once we are willing to make the descent into our own psyche and connect with whatever forms are sleeping there so that we can begin to live our own power. When these connections are made she is present too. She teaches us by her presence alone to become deeply and spontaneously sexual, assertive, straight, incorruptible, prophetic, intuitive and free. All of these qualities are asking to arise at menopause and all are gifts of the crone. They are, it must be said, also the qualities which most terrify the patriarchal culture in which we live.

Inexorable Nature

The crone is the irrational power of nature which causes all things to decay and be changed. The experience of change is terrifying to both men and women who have lived their lives believing that material reality is all there is and that reason is the ultimate means by which all our problems will be solved. Whatever else she may be, the crone is most certainly not reasonable. No more reasonable than the forces which cause leaves to decay when they fall in autumn, transforming them into leaf mould that will eventually bring new life to the forest. No more reasonable than the hurricane which, irrespective of man's wishes or longings, blows its course through city and countryside. No more reasonable than the earth herself as she quakes and trembles with the shifts taking place in the continental plates of her body.

It is little wonder that male-centred religions have diabolized the crone. For she is the ultimate destroyer, the emasculator of male reason. Nature and the crone aspect of the Dark Goddess become in men's minds the castrator – so much so that during the Inquisition witches were accused of collecting severed penises in boxes or birds' nests. Yet even the male penis itself represented – and still represents – an instinctive power to the male which most western men feel uncomfortable with. For the penis seems to have a life of its own, quite separate from the man to which it is attached. Like the Dark Goddess it defies man's sterile reason. As Barbara Walker says in *The Crone, Woman of Age, Wisdom and Power*: 'The conviction peculiar to males that sex organs have an uncontrollable, independent life of their own, is expressed in the churchman's belief that the stolen penises moved about and ate food in their captivity like animals.' The penis, too, is an instrument of the Dark Goddess.

The Dark Goddess lives at a woman's core. She guards the self. She is the friend of the soul whose purpose in your life is to fiercely protect and further the whole process of your learning to live authentically from your core. She never trades in deceit, she never lies, nor does she veil her power. She refuses to uphold any relationship that doesn't work and she tears away at anything within us that is greedy or grasping or infantile. She continually urges us to reclaim our own power – the power to set limits and to shout 'no', and the power to say 'this is what I will do and this is what I won't do' when we are faced with any sort of abuse or anyone trying to steal our power or dominate us.

Madness of the Imprisoned

But she is far more than this. The Dark Goddess is the female power so long rejected and repressed by western civilization that when it rises to the surface it may break forth in fury to devastate a woman's ordinary world. Sometimes when she forces her presence to be felt at menopause she can well up inside and make us hysterical. Her frenzies – which in the male-dominated world of linear thinking are looked upon as something for which a woman should be tranquillized and kept under control – were once treated with the deepest respect as visitations from the gods. It was in such a state that the Pythia or Sibyl at Delphi prophesied the future and told secrets capable of turning those who sought her help into conquerors of nations. When we forget the power of the Dark

Goddess – when we separate ourselves from her essential nature – then we experience her as the destroyer who arrives like a great snake to break up the structure of our lives, devour our relationships and make mincemeat of our most precious self-deceptions. She can quickly cut through the patriarchal feminine image of being 'pleasing', 'submissive', 'gentle' and 'nice'. If a woman has so much control of her own behaviour that the Dark Goddess is unable to arise when it is time for her appearance to be made, if she remains deeply suppressed, then a woman can experience her energies in the form of a life-threatening disease, depression, hopelessness or despair. Or she may find herself living in a wasteland and feel her life to be meaningless and without direction. It is only by finding ways to reconnect with her energy within that the powers of transformation are set free to work their magic and lead each of us on our own individual path towards freedom. As Demetra George says in *Mysteries of the Dark Moon*: 'Whether we see the Dark Goddess as dancing ecstatically in a swirl of red flames, or enveloped in mist gazing into the inner pools of her psychic awareness, or throbbing with her orgasmic, magical creative energy, or embracing us in our grief, or furiously raging, screaming, crying, or desperately withdrawing into a stupor of denial or numbness, her ultimate purpose in each one of these guises is the same. She destroys in order to renew. The Dark Goddess of the dark moon is the mistress of transformation, and she exists everywhere there is change.'

At the time of her appearance at menopause the Dark Goddess demands that each one of us clears out of our lives whatever is no longer essential to our inner being, whether this be possessions, relationships or jobs – anything that does not help us grow and fulfil our deepest needs. If we ignore her demands, like the wild and unruly creature she can be when thwarted, she ruthlessly tears apart whatever in our own lives is restricting the full expression of our souls. Her rise can threaten everything which in ordinary life we try desperately to hold on to – our self-confidence, our self-image, our sense of accomplishment, our material possessions. All of the things which for many years may have supported us now come under the scrutiny of her gaze and the ruthlessness of her sword.

What can be hard to realize, while all this is happening, is that everything she does is done with love. We see such things as the breakdown of a marriage, the loss of a job, the physical illness that can come at times of enormous change as evil and negative. We spend most of our lives trying to avoid a crisis at all cost. Yet crises are often the only means by which we can be thrust forward to a new life. Were the energies of the Dark Goddess not to rise we would remain stagnant. We might continue living out an artificial existence while all the time trying to fill up the emptiness within with whatever we can lay our hands on, from drugs and sex to success and power in the world – yet never succeed. It is the Dark Goddess that gives us the motivation to change and brings us the power to be able to carry it out.

Migration of Power

She also pulls us away from the external world, asking us to withdraw to a place of stillness in which we can begin to hear the echoes of our own souls – sounds which for years may have been ignored or forgotten. She stirs our being at the deepest level. She asks us to enter our own personal darkness, calling us to make a vision quest, presenting us with pain over any issues in our lives that we have been denying. She asks us to face our fears and taboos, whether they be addictions, dependencies or inadequacies, so that we can bring them into the open where they can be looked at and healed. Like the crone who is her messenger, the Dark Goddess has no adornments. She is naked and raw in her confrontations. She arrives to lead us into the labyrinthine recesses of our own being and, if we consent, she offers us the courage and the strength to face our own personal demons. Either we acknowledge her call, retreat from the outer world and begin to make our descent voluntarily, or she grabs us by the throat and drags us under. And, just in case we might be tempted to think when menopause arrives that sexuality is dead, she makes us think again. It has not died but rather been transformed.

The sexuality of the postmenopausal woman is the sexuality of the crone. It is the sexuality of sheer instinct – wildness set free. It is she that calls a woman into the secret places of the woods and provokes her to dance naked in wild abandon. Hers is a sexuality to be used in any way a woman chooses – in union with another or alone to generate the alchemical meeting of male and female within her own body. The sexuality of the crone belongs to herself alone. She will be what she is, she will have what she wants. She is neither passive, nor submissive, and her sexuality has nothing whatever to do with bringing physical children into being. The crone's eroticism is sheer ecstasy, lived for its own sake, and sheer creativity. She creates in an uninhibited, animated, fiery way which emanates from the soul of a woman. Such sexuality is the fuel for all creative powers in the world. It carries with it the energy of regeneration and of healing, not only for a woman herself but for the world. It is the kundalini power – the rejuvenating cosmic illumination, the power of the serpent, the sacred fire which heals. As the crone gains entrance into the body and psyche of the menopausal woman she illuminates one dark corner of her psyche after another, lifting away all that is old and dead and without meaning, the way kundalini energy rises up within a woman's body to illuminate each of the chakras. Her power becomes the power of the menopausal woman. It lies in her dark blood – the blood of creation which now for ever more will be retained within a woman's body.

Today is Almost Over

Before menopause, before the Dark Goddess makes her appearance in our lives, our energies are occupied with the challenge of adjusting to the world and caring for others. At menopause these energies become set free to shine forth with their own brand of pure beauty. A woman becomes aware of herself at menopause – as a living being separate from the collective life of work, of the family and the community. Until menopause most women in the so-called civilized world have lived under the guidance of the ego. We have sought to gain power over our external world and over nature in order to fulfil our personal needs. And to a greater or lesser extent we have succeeded. What happens at menopause is that suddenly the way we have been living and the skills we have learned – getting on with people, getting ahead in the world – no longer work, or if they do work and we continue to get what we think we want we often find that it no longer nourishes us.

Then all of a sudden as the moon reaches its fullest peak, like the woman who is coming to the zenith of her power, a shadow appears. The ancient Chinese insist that when the moon is almost full and at its brightest, this is the moment at which the powers of darkness are strongest within, readying themselves to break forth. So it is with a menopausal woman. Suddenly, the strength, the power, the sense of control, seem doomed to slip away from you. The ordinary world in which you have lived and been comfortable with no longer works. The world of safety begins to dissolve. As it dissolves this rising of the shadow reflects in a stark way any weaknesses, deficiencies, or parts of us that still remain ungrown or unlived.

I was the daughter of a jazz musician. As a child I didn't go to school. I grew up on the road with my father, travelling hundreds of miles a day from one job to the next. Many of the places where his band played were amusement parks. Amusement parks are wonderful places, full of all sorts of bright lights, games to play, things to do and prizes to be won. However, I remember noticing, at the age of six or seven, that amusement parks in the stark light of dawn revealed every hidden scrap of paper, every surface whose paint had worn. A funfair the morning after is quite a different place to the one it was only hours before. Often a woman's experience of menopause is like this. An amusement park in the stark light of dawn can be terrifying to someone who wants to go on, entranced by the illusory games it offered a few hours before. But to others who have grown tired of the games, it offers new textures and colours – a far richer and starker experience of reality and aliveness than any number of neon lights and whirling wheels could ever hope to mimic. 'The party's over' the song says, 'the candle flickers and dims . . . now you must wake up.' This is the challenge of the menopausal woman. In this challenge lies a choice – try to run back into the world of

Chapter Sixteen

Call to Adventure

The joy of menopause is the world's best-kept secret. Like venturing through the gateway to enter an ancient temple, in order to claim that joy a woman must be willing to pass beyond the monsters who guard its gate. As you stand at the brink of it, it can appear that only darkness, danger and decay lie beyond. And in a way this is true – although most certainly not in the way most women believe. For having passed through the doorway of menopause into the realms beyond, I have come to believe, as thousands of women from all cultures throughout history have whispered to each other, that it is the most exciting passage a woman ever makes.

Of course nobody told me this beforehand. It was a secret I had to discover for myself. Like most modern women my head had been filled with the horrors of hot flushes, fainting spells and dry vaginas; with memories of my mother's tears shed over a wrinkle that appeared one day to mar her perfect face; with the prospect of enforced celibacy – after all, no man can feel lust for an old woman, or can he? It was partly by accident, I think, and partly because – despite good health and secure family circumstances – my own journey through menopause was not an easy one, that I discovered the secret which throughout history women living in patriarchal cultures have guarded close to their hearts. The doorway of menopause which each of us is invited to pass through is a call to adventure. It connects the ordinary world in which we have been living to a numinous zone of magnified power. Within that zone are hidden treasures to match our wildest dreams. But, like every prize worth having, these riches can only be claimed and brought back if a woman is bold enough and persistent enough to answer the call. What is calling? Nothing less than her own soul.

Hero's Journey

This call to adventure which a woman hears at menopause can arrive in as many different forms as there are women to hear it. But, whatever shape it takes, its purpose is the same. It is asking her – imploring her – to leave behind the comfortable world of her ordinary existence and for a time to venture into a challenging unfamiliar place. It is asking her to set out on her own hero's journey – a journey which is completely unique to her. Sometimes this entails making an outer journey to a real place, moving to a new job, or leaving behind a marriage which has outlived its usefulness. For many the journey only takes place in the mind, the heart and the spirit. Either way it is primarily an inner journey which takes a woman out of her ordinary world with all its ordinary assumptions to transform the way she thinks and lives – from weakness to strength, from grief to purpose, from despair to hope – and then brings her home again.

The word *hero* comes from a Greek root which means 'to protect and to serve'. Like 'poet' or 'teacher' it is a word which refers equally to a woman or man. A hero is someone willing to move through and beyond narrow thinking and familiar landscapes in order to discover the larger world of meaning – someone willing to sacrifice or to transmute her own fears and hesitation, anger and sorrows into creative power. From a psychological point of view the hero archetype corresponds to what Freud called the ego – that part of a woman which, in separating from the infantile bond to the mother, establishes her ability to function as a unique member of the human race. The hero archetype also represents the ego's search for its true identity – the self – and for wholeness. The task a woman faces at menopause is to call forth the hero within and, by journeying with her, to identify and resurrect whatever parts of her own being and whatever creative potential is still waiting to be lived out. It could be said that the hero's journey as a whole is the process by which the ego (the hero), believing herself separate from the other parts of herself, comes to incorporate them in order to become the self. Well travelled, such a journey enables a woman to turn her potential into power and her dreams into reality. And on every woman's hero's quest it is the Dark Goddess who is her handmaiden, her sister, her guide, her destroyer and her midwife.

Language of Myth

The transformation involved in a woman's passage to power is profoundly mysterious. It is an experience which, although a few things can be said of it in terms of psychology, ultimately defies analysis. One cannot speak of it in the same language we use to discuss the biochemistry of hormonal changes or the relationship between essential fatty acids and brain chemicals. This is because the linear, denotative language of science fragments and separates and therefore only helps us to scrutinize the surface of reality. It won't enable us to take even the first step past the guardians of the threshold when menopause arrives, let alone empower our journey. To speak of the nature of the hero's journey at menopause we must leave behind the words and concepts of science and find a new language – or perhaps resurrect a very old one. For this we need stories, tales, rituals and dreams. We need to call on the language of myth for only myths reveal the eternal patterns of our souls.

Thomas Mann speaks of what it is like to look at the world through mythic eyes, about the way that a human being becomes conscious 'proudly and darkly yet joyously of its recurrence and typicality'. 'Myth', Mann says, 'is the legitimisation of life. Only through and in it does life find self awareness, sanction and consecreation.' Joseph Campbell puts it another way: 'Myth is the secret opening through which the inexhaustible energies of the cosmos pour.' 'The wonder is,' he says, 'that the characteristic efficacy to touch and inspire deep creative centres dwells in the smallest nursery fairy tale – as the flavour of the ocean is contained in a droplet or the whole mystery of life within the egg of a flea. For the symbols of mythology are not manufactured; they cannot be ordered, invented, or permanently suppressed. Myths are spontaneous productions of the psyche, and each bears within it undamaged the germ power of its source.' Myths live forever in our fantasies, dreams and relationships.

Mythological archetypes, symbols and rituals are the stuff on which we need to draw and to which we can relate when exploring the meaning implicit in the changes which each woman is impelled to make when menopause arrives. By coming in contact with appropriate myths – myths which address the challenges we are facing and help us to experience the flavour of the worlds we are preparing to enter – the seeds of new awakenings can be sown. 'If a story is seed, then we are its soil. Just hearing the story allows us to experience it as though we ourselves were the heroine who either falters or wins out in the end. If we hear a story about a wolf, then afterward we rove about and know like a wolf for a time. If we hear a story about a dove finding her young at last, then for a time after something moves behind our own feathered breasts,' says Jungian analyst Clarissa Pinkola Estés in *Women Who Run With the Wolves*. 'If it be a story of wresting the sacred pearl from beneath the clay of the ninth dragon, we feel exhausted afterward and satisfied. In a very real way, we are imprinted with knowing just by listening to the tale.'

THE FROG PRINCE

Once upon a time there was a king who had three fine daughters. The youngest of these was so beautiful that when the sun shone upon her it smiled. She liked to play with her favourite toy, a little golden ball the queen had given her. Now gold is the incorruptible metal and she loved her golden ball more than anything in the world. A golden sphere. The perfect circle of her soul.

Every day she would steal away from the castle, take her little ball and wander down a path through the woods to the edge of an old well – the entrance to the underworld. There she loved to sit beneath a feathery willow tossing the golden ball into the air and catching it as it fell. Tossing and catching. Tossing and catching. One day while playing her little game and tossing her soul around, a shimmery dragonfly buzzed by. For just an instant she took her eye off the ball. But that was all it took. Whoosh. The golden sphere flew straight past the lovely hand held out to catch it. Splash, it hit the water. Down, down it went until the dark water swallowed up her beloved soul completely and carried it who knows how far beneath the earth. Gold is a heavy metal.

Heartbroken, the princess weeps. She wails. She cries. She stamps her feet. Alas, nothing will bring back her beautiful golden ball. Her soul has sunk to the bottom of the well. Of course everybody knows that when something gets swallowed up in the underworld one of its inhabitants is sent to the surface. Sometimes it is a dragon, sometimes a wolf, sometimes a monster or a bear. This time it is a little frog which comes plopping up out of the water. 'What's wrong, princess?' he asks. 'Why are you crying?' 'I've lost my golden ball, funny frog,' she says. He replies, 'I'll go and get it for you.' The princess is delighted. 'But what will you give me in return?' demands the frog.

Of course, why did she not think of that before: every kindness must be paid for. 'I'll give you anything you want,' she says, 'my clothes, my jewels, even the golden bracelet I wear.' 'I don't care for your clothes, your jewels and your golden bracelet,' the frog says. 'Well then what *do* you want?' she snaps. 'I want to be your playmate,' he replies. 'I want to sit at your table and eat from your golden plate. I want to hop on to your bed and sleep at the side of your pillow. Promise I can do this and I'll swim right down and fetch your ball.' The girl doesn't even stop to think about the deal. After all, she supposes he is only a useless frog and there is no way a frog can be the friend of a princess. So she says, 'All right, you can do that.' True to his word the frog dives.

* * *

Now he has become the hero on an adventure. And so the story goes . . .

Every hero's journey begins as we meet the hero in her ordinary world. The ordinary world is the place where you know who you are, are familiar with how you have been living, and with the various roles you have been playing – mother, friend, worker, lover. Yet we know before a dozen words are spoken that this ordinary world is going to change, just as a woman in her late thirties and forties begins to sense something pretty fundamental is about to shift. The hero never knows what it is, but we who are listening to the story know that her ordinary world is bound to be a vivid contrast to the strange new world she is about to enter. In *The Wizard of Oz* we are introduced to Dorothy's boring day-to-day existence in Kansas. In *Romancing the Stone* we meet Joan Wilder at her desk in her drab little flat finishing off yet another romantic novel with not the least hint of romance in her own life. For the princess, living her ordinary life means sitting beside a well playing with her toy. Then something happens to disrupt a woman's life. It can be an illness, a death, the loss of a job, a love affair or unendable ennui. Maybe the Fisher King has been wounded and the land is dying, as in the Grail Legends, maybe some wrong has been perpetrated that needs to be put right. Maybe, as happens to the princess, the hero's attention is stolen momentarily and her beautiful golden soul is lost.

Maps of Unknown Territories

A prime function of mythology is to supply the symbols that can transport a woman onwards. Whether they echo through the tale of Persephone and Demeter, the story of the Loathly Lady from the Grail Legends, or films like *An Officer and a Gentleman*, all myths are like maps which guide you off their edges into unknown territory. Each story, like each woman's life and journey, is unique yet the archetypes which underlie it are universal. They cannot be ordered or invented. Neither can they be repressed forever. When the time is ripe they spring forth spontaneously from the human psyche, each bringing with them intact transformative power. At that moment a story such as Beauty and the Beast, or the tale of Greek earth goddess Demeter and her daughter Persephone, becomes soul food to nourish, inspire and focus a woman's energies in a way that reconnects her with meaning. Myths and rituals help us define our rites of passage. In primitive societies they are the ceremonials connected with birth, the naming of a child, puberty, marriage, menopause and death. Each transition in the tribe was associated with specific rites and myths which went with them and would function as a formal exercise for severance. By letting a myth echo through one's being it becomes easier for the mind to be radically pulled away from whatever attachments, attitudes and patterns of living at any particular stage need to be left behind.

The Dark is Rising

One of the curious things about mythic stories and rituals is that, if they are not supplied from the outside in the form of stories that carry power for transformation or rituals which help us gather these transformative powers and direct them, then they will come from within in the form of dreams or images. At the brink of a significant shift in my own life I dreamed I was on a desert island. There were priestesses dressed in white robes carrying a bier on which lay a mummy wrapped in white gauze. They moved slowly under the sun. Dazzled by the light upon the sea, I watched them carry their burden across the sands towards me. It was as though I was mesmerized. As they drew near, one of them raised her hand. They stopped. They set down the dead body on its bier right before me and began to unwrap it. One of the priestesses glanced up at me. Her eyes were dark and piercing. Suddenly I knew with absolute horror that they were unwrapping the cadaver because I was supposed to eat the dead body – something so absolutely repugnant to me that I would do almost anything to avoid it. I awakened trembling and swimming in sweat.

The dream which so frightened me was a unique product of my own mind yet within it lay the archetype of transmutation – the same experience you find within the holy eucharist or communion rituals of the Catholic Church during which wine and bread are transmuted into the blood and body of Christ. The deeper layers of my being were sending me messages through the language of dream that something in my life which had died and been embalmed now needed transmuting. The idea of eating a dead body was anathema to me. Yet through my dream my soul was calling out to me, telling me not to run away but to face the task before me and learn to look at things with new eyes. Once I got over the first shock I realized it was teaching me that in 'eating' a dead body, that is in consciously welcoming into my awareness what was moribund in my life and devouring it (instead of trying to avoid it as I had been doing), the old and dead could be transmuted into new life just as the dead parings from vegetables become compost to nourish spring flowers.

Whether they appear in dreams or stories, such myths and rituals that are available to us contain the symbols we need to carry our own lives forward. Without them it is far too easy for a woman to become crystallized, transfixed in the habits of her past which tie her down and hold her back. At puberty we need to break away from the absolute dependence we have known as children. If we do not do so we find ourselves trapped in neurotic patterns which make it impossible for us to enjoy our lives and find meaning in them. Motherhood, too, has its myths. Like the youngest child in the fairy tale, we must set out to find our fortune. So does menopause. Mythic symbols – the snake who forever sheds its skin and is born again, the Beast who becomes transformed through the love of Beauty, the Medusa's head which when looked upon turns men to stone – do not refer to something that is in any logical sense knowable or known. They speak of spiritual powers which move through our lives and can only be known by the effects they bring about. The function of the archetypal journey of the hero – so important in a woman's life at menopause – lies in its ability to help a woman blinded by the emptiness of material existence become transformed into someone who knows that in choosing to live for cultural and spiritual ends she becomes connected at the deepest level with her own values and nourished by her own soul.

THE TALE CONTINUES

In a jiffy the frog is back with the ball in his mouth. The princess, without so much as a by your leave takes it from him and skips back up the path home. The frog, in his floppy-frog way, follows behind her crying, 'Hold on. Wait for me.' Plop, plop, plop. But of course, being a frog, he is very slow. The princess and her family are at supper when at last he arrives at the castle. Plop, plop, plop, the king hears something coming up the steps. The princess squirms in her chair. 'What is that?' her father asks her. 'Oh, nothing,' she replies, 'just some silly frog I met.' 'Did you make him any promises?' the king wants to know. (All at once morality enters on the scene.) 'Yes,' the princess replies. 'Then he better be let in,' her father answers.

The small spotted creature comes galumphing through the door then leaps up on the table, plopping his funny feet on the edge of the princess's lovely golden plate and completely spoiling her dinner. Finally, she gets up after eating nothing and goes off upstairs to bed. But guess who is following her – plop, plop up the stairs – right up to the heavy door to her bedroom which is shut tight. So the frog hurls his little green body against the door crying, 'Hey, princess, I want to come in.' She opens the door. 'I want to sleep in your bed with you,' he says. By now the princess has had enough of this disgusting intruder even if he did rescue her beautiful golden soul for her. So she picks him up and dashes him against the stone wall with all her might. The frog's body splits open. Out of it steps a handsome prince with eyes as blue as the summer sky. It seemed that he had been cursed by a hag who had turned him into a frog.

(Like the princess he, too, had been stuck at the brink of adulthood unwilling or unable to move onward. One of the reasons I so love this tale is that in it each of them in a funny way is able to rescue the other.)

The next day, after the princess and the frog prince are married, a mysterious coach arrives at the castle gate to fetch them and take them back to the prince's land. They get in it and set off when suddenly there is a loud ping. The frog prince shouts to the coachman, 'What is that? What has happened?' 'It is just the sound of an iron band breaking,' he replies. 'It has been around my heart ever since you have been gone.' The coachman, like the land the prince left behind when, cursed by the hag, he was forced to descend into the underworld and become a frog, has been suffering. His heart has been bound up while the land itself, deprived of the generating and governing power of the prince, has lain barren. Now that he is on his way home the band is broken and the land is beginning to be fertile again. And the prince brings an even greater boon gathered on his descent – a wife as a gift to the world which has been longing for his return.

* * *

A myth is a special tale that can be told ten thousand times in a thousand ways without losing its power. It is a tale which will be received differently by everyone who hears it yet will carry the same archetypal hook for all of us. In every myth, in every tale of power, each character represents a different part of the psyche. The maiden is the unawakened, innocent, sleepy female beneath which is to be found a warrior's heart and the ability to bear the pain of loneliness, difficulty, hurt and betrayal in order to triumph. The king is the moral principle. He has a full knowledge of the underworld into which the hero falls or is dragged, as well as skills that can advise her and spur her onwards in her journey. The frog represents the nursery version of the great serpent which inhabits the underworld. He is consort to the Dark Goddess who carries the life-generating powers of death and resurrection up from the abyss. He also represents all that has been rejected by the proud princess in her callow youth – all that is unadmitted, unknown and undeveloped in the depths of a woman's consciousness, the treasures hidden in submarine palaces, the glittering diamonds waiting for the hero if only he or she will descend and claim them. The prince is the formative power of the hero destined through perseverance and single-mindedness to reclaim his power and regenerate his land.

Listening to the Whispers

Until recently, when the power of stories and rituals has begun to be recognized (thanks to the work of people such as Joseph Campbell, storyteller Clarissa Pinkola Estés and astrologer Demetra George), the myths needed to help guide us had been all but forgotten. Sadly they still play no part in our linear left-brain education. Yet they are essential to our growth. Myths help us to see who we are and what we can become. They connect us to the archetypal or universal dimension of human experience. In doing so they help free us from our own sense of personal limitation and from habit patterns that imprison us. For somewhere in the depths of our humanness the echoes of mythic archetypes which can empower us still sound. Hearing such stories help us learn to stop and listen. Without the right myths women at menopause can easily become trapped in an obsession to restore youth and to continue our blood cycles, even if only artificially by taking artificial hormones. Then, instead of taking up the call to adventure and facing our fear, like a prince and princess at the brink of adulthood, we refuse to move forward.

Thousands of women today are being denied the experience of a natural menopause. They have been seduced into believing that what is happening to their body and psyche is a disease, something terrifying which can only be handled by medical intervention. They have become disempowered by elements that would steal a woman's power for their own commercial ends and they have become frightened by information in the media, advertisements, and by doctors, whose only knowledge about menopause comes from 'facts' disseminated by the manufacturers of hormones designed to 'treat' it. So much fear surrounds the menopause – fear of losing one's attractiveness, of getting old, of no longer having the right to be called female. Like the Gorgon's head or the Medusa, menopause looms large in our society as something that must not be looked upon directly lest we are turned to stone. For when we lose touch with the myths of menopause's hero's journey, we lose touch with its meaning.

This journey both echoes and is an echo of the hormonal, physiological and biochemical changes taking place in a woman's body. So it is imperative that we become aware of how to balance our hormones and nurture our bodies. Then the years beyond menopause can be lived in optimal health and we are able more easily to manifest in the world the treasures we return with.

I have come to believe that the hero's journey we are called upon to make at menopause is the most important journey a woman ever takes: first because, given her age and maturity, it is taken with the greatest awareness and, secondly, because at the end of the childbearing years in a biological way a woman has become free of the need to channel her creative energies into propagating the species. Now, at last, she is free to use her creativity in any way her soul dictates. The power of creation has always been centred in the feminine. That is why poets turn towards the muse for inspiration. Yet few women in the last few thousand years have succeeded in making full use of those creative energies except in a biological way. We have been far too busy giving birth, raising children and nurturing the creativity of others to be able to explore our own at very deep levels. The hero's journey at menopause offers the possibility of changing these patterns in our lives once and for all – first by reconnecting with the creative fire within each of us and, secondly, by honouring our right to use it to accomplish whatever we want.

Chapter Seventeen

Hero's Journey

The hero's journey each woman takes is unique. Yet every hero's journey told throughout history follows the same archetypal patterns. The story begins in the ordinary world. We meet the Princess doing what she always does – sitting in her favourite place playing with her golden ball. Then comes the call to adventure. Something happens to turn the ordinary world on its head. The hero is faced with a problem, a challenge or a difficulty to overcome. Sometimes the call can come by what would appear to the linear male world to be sheer chance – a blunder – the way the Princess's golden ball falls into the well. Except, of course, there are no chances in the cyclical realm of the female where the interconnectedness of all things is recognized. There are many ways in which the adventure can begin.

Frequently the call comes in the form of a challenge. It can be physical. Suddenly you wake in the middle of the night with hot sweats. It can also be psychological. You find one morning that your life no longer means anything to you. You wonder where you have got to and where you are going. Something is definitely not right. In whatever form it comes the call heralds the beginning of adventure. From now on things are never going to be the same again. It puts us on notice that destiny has summoned us and our spiritual centre of gravity has suddenly shifted out of the familiar world of society towards realms unknown.

Refusing the Call

Invariably, following closely in the call's wake, fear raises its familiar head. We want to run back into the past and hide. We want to pretend that we didn't hear the summons in the first place. The princess wants her ball and the frog fetches it but she is not willing to honour the bargain she has made with him for she finds him repulsive and only wants to get away. The hero now becomes a reluctant hero. The greatest fear that any of us ever have is fear of the unknown. And what lies ahead is completely unknown. So we try to pretend that everything is all right, we try to hold things together, we go and have a facelift, or go on another of those slimming diets. Or maybe we work even harder and start to lean heavily on our emotional crutches and addictions. At the beginning of any hero's journey the world sings sweet seductive songs and sends up countless distractions to bewitch us so we go no further. In detective novels the private eye tries to refuse the case being offered him only later to accept it although he would rather not. Somehow he gets a little push over the edge and the tale begins to unfold. The frog follows the princess, refusing to take no for an answer. In *Star Wars* Luke Skywalker turns away from Obi Wan Kenobi's call to adventure to run home to his aunt and uncle only to find that the farm has been destroyed by the Emperor's storm troopers. His hesitation is overcome by the evil that has been perpetrated on his ordinary world. Now he begins his personal quest.

Gritting our teeth and battening down the hatches is one way of refusing the call. So is being a servant to social niceties. Women who have forced themselves to live by such rules never have the rich relationships they long for because they cannot share their soul. This in turn creates a wasteland and loneliness – the loneliness of a soul which has been banished to the dungeon lest it challenge the rules. When the call comes, a woman is being asked to enter into the loneliness she feels and to walk forth into her wasteland with eyes wide open. If the loneliness we experience cannot be brought into the ordinary world and shared with others then probably we are spending time with the wrong people. We also may need to do something on our own.

At this point in the journey a mentor usually arrives to help us out. The mentor is often a Merlin-type character, a book, or an older woman who knows more than we do and who can help us find out what we don't yet know. The mentor's purpose is to help make the hero ready to face the unknown. He or she represents the tie between mother and child, goddess and woman, healer and the healed. The helpful crone and the fairy godmother are common mentor figures in European folklore. They provide the hero with the talisman she will need against the unknown forces she will have to meet. Glenda, the good witch in *The Wizard of Oz*, gives Dorothy her wisdom and a pair of ruby slippers for her journey. Then she sends her on her way. The adventure has begun in earnest and the presence of a mentor helps to push the hero forward.

Guardians of the Threshold

Now, armed with the powers of destiny bestowed upon her by her mentor, our hero approaches her first passage. Here she meets the guardians of the threshold whose purpose is to prevent the faint-hearted from entering the magical realms that lie beyond. Before she leaves New York, in *Romancing The Stone*, Joan Wilder has to face her publisher who scathingly warns her not to go to Colombia to rescue her sister because she is not strong enough to handle the challenge. Like a nasty old witch she even pronounces a curse that something disastrous will certainly happen. As women approach menopause their lives are suddenly full of guardians of the threshold. Often these are well-meaning people who prey upon our worst fears – fears of inadequacy, of failure, of hopelessness, of illness and of death. Whatever they are they need to be faced before we can go on. Face them head on and you pass through the gate. Now, at last, you are committed to finding out who you are and what your life is about. Crossing the threshold is the first step we take into the sacred realm of the Dark Goddess's world – gateway to the universal source. As Joseph Campbell says in *The Hero With a Thousand Faces*: 'The adventure is always and everywhere a passage beyond the veil of the known into the unknown; the powers that watch at the boundary are dangerous; to deal with them is risky; yet for anyone with competence and courage the danger fades.'

Tests, Allies and Enemies

Now comes the exciting stuff. Now it is time for the hero to deal with the tests, allies and enemies she will meet along the road. Obstacles to change are always in our way – insufficient money, physical problems, fears that we have no possibility of ever fulfilling our dreams. New challenges arrive, new things need to be learned. Yet each obstacle overcome, each puzzle solved, each difficulty embraced brings us more power for what lies ahead. And we meet new people, new ideas or make new relationships with nature, with animals and with the unseen world. In *Star Wars*, Obi Wan develops Luke's skill in using The Force by insisting that he fight blindfold. Before long Luke faces minor battles which serve to hone his abilities further and help to prepare him for the supreme ordeal that is to come. Joan Wilder – the timid little lady from New York – is forced to face gunfire, sinister men in black gloves, the loss of her belongings and threats to her life. Along the way she picks up an ally – Jack – who will be her companion for most of the remainder of her journey. Dorothy picks up her friends, the lion, the tinman and the scarecrow, while passing her tests. She oils the tinman's joints. She coaxes the lion to face his fear. She unhooks the scarecrow who has been unable to move. With each challenge she meets, the hero develops her strength and collects more support from companions both in the seen and the unseen world. They will turn out to be very useful to her purpose as she approaches the innermost cave.

The Innermost Cave

Now she approaches the entrance to the most dangerous place of all. Here the goal of her journey awaits her. It is the innermost cave. In Arthurian stories this is the Chapel Perilous – the dangerous room wherein the Grail is hidden. For every woman her innermost cave is the inner sanctum of the Dark Goddess. The hero entering the cave comes prepared. If he is a man he knows that this is where the dragon will eventually need to be fought if he is to win the treasure. The same can be true for a woman too. But more often than not, instead of having to slay a dragon, a woman will need to remain in solitude in this inner Goddess realm, enduring what seems unendurable silence. She will listen and need to learn before she can find her treasure. In stories of male heroes the central image for what is sought is often a gem or a radiant jewel. For a woman it is frequently the image of a child – the offspring of her spiritual birth.

It is now on the hero's journey that a woman makes her descent into the underworld. The journey a woman makes at menopause is usually fraught with confusion and grief, and filled with loneliness and anger. In this place of bone-chilling darkness within the earth she may feel turned inside out, naked and exposed. All the things she thought she knew don't seem to apply here. Far away the comfort and companionship of the outside world – which by now she may only vaguely remember anyway – have gone. Silence pervades. Endless tears without name can be shed. There is no place of comfort, nowhere to turn. When a woman enters her inner-most cave she may not even have the strength to get dressed, let alone cook or clean or buy food. To her friends and family she often seems like a creature lost. She may go to bed and stay there. She may forget things, she may dig in her garden or wander in the woods. All these things are wise work. For the route that will eventually lead her out of the underworld and return her in a transformed state to the land above is not the same as that of a man. He may need to move up *away* from himself out into the light. But to find her treasure a woman is asked to lay aside any fascination she has with culture or games of the mind and turn within – to come instead to know her body, her sexuality, her dreams, her images and her desires. She moves down even further into her depths to reclaim the parts of her that have been lost. It is here that she will face her supreme ordeal, confront her greatest fears and undergo the psychological life-or-death moment which is the central crisis of her hero's journey. She tastes death and faces the shadow of herself. When at last it is all over the Dark Goddess awaits to bless her and bestow upon her the greatest treasure of all – her soul.

The Road Home

Yet this is not the end of the hero's tale. Once she has made her descent, and won her treasure in a life-or-death struggle, she has the task of bringing it back. It is a job easier said than done. Dorothy escapes from the castle of the wicked witch, Luke rescues Princess Leia and gets the plans of the Death Star, the princess throws her frog against the wall and he turns into the beautiful prince. But the game is far from over. Having survived the ordeal, withstood the pressure, slain the monster and taken possession of the treasure a hero now has to make her way home. The underworld is not a place that anyone must remain for too long. For when Persephone is raped by Pluto and dragged kicking and screaming into the underworld, where she remains for a seemingly endless period, the crops on the earth above fail, the flowers wither and the land becomes barren and desolate. Only when she returns will her mother Demeter allow the crops to grow again and the birds to sing.

Further difficulties invariably appear. Dorothy finds that the hot-air balloon which the Wizard has provided to take her back to Kansas is not the sure form of transport she had hoped it was to be, Toto runs off after a cat. In trying to bring him back the balloon takes off without her and we fear she may be trapped forever in the underworld. Luke Skywalker and Princess Leia are pursued by Darth Vader as they make their escape from the Death Star. Joan Wilder, having defeated the evil men who wanted to kill her and steal the stone, returns to New York where she faces the arduous task of turning what has happened into her next romantic novel. It is not easy for any hero to pass back and forth between ordinary and non-ordinary reality. Much energy has been spent during the supreme ordeal and the hero may not have finished off the enemy completely. There still may be shadows lurking – old ideas, old ways of doing things. But the game has changed now. There, in the inner sanctum, some kind of alchemical process has taken place in us. We are no longer the women that we were. So we need to learn new ways of living and new methods of returning to the surface since most of the rules we lived by before no longer apply. Sometimes on the road home the hero can experience a sudden reversal of fortune just when it seemed that the worst was over. Here, too, the hero has the chance of testing out her new-found powers in overcoming it.

Resurrection and Elixirs

In primitive societies whenever a woman had entered the Moon Lodge for a few days or whenever a man had returned from a hunt, he or she was required to be washed and purified before they could re-enter the community. For they had visited the underworld of non-ordinary reality; they had walked in the land of the dead. The blood that had stained their hands and the mud that remained on their bodies needed to be washed away. The woman's soul that has taken birth is ready to emerge from the womb reborn a new creature. But first it must be blessed with water. So on her return from the underworld of menopause a woman will often feel the need to regenerate herself using a diet that can spring-clean her body. She may also want to listen to music for hours on end or to awaken at dawn and take long walks or to carry out some ritual or meditation that can help her energies and refocus her life as she returns to the ordinary world.

At last the hero arrives back with her elixir: the treasure, or wisdom, or the knowledge that the non-ordinary world exists and that trials can be faced and overcome. She has made her connection with her soul. Dorothy gets back to Kansas having learned that she is loved and finds that after all is said and done, 'there's no place like home'. Luke Skywalker destroys the Death Star so peace and order can return to the galaxy. Joan Wilder writes her book, keeps the faith and gets her Jack complete with alligator boots and a boat in which she can sail around the world. The hero's journey has come full circle. She has returned to the place where she started. Yet somehow it is not the *same* place for her. For, having carried her elixir intact from the special realm of numinous power all the way home, she is reborn. The world has been renewed.

The woman who completes her passage into the underworld and returns finds within the darkness and confusion and loneliness a new joy, a new sense of meaning, a knowledge that the world which once seemed fragmented all fits together. She also discovers her own power and freedom – that she no longer has to live by other people's rules. Indeed, it is likely no longer even to be possible for her. She is no longer 'seducible' by those who would make her feel inadequate so they can sell her another body, another prestigious car, another love affair, just to fill up the emptiness that was once there. She has been released from it all to learn the new art of living as mistress of her own life.

And so the hero's tale ends. Yet one big question remains for every woman who has made her journey. What will she do with the treasure she has brought back? In most of the male myths there are said to be two choices. Either he takes his treasure into his castle and lives happily ever after or, like Percival, having found the Grail he shares it so that the Fisher King's wounding is healed and the land devastated by barrenness becomes fertile again.

It's My Nature

It is my observation that, having completed her journey, the female hero has no such choice. A woman by her very nature is so much more connected with fostering the energies of life and the powers of the earth, and so much more aware of the inner relationship of all things, that sooner or later she has no choice but to share the boon of her wisdom. She has experienced the power of the Dark Goddess, been given back her soul and come face to face with the crone – the most essential and generous, wise and powerful of all the faces of woman. Once the crone has touched your heart something of her generosity seems to be imparted to you. She teaches you without words that you *are* the wisdom that men seek, the bounty that battles are won and lost for – and the power and the joy. Once a woman learns this truth, like the crone who helped her discover it, she must bring her elixir to the world, fostering both her own life and the lives of all other living things. She seems to have no choice. It is her nature to do so – something so deeply entrenched in her genetic material it cannot be denied.

* * *

Once upon a time there was a scorpion who needed to cross the river. She could not swim and the river was wide and deep. Sunning himself on the bank was a beautiful red fox.

That fox, the scorpion thought, could easily carry me across the river on its back. 'Hey Mr Fox,' says the scorpion, 'what about giving me a ride across the river on your back.' 'What?' said the fox. 'Do you think me a fool? You are a scorpion. If I were to carry you on my back you might sting me.' 'Oh, don't be ridiculous,' replied the scorpion. 'I am not going to sting you. If I did that then we both would drown.' The fox thought about this for a few moments, then raising himself to his feet he replied, 'Okay friend scorpion, a swim in the cool water would be pleasant, hop on my back.' And so they started off. Halfway across the river the scorpion stung the fox. Stunned, and in terror for his life, for everybody knows a scorpion's sting means death, the fox cried out, 'You fool. Why on earth did you do that?' 'I don't know,' replied the scorpion, 'I guess it's just my nature.'

* * *

Doing what somebody else wants you to do is living by a slave mentality. It is the perfect way to encourage physical degeneration and to lose one's soul. Doing what you do because the desire to do it springs forth from your soul is living with the crone's generosity. It is living with enthusiasm. Enthusiasm is central to living in power. The word *entheos* means 'god-filled'. When you reach out for whatever fills you with enthusiasm – a sense of the divine – then what you do flows freely from your being without effort. You can not only help transform the world around you, you have set yourself free.

Chapter Eighteen

Soul Loss

When a woman takes up the challenge of her own passage to power and commits herself to her own journey, often the first message from her depths to surface is a sense that there quite simply is no one there. This is the experience of *soul loss*. And it is a common one. Women have throughout history been schooled in self-denial. Take a look at every acceptable female image in patriarchal societies – the mother, the coquette, the devoted employee. You will find that they all have one thing in common: all put the needs of others before their own. Most of us, regardless of how emancipated we think we are, fit into this way of being all too easily. It is almost as though self-sacrifice has been encoded so deeply in our flesh that it becomes automatic. Often the first inkling that a woman has that she has misplaced part of her soul comes when she stops serving others just long enough to ask herself the question: 'But what do *I* want?' Not only is it a difficult question to answer. For many women it seems difficult even to locate an 'I' at all.

Soul loss occurs in each and every one of us to some degree or another. It is the sense that we cannot see who we are, that somehow we have lost a crucial part of ourselves which provides us with creativity, with vitality or with a sense of meaning in our lives. Primitive people have long lists of experiences that can cause soul loss. They consider it a spiritual illness that in turn can produce physical disease. In tribal cultures it is believed that soul loss can occur from all sorts of causes: meeting a particular animal in the woods; entering a house where someone has died but the whole house has not been re-blessed for life. In modern times soul loss occurs in what is called in psychology 'disassociation', which in its minor forms is where one part of a woman feels split off from the rest, and in its major forms includes the true multiple-personality experience.

The word soul is one which most primitive people have no

trouble understanding. Yet it is a word which in our material-istic culture is easily misunderstood or dismissed as a figment of imagination. Look the word up in *The Shorter Oxford English Dictionary*. It will tell you that 'the soul is the principle of life . . . the spiritual part of man in contrast to the purely physical . . . the seat of emotions, feelings or sentiment' and, perhaps most important of all, '. . . the essential part or quality of a material thing'.

There is a belief in classical Jungian psychiatry that soul loss becomes conscious in or around the time of menopause, somewhere between the age of 35 and 50. 'Soul loss can be observed today as a psychological phenomenon in the every-day lives of beings around us,' writes Jungian analyst Marie von Franz in *Projection and Recollection in Jungian Psychology*. 'Loss of soul appears in the form of a sudden onset of apathy and listlessness; the joy has gone out of life, initiative is crip-pled, one feels empty, everything seems pointless.' A woman continues to do her duty, to carry out the obligations of her life from day to day while putting off her own inner desires so successfully that in time she no longer hears the inner voice that says that she would rather dance or dream or build bridges or wander through the woods. When a woman has ignored her soul voice for long enough it can grow very small, so small that it takes a lot of patience and stillness to make out the words that are being whispered.

There are many different experiences of soul loss that can surface as a woman approaches menopause. But whenever soul loss has appeared and in whatever guise, the challenge facing a woman is always the same: she is being called upon to heal the internal split that has occurred between herself and her own feminine nature.

Gilded Cage

A woman marries and is provided by her husband with the home and the material possessions. They have a family. She is allowed to do pretty much whatever she wants to do provided the family is well fed and provided she continues to be a pleasant, decorative addition to the husband's life. From the outside such a woman appears to have everything. She is often a source of envy to other women who face material struggles – rather like a bird in a gilded cage. The years go by, then one day, around the time of menopause, she begins to realize that she has become disconnected from her own sense of meaning, her soulfulness and her passion. She has allowed herself to be swept away and seduced by the promise that someone will love her, or by material possessions, and she has embraced ideas supported by the patriarchal society she grew up in – a society which would have her believe that woman's fulfilment should come from being a good woman and good mother. For some women it mostly does. For others such an imperative only strangles the very life out of them.

My mother was such a woman. An archetypically beautiful Californian blonde she was a *prize* for any man. She also happened to have a passion for life, a belief that anything was possible if only you put your mind to it, and a great deal of talent. But, like a lot of women of her time, and for that matter like many women of our own, she never really questioned the cultural assumptions about women nor the sacrifices they were asked to make in an attempt to live up to them.

My father was a piano player. Like my mother he came from a poor family but had big dreams. They were married when she was twenty years old and he twenty-three. Since he could only eke out the barest of livings in the early days of their marriage – at one point they had only twenty-five cents a day to spend on food and ate baked beans every day for weeks – my mother went to work for a tailor. Before long, thanks to her ingenuity and energy, the tailor's business had quadrupled. He offered her a partnership in the business. She loved what she was doing and wanted to take him up on the offer but my father insisted it would be too much for her. He needed her, he said, and so she put aside her own wishes to support him – both emotionally and in his career. In fact she put all the energy she had into making my father a success, day after day, year after year. She encouraged him when he felt hopeless, looked after him when he fell ill, did his books for him when he began to make a bit of money, as well as doing his publicity. And she stood by his side. Successful he became. Not only was he able, with my mother's support, to start up his own band, within a few years he had become one of the most well-known jazz musicians in America. Yet when anything went wrong or he was scared, he ran to my mother. She wiped the sweat from his brow and bound his wounds. While all of this was going on there was never any time in my mother's life to even consider what she wanted to do. Before long she gave birth to her first child so that now she had *two* people to sacrifice herself for – two people who needed her support and care and encouragement, which by now she knew superbly well how to give. That is to everybody but herself.

Fair Rapunzel

Finally her marriage to my father ended because she desperately wanted a husband who would stay at home and help her raise a family. Having got to the top in his career all he really wanted was to stay there. At the age of 35 she married a man whom she believed would give her the home and stability she had always longed for. He did, but at a price. The price was her soul. Like the golden-haired Rapunzel he locked her up within a magnificent house built, it must be said, with the money she brought to the marriage and indulged her wishes to do yoga, to go to this or that restaurant. Yet he never really took her desires seriously. Nor by now did she – when she could still hear what they were clearly enough to follow them. And before long she had another child, another person to serve and care for.

Every so often my mother would drink a little too much and verbally abuse her husband or her children but that was generally dealt with by all concerned as one of 'Mother's little spells'. Meanwhile, not fully understanding what was happening to this woman who by now had given everything she had to those she loved, I saw my mother show more and more signs of severe stress. It was very much like the stress an imprisoned animal demonstrates by pacing up and down in its cage, tearing at its fur and spending long hours staring emptily into space.

When her call to adventure came at menopause she began

to have fainting spells. Her mouth would fill up with water and then she would black out. Her family dealt with them, as most upper-middle-class American families would, by calling in the doctors who could find nothing physically wrong. They decided it must therefore be 'all in her head'. She also suffered, as she had periodically throughout her life, from bouts of irrational fear. Then an opportunity presented itself for her to work in a shop owned by her best friend from childhood. She took it, working a few days a week, despite her husband's disapproval. He said he would rather she be at home. Before long his 'need' for her wore my mother down and she gave up work. She had also developed a passion for painting and, although she had no confidence in herself, she began to attend a weekly class. She discovered there that others, including her teacher, believed she painted rather well and she loved it. But before long again subtle pressures from the family, coupled with new symptoms she had developed which gave her difficulty in breathing, forced her to cut down on the painting. Again she was sent to the doctor. This time she was told she had emphysema and was put on medication.

It took four and a half years, with one drug prescribed to combat the side-effects of a previous drug, before her strong body and magnificent spirit succumbed to death. Yet even then she seemed to have made a deliberate choice to sacrifice herself so her husband could live. The final eighteen months of her life were for her full of terror and extremely demanding in terms of the care she needed. It took its toll on my stepfather, so much so that he had a heart attack. Soon afterwards my mother was told by the doctor that everyone needed to be careful not to put too much strain on him. Within thirty-six hours she was dead. So far had my mother become separated from her own feminine nature that the call of her soul could only be heard in the form of physical illness. And by then it had been too late to heed it.

The Madness of Woman

Her story is not so extreme or so unusual. Fine novels have been written about such women, such as *The Madness of the*

Seduced Woman by Susan Fromberg Schaeffer. They describe what happens when women of passion have become so separated from their wild nature that the only possible triumph left to them is a triumph of spirit that ends in death or at the very least destroys them. This is an extreme example of soul loss. It is also, in my view, an inexcusable waste of a woman's life as well as something that no amount of ranting and raving against the male world for what it may or may not have done to women is going to change. The only thing that can change it is each one of us coming to an increasing personal inner awareness of how to one degree or another soul loss may be operating in our own lives and then taking steps to correct it.

I was young and did not understand what was going on with my mother at the time but I remember sitting for long hours and listening to her speak in confusion about herself. I was aware that she never really appreciated her own strength, and I know that she was forever giving the power that she had away to others. I also watched her at the age of 50 become increasingly embittered. Without ever realizing it she had made an unspoken 'devil's bargain' with the world. It was this: if only she were good enough, if only she gave enough, if only she cared enough for those around her, then life would reward her. Of course it didn't, it never does. And when she realized it didn't, the agonized fury of the soul which had become separated from her turned against her and eventually destroyed her. I don't think she ever even realized what had happened. All she had was a sense that somehow she must be the one who was at fault and that whatever she had done she had not done it well enough.

Into the Desert

With the experience of soul loss, no matter what its cause, comes a sense of desiccation – a feeling that there is nothing inside you or that whatever is inside you is likely to be of no real value. Living in such a barren landscape it is virtually impossible for a woman to create anything other than frustration and fear. For other women their sense of soul loss comes as a sense that it has gone into hiding, because there is too much pressure from the outside world and there is no place for the soul to live. This is often connected to the idea that a woman is basically on the earth for the purpose of serving others. So deeply ingrained is this notion in the female character that one of the few alternatives a woman has available to protect herself is for her soul to be 'absent without leave'.

Someone Else's Dreams

For women who have rebelled against the idea that a woman's place is in the service of others, the experience of soul loss comes differently. Yet it still brings with it a sense of emptiness, sterility and dismemberment. Every culture has its own set of underlying myths and values within which its society functions. In our western world these myths are almost entirely male-defined. We value accomplishment, success, winning authority, worldly power, glamour and prestige. Daughters of the father, unwilling to become the all-serving females, opt instead to play by the masculine rules of the game and, although they are usually not fully aware of it, do all they can to win masculine approval. Daughters of the father have bought into the stereotyped male values lock, stock and barrel. They tend to spend their lives seeking (and often attaining) power in the world, financial success, or artistic or academic achievements. Sometimes they wake up somewhere between the age of 35 and 50 to find that the dream that they have been dreaming is not their dream but someone else's – i.e. the values of the male culture in which they have been raised. Why do I have this sense of emptiness, betrayal or dislocation, a woman asks? The answer is simple – because in her effort to succeed, to get things done, she has not had time to listen to her *own* instincts or followed her *own* dreams. As a result she has lost touch with the deep relationship to her own wild female nature which is the only thing that can feed her at the deepest levels. And she is hungry.

Any woman experiencing soul loss, whether she lives in a golden cage, has become a successful daughter of the father, or has gone into hiding, finds herself living in a world that has lost its moisture – a desert known too well by any captive creature. However soul loss has occurred, once a woman crosses the threshold to begin her hero's journey, like the princess with the golden ball, she is faced with a reflection of herself which is inevitably fragmented, distorted or simply not there.

Way of the Shaman

The group of people who understand most about soul loss are not the psychologists or the priests but rather the shamans. Shamanism is a tradition of healing which has been practised for tens of thousands of years by tribal communities throughout the world – in Africa, China, Australia, North and South America, Lapland and Europe. The word shaman means 'healer' or 'one who sees in the dark'. It is a Tungus word that originated in Siberia and Mongolia. It describes someone who, through drumming, dance or some other meditational technique, places him or herself in an altered state of consciousness and who then, by leaving the body, travels to a parallel universe that is outside time and space in non-ordinary reality in order to heal, to gain wisdom for the tribe or locate and bring back a lost or stolen part of the human soul. A shaman is a healer who himself or herself has been profoundly wounded. In fact it is through the experience of wounding that a shaman develops the power to journey into the unseen world for the benefit of others. A shaman believes that – as a result of trauma or difficult life circumstances – a part of a person's essential nature will leave the body and move into a non-ordinary reality, usually as a means of protection so that the person is able to survive an otherwise devastating or life-threatening experience. This is soul loss. It is the shaman's job to retrieve that lost essence or soul and bring it back to the person who lost it. It is also the shaman's job to heal both the living and the dead. To accomplish this he or she works with helping spirits in non-ordinary reality. Some of them are what are known as power animals. They are the shaman's constant companions on his or her journeys into the unseen world.

What makes a shaman different from the priest, psychologist, witch doctor or other healers is the fact that he or she makes a journey in the non-ordinary world in order to discover both the cause of a person's illness and also in order to retrieve the parts of someone's soul which need to be brought back into that human being for healing to take place. Such splits can occur as a result of trauma and in their most exaggerated forms appear to be the underlying cause of the multiple-personality phenomenon, where the basic integrity of a person's being is literally split open so that not only does soul loss occur but the person can even be inhabited by spirits from other dimensions. Or it happens because a person is forced to live in circumstances either as a child or an adult which literally create no space for the soul to be in, so fragments of it leave in a bid for survival. American shaman Sandra Ingerman has written a compassionate and wise book called *Soul Retrieval* in which she describes what the shamanic journey looks like as well as the various causes of soul loss and the experience of having one's soul fragments returned. 'One can return only a certain number of soul parts at one time,' she says. 'The reason for this is simple. When the soul returns, it comes back with all the pain it experiences on leaving. The memories surrounding the trauma often take a while to return. I don't want to overwhelm a person with too many memories of physical and/or emotional pain. The way I know how many parts to bring back is by following directions from my power animal, whose judgement I trust implicitly. When he says, "That's enough for now," my search ends,' says Ingerman. 'Integration of the returned soul parts takes some time.'

So widespread is shamanism in primitive cultures, so long has it been practised – thousands upon thousands of years – that it is believed to be the oldest and most widely used system of healing in the world. In our western culture shamanism was for many centuries suppressed by a materialistic culture which sought, despite its rhetoric to the contrary, not to free people so that they could live from the soul but rather to make use of them to maintain the structures of social, political and economic control regardless of the cost to the soul. In recent years, however, shamanism has undergone a considerable revival. It is becoming a useful part of a holistic approach to healing and growth that respects human individuality and nurtures creativity. In the hands of a developed and highly trained shaman, the process of soul retrieval can be a tremendously important part of a woman's journey at menopause. Shamans also concern themselves with retrieving the soul energy lost from forests and mountains, houses and cities as part of a wider intention to bring healing to the planet. For soul loss is a spiritual illness that can result in a physical disease. What impresses me about shamanic journeying for soul retrieval is that it is so simple yet effective. It can often do in a couple of hours what years of psychotherapy has been unable to accomplish, probably because it cuts quickly through concepts and intellectual ideas and goes to the core of a person in a way which is non-threatening and respectful of human life.

Whether you think of soul loss in a metaphoric sense the way many psychologists do – as parts of oneself which are not accessible for use because they are repressed in unconscious material – or whether you prefer to think of soul loss as primitive cultures do in a more literal sense as fragments of the soul (in the case of someone in coma the entire soul actually leaves the body to dwell in other dimensions which are more comfortable for it), this makes little difference. After years of exploring the soul-loss phenomenon, I have come to believe that both points of view are valid – like two sides of the same coin. The important thing is that soul loss occurs regularly.

And how does one retrieve lost fragments of oneself? The first step is by being aware that they are not there. American shaman Sandra Ingerman lists a number of factors in someone's life which are thought to indicate possible soul loss. They include addictions, chronic illness during childhood, gaps in memory, chronic depression, a feeling of numbness or deadness, a difficulty in staying 'present' in your body or a feeling that you are sometimes outside your body, a longing for something to fill up a sense of emptiness in your life, multiple-personality syndrome, a sense of possibly having blocked out traumas, difficulty simply moving on with one's life. All of these experiences can be an indication of soul loss. The menopausal hero's journey is one of the means by which the missing pieces can be found.

Chapter Nineteen
Girl without Hands

The soul of a woman gets wounded in a very different way to that of a man. Where soul wounds in a man interfere with his ability to *feel*, those of a woman most often render her unable to *do*. She can feel, she can dream her dreams, she can have great visions, yet somehow generations of soul imprisonment may render her unable to act on those feelings, unable to trust her instincts and desires. She is like a girl without hands.

There are many wonderful tales of the female hero's journey to inspire and comfort, to encourage and guide a woman who has heard her call. The myth of the ancient Sumerian goddess of heaven and earth, Inanna, is one. Inanna makes her descent to attend the funeral of her dark sister Erishkigal's husband in the underworld and has to remove her every adornment in the process. But Erishkigal, jealous of her sister's beauty, tries to kill her and hangs her from a meat hook to rot. The tale of how Inanna is finally rescued by humble creatures fashioned from the parings from the nails of a lesser god holds many secrets to be learned. So does the story of Demeter whose daughter Persephone is raped and dragged into the underworld by Pluto. Demeter wanders in the wasteland until she finds a means of reclaiming Persephone and restoring fertility to the earth. Of them all, there is one tale which I like the best. I suppose it is because it seems most relevant to women now. It is called 'Silverhands' or 'The Handless Maiden.'

Told by the Brothers Grimm and hundreds of others in one form or another, this is a story of a girl whose father makes a bargain with the devil. It addresses the soul wounding of the woman who at menopause cries out in pain, 'I feel so useless. Who am I? What can I *do*?' It also speaks of the damage done to the human spirit in both men and women by the mechanical world which we have created out of the Industrial Revolution. Like all good myths, it also points the way towards healing.

THE HANDLESS MAIDEN

Once a miller lived with his wife and his lovely daughter deep in the forest. A good and honest man, the miller had been grinding grain to make bread for the villagers for two score years with the help of his faithful ox and by the sweat of his brow. But grinding corn is hard work and the miller had grown weary of the toil. One afternoon, as he is chopping wood at the end of a long day, a dark stranger appears and says, 'Why do you waste your time with all this chopping and grinding? Give me what stands behind your little cottage and I will turn your grindstone for you and chop your wood by magic. I will also change your humble house into a great mansion.'

It all sounds like a great idea to the miller. After all, the only thing that stands behind his cottage is an old apple tree. Who in their right mind would not trade that for a life of luxury and the freedom to spend his time as he chooses? So he agrees. 'Good,' says the dark stranger, 'then you shall have your riches and your freedom from toil. And I? I shall return in three years to claim what is mine.' Then he disappears as mysteriously as he arrived.

The miller picks up his shining axe and begins to make his way back through the woods to his cottage. But who is this running towards him? It is his wife, except her simple housemaid's apron has gone. In its place is the finest velvet dress of crimson that he has ever seen. 'Husband, you should see what has happened,' she cries. 'Our house is gone. In its place stands a great mansion with glittering turrets and a herb garden woven like a braid into the meadow.'

Pleased with how shrewd he has been to do his deal the miller tells his wife of the bargain with the dark stranger. 'But what did you promise him in return?' she wants to know. 'Only that which stands behind our cottage – the gnarled old apple tree that I should most certainly have cut down soon anyway.' The woman throws up her hands in horror. She wails. She shrieks. 'Oh, husband what have you done,' she screams. 'It is our daughter who stood behind the cottage this afternoon sweeping the path. You fool, you have sealed her fate forever.' [Alas, terrible things happen when in his thirst for mechanical devices and in his lust for gold a man is willing to win it at the expense of the feminine.]

The miller and his wife return home weeping despite their

finery. They tell their daughter what will become of her in three years' time. The girl bears the news with patience and in silence. And for three years she awaits her fate. Then one day, sure enough, the Evil One appears to claim his due. The girl washes herself, dresses in white linen and draws a circle around her body with a chalk. But when the stranger reaches out to take her by the arm he cannot bear her purity. 'Keep her away from water,' he orders, 'or I shall have no power over her. I will return tomorrow.' The miller does as the stranger bid him to do for he is terrified of the Dark One's power and can only tremble in his presence. The next morning, when the stranger comes back, he finds the girl has shed tears all through the night. Because she is clean and pure again he cannot approach her. By now he is furious. 'Chop off her hands,' he orders the miller.

Horrified, the miller refuses. How can he chop off the hands of his only daughter? 'If you do not do exactly as I say,' hisses the Evil One, 'then I shall take you away with me forever.' So, in tears, the miller approaches his daughter, 'My child,' he says, 'the Devil will take me far away unless I chop off both your hands with my axe. Forgive me the injury that I will do to you.' 'Father,' replies the girl, 'I am your child. Do what you will.' And she holds out her hands. One swift slash with the axe and they lie bleeding in the soil. Now the stranger arrives for the third time to find her stumps all bandaged in gauze. But again the girl has wept so long and freely that they too are washed pure with her tears. Defeated, the Evil One now knows he has lost all right to her and so he leaves.

The miller tries to make up to his daughter what he has done. After all he is rich now and can offer the girl anything she wants. She will be able to live in comfort for the rest of her life. He will feed her and take care of her and she will want for nothing. But the girl replies, 'I cannot stay, father. I must go away. The kindness of people will provide for me.' So her mother ties her maimed arms in fresh gauze and the girl sets out on her journey – but to where and for what she does not know.

All day she walks. At dusk she comes to an orchard full of trees heavy with wonderful smelling fruit. Oh, how hungry she is. 'If only I could get some of that fruit,' she thinks. But she cannot enter the orchard. It is surrounded by a moat that is filled with water. She kneels upon the ground and says a prayer to the earth, her mother, 'I shall die, sweet mother, if I do not taste of that fruit.' Suddenly an angel appears and clears the water. The moat goes dry, the girl crosses and, reaching out with the gauze-bound stumps, she plucks a pear from the tree, holds it and eats it.

The orchard belongs to a king. He is a good man but somewhat miserly. He has his servants number every piece of fruit and keeps a gardener on constant watch to make sure none is stolen. Of course, the gardener sees the girl. But he also sees the angel and so he is afraid that the girl may be a spirit. He decides not to report the loss to the king. The next morning when the king comes to count his pears, however, he discovers that one is missing. 'Your Highness', says the gardener, 'I saw it go but I know not if it was taken by a maid or by a spirit with no hands.' 'And how did this spirit cross the moat?' the king wants to know. The gardener has no answer. 'Where did it go?' the king asks. 'Why it disappeared into the thicket,' says the gardener. 'Then I shall watch myself to see if it returns tonight,' says the king.

So that evening the king and his magician conceal themselves behind an old wall and wait. Sure enough a figure dressed in white comes creeping from the thicket, approaches the tree, takes another pear and starts to eat it. The magician reveals himself. 'Are you of this world or another?' he questions the girl. 'I was once of the world, yet I am not of *this* world,' replies the girl, 'it has forsaken me.' The beauty of the girl's face and the strange simplicity of her manner touches the heart of the king who falls in love with her and rushes forward. 'Sweet maiden, you may be forsaken by the whole world, but I will not forsake you.' So he leads her to his palace and there he marries her and commands his craftsman to fashion silver hands to replace the ones she has lost. But what good are silver hands to a woman who longs to make use of them?

A year goes by. The king is called to war. The maiden, who is now the queen, awaits her first child. So the king goes to his mother and asks her to care for Silverhands while he is away. When Silverhands is brought to bed, he tells the mother she must send him word of his wife's state of health and of the child. Not long after the queen gives birth to a boy. True to her word the king's mother sends a letter saying that both are well and wonderful. But the messenger carrying it is waylaid. He grows tired at the bank of a river, stops to rest and falls asleep. This is the work of the Evil One who has come to substitute the letter with another announcing that the queen has given birth to a child half-man half-beast.

When the king reads the forgery he is much distressed. Yet he writes back to say that his mother should care for them both until his return. On his way back to the castle once again the messenger is overcome by drowsiness. The Devil comes, takes the king's letter from his hand, and switches it for another telling the mother she must kill the queen and her child. Horrified, his mother reads the letter. She writes back, sure there must be some mistake. But yet again the letters are switched, and yet again. Finally the last letter arrives from the king insisting his mother must kill the queen then cut out her eyes and tongue for him to see on his return.

The queen cannot bring herself to carry out his orders. So she packs up Silverhands and the babe and sends them out into the world, saying, 'I cannot kill you, but you must go far away and never return.' She ties the child to the queen's back – for the queen's useless silver hands cannot perform even a simple task like carrying her own child. In tears, poor Silverhands wanders away and goes deep into the woods. Now in despair for the second time she falls upon her knees and prays. Once again the angel appears. 'You are welcome, fine queen,' the angel says, leading her into a lovely cottage. There she unties the child from Silverhands' back and it begins to nurse. 'How did you know that I am the queen?' asks Silverhands. 'I am a handmaiden of the Dark Goddess,' the angel replies. 'I have been sent to care for you and your child.' So Silverhands stays in that little house and is happy with her child and with her life. Gradually her hands grow back. In the beginning they look like baby hands, then like the hands of a child. Finally they grow into the beautiful hands of a woman.

Not long after Silverhands leaves the castle, the king returns having won his war to find his wife gone and the eyes and tongue of a deer in their place. His mother tells him of the letters and admonishes him for his cruelty. But no, it was not he who sent them. 'How could you kill my wife and child?' he insists, trembling with grief and rage. 'I could not kill them either,' his mother confesses. 'I killed a deer and sent them far away.'

So for seven years the king wanders in search of his family. In all that time he neither eats nor drinks. His hair grows long and his beard becomes tangled with brambles. Then one day he arrives at the cottage in the woods. The angel greets him at the door and invites him in. He is so tired after his wandering that he falls immediately into a deep sleep and the angel places a fine linen handkerchief over his face. But the child – his very own child – comes into the room. Finding a man lying on the bed he lifts the piece of linen to see what is beneath. The king awakens and finds this beautiful child and his lovely mother gazing down on him.

'I am your wife,' says the queen, 'and this is your son.' 'Alas, that cannot be,' says the king. 'My wife is called Silverhands for she has no hands of her own.' 'I was once she,' his wife replies. 'Through my dreams, my silence, and my care these hands have grown back. I am no longer the handless maiden you once knew.' She who had once been Silverhands now goes to fetch the same silver hands and shows them to the king. Brimming with joy after his long years of wandering the king embraces his family. They return from the forest that very day while all the angels and the people of the forest celebrate with a great feast. When the king and his family arrive back at the castle another wedding is arranged. The queen mother rejoices. They have many more children and all is well.

* * *

I love this story. It holds within it so many of our secrets. It tells of the terrible bargains we women blunder into. The miller who trades his apple tree in a bargain with the Devil then finds he has sacrificed his daughter's hands. Like our culture of the western world, he is seduced by wealth and the technology of magic and so he gives away what he loves most.

The miller betrays his daughter as we in all innocence betray ourselves – bargaining away our freedom and our wildness for what we think will bring us safety or for some bauble that catches our eye. We marry when we should not. We force ourselves to live lives that do not feed us. All such trades are Devil's bargains. In making them we lose our hands, our claws, our ability to do and make what deep within we want most to do and make – and our ability to protect ourselves. Meanwhile the simplicity of human life has lost its flavour and the Devil stands forever by – ready to offer us another bargain we cannot afford to refuse.

The light of a young woman's soul which slumbers invariably attracts a predator. No evil creature can resist such sweetness. The girl's initiation, like our own, comes with the loss of her hands. She has given up dominion over her own soul. Yet in her innocence – knowing not what she has done, her tears of grief wash her clean so the Devil cannot take her. And her loss, tragic though it is, is also her salvation, for it is the beginning of a hero's journey which, after many trials and tribulations, will lead her deep into the forest where in silence and in the presence of an angel sent by the Dark Goddess she will regrow her hands, regain her power, and her wholeness. It is the first betrayal that sends us on a journey which will awaken us. And when our soul no longer slumbers then the dark stranger has no power. Evil cannot touch us.

The girl is lovely. Her beauty draws pity from the king and a certain kind of love. He will, he promises, look after her forever. Some would say a girl in such a condition is lucky to have the offer. Yet what woman can live her life, what woman can nurture her child, or paint her picture or move her mountain with a useless pair of decorative hands bestowed upon her by her husband? There has to be another way if only we wait long enough, if only we can find somewhere deep within the woods where we can rest and listen and let our hands grow back – if only we can pray for that. And in those darkest times and in the deepest forest, prayers can be answered. We find our place. It is a place of stillness deep within the forest. There a woman is safest. It is her realm. Here she is happy amidst the ancient trees and amongst the beasts, amongst the flowers. There is no devil who can touch her here with his sinister bargains and his thieving ways. Like all women, Silverhands has several initiations in her life. Each brings its lessons and its comforts until at last she finds her place and rests. Then, in time, she rises from the underworld of her magic forest peopled with sacred trees and beasts both wild and tame. She returns to the world no longer crippled but with soul intact and hands ready to do whatever she may ask of them. At last she has reclaimed her wildness.

Chapter Twenty

Crone's Retreat

The first step in any initiation is isolation, some kind of withdrawal from our ordinary lives so that we can confront the changes taking place in our bodies and the transformations in our lives, and so that we can come to terms with what within us is dying and make way for something else to be born. In primitive societies, when the signs of menopause arrived to herald the dark phase of the moon in a woman's life she was allowed to leave the tribe and go away for a time. Rather like a modern sabbatical, this year away was known as the crone's retreat. It is an important ritual. Although few women these days can take off for a year's holiday all expenses paid, it is always necessary that a woman initiate some form of retreat in her own life around the time of menopause. It may mean giving up certain responsibilities, or arranging your life so that for at least two or three hours a day you are left alone simply to *be*. Like many ancient rituals, the crone's retreat developed out of a need that is universal in menopausal women: when menopause arrives every woman needs the time and space to turn around and discover what is stalking her. Women who refuse to honour their inner demands for time alone often get sick and have it forced upon them.

When my own perimenopausal years arrived, I had never heard of the crone's retreat. I had hardly ever heard the word crone – except to refer to some terrible old witch on a children's television programme. But what I did hear loud and clear from within was a demand that I turn away from the outside world. I could not silence it. The call to retreat can come in as many different guises as there are women to hear it. In my own life it came as a demand from somewhere deep inside that I stop everything I was doing and sit down to write a serious novel. This was something I hardly dared to dream was possible. It was responding to that demand – and I had little choice of not responding to it so insistent had it become – that led me into my own crone's retreat, taught me first hand about the nature of the hero's journey and took me through my own initiation of the dark moon. Whatever else it was, it wasn't easy.

To anyone who has never done one, the idea of going on a retreat can conjure visions of saffron robes and jasmine flowers or medieval cloisters filled with pious nuns in black habits gently wending their way to evensong. To some, the idea of retreating from day-to-day communications for a time may seem like an extended holiday during which life's stresses are sloughed off. The reality, to say the least, is somewhat different. Crone's time away does something quite different than simply lift you out of your ordinary world and transport you into a comfortable realm of spiritual peace. It brings you face to face with the deepest layers of your own being. This is never a comfortable prospect. It always makes me laugh when someone at a dinner party begins to criticize recluses, monks and nuns, saying that they should have the courage to live in the world. In my experience, living in the world can be an easy task next to entering the realms of the soul.

Charnel Ground

In the twenty years before menopause I had carried out a number of short retreats including one of several weeks in a Tibetan monastery in the Himalayas where (among other things) I learned that my greatest attachment was to porcelain lavatories and my worst karma was with fleas. Each of them was some preparation for my lengthy crone's retreat during which I gave up all my connections to the outside world to wrestle with the question of whether or not I could find new meaning in my life by writing my first novel. The task took me deep into the recesses of my own psyche. It was an experience which – only now that the period of withdrawal has come to an end – I realize had echoes of the cold dark isolation which St John described and the bleakness of wandering in Vajragini's (one of the great goddesses in the Tibetan tradition) charnel ground.

It is a funny thing how a crone's retreat usually comes about. It is quite different to setting aside a long weekend or a fortnight to go to a meditation centre as a means of breaking out of your routine and deepening your spiritual insight. You do not choose it. It chooses you. In the beginning you are rarely aware that this is what is going on. All you know is that something inside is demanding that you listen to it. It is a demand which often comes with ruthless insistence, even if listening to it means turning away from a life which on most levels seemed to be working well.

Ancient Dreams

My own retreat began when I was perimenopausal. It was to last more than three and a half years and only came to an end the same month I had my last period. Strangely enough the first inkling of what it would be about had come twenty years before in a dream. I dreamed I was standing in the midst of a magnificent garden. It was like a garden in one of those Persian miniature paintings, filled with masses of flowers in luminous colours and trees all covered with fruits. There was a great pond in the midst of the garden and Beethoven's music was playing. It was nothing of Beethoven's I had heard before and yet I knew that it was by him. I stood in the centre of this garden entranced by the colours, the sounds and the beauty around me. As the music reached a crescendo, suddenly the trees and flowers, fruits and sky became transfigured with light. Then the hand of God – it looked like Michelangelo's God who reaches out to Adam on the ceiling of the Sistine Chapel – came down from the heaven. Its index finger touched the centre of the pond sending ever increasing circles outwards. This was more than I could bear. I closed my eyes and put my hands over my ears. Moments later, as the music began to descend from its climax, when I removed my hands and opened my eyes, I saw that the garden was returning to its previous colours and state. A voice within me said, 'It is all right – the next time such beauty comes you will be able to bear it.'

That was all. The dream had occurred in my mid-twenties. I had no idea what it 'meant'. All I knew was that it felt like some kind of a blessing had been offered or something fundamental had shifted in my life – at least in my *inner* life for my outer life was full of trying to care for three children on my own and earning a living for all of us. I suppose that I learned something pretty fundamental about myself from the dream. It was strange and I could make little sense of it: I learned that the thing which frightens me most is not the horror of pain, deprivation or loneliness but rather the intensity of a profound experience of beauty. Real beauty, like great joy, carries with it a devastating quality of truth. This, I learned from the dream, was what I have always feared most.

Then for many years I forgot about it. I immersed myself in earning a living, writing books, making television films, and doing all the things we women do every day in the middle period of our lives when the responsibilities of a householder sit heavily on our shoulders. Some fifteen years later, the dream came back to me and with it this strange imperative: *You must put everything aside to write a novel about Beethoven.* I had never written fiction. I had never dared to dream I could. I fought the inner command with the vehemence of a trapped animal. It terrified me. At first I thought the fear was a fear of failure. Like many women I have never suffered from an abundance of self-confidence. It was only much later that I was to realize it had another – far deeper – cause as well.

Into the Silence

My retreat began by withdrawing from my outside work. Having raised four children – by then I had had another child – I had been forced to spend quite a lot of my time earning a living; in fact virtually all of the time not spent being with my children. Early on in the years of my research for the novel, I began to see that there was no way in which I could write it unless I could give up my work in the media and not have to earn a living until it was finished. I began to pray that this would be possible although I saw no way in which it was going to happen given my financial responsibilities.

The trouble with prayer is that it can be dangerous. Often you end up getting what you pray for – which means it is a good idea to be very careful about what you ask for. Many of us would like to convince ourselves that the only thing that is stopping us from doing what we want is money. It is only when such a prayer is answered that you realize the impediments to your moving ahead to do whatever you longed to do lie not in a lack of money as you have always assumed but rather in an unwillingness to embrace the absolute freedom of choice each of us has. This is exactly what happened to me. Until then I had been able to see myself as a conscientious and caring mother – if somewhat long suffering – who was willing to sacrifice her own desires to earn a living and care for her children. Suddenly I found this was no longer necessary. In my forties, to my surprise, I found myself with all the material resources I needed to do exactly what I had been saying for several years I wanted to do and, just as the beauty in my dream had overwhelmed me all those years before, this new-found freedom terrified me. So began my crone's time away for which I was ill prepared. The short retreats I had done before had been well structured within religious traditions: you went into meditation, you kept silence, you ate one meal a day and so forth. All of that had been easy compared with what I now faced.

Wild Energy

In the Hindu and Buddhist tradition there is an unusual spiritual path known as *left-handed tantra*. There is, I think, something decidedly *female* about the energy connected with it. It is *wild* energy – the energy of nature which refuses to fit into the shapes we would impose on it. Left-handed tantra is not much written or spoken about and it is not much practised. It differs from other spiritual pathways in that the empowerment which is believed to come to the individual from the divine (an intense energy which is highly volatile) in most religious traditions comes carefully packaged and structured within ethical and meditational rituals. Usually they are carried out under the wise gaze of a teacher who has already trodden the path. In the case of left-handed tantra all this numinous energy suddenly pours through you with no conceptual framework, no spiritual guidance and no useful practices designed to render it more bearable. It was only after my lengthy retreat had finally come to an end – as had the novel which engendered it – that I realized I had unwittingly been thrown into the seemingly chaotic energies of left-handed tantra.

Somehow, a wild spirit – a ruthless manifestation of my own life force – had arisen from within demanding that I follow it no matter how difficult or frightening that might become. It seemed to have an almost total disregard for my personal comfort or for the wishes of my ego. Like a disciple who attaches himself to the guru and follows his master's every whim, I found myself in the service of creating this book. At each moment during the years which it took to complete, I had a choice to make – either to honour my commitment or to run away. The experience turned out to be nothing like what I had assumed the writing of a novel would be about. For one thing it was not at all a question of 'making it all up'. It was more a process of uncovering layer after layer of truth and meaning as though the form and shape of the book was already there and it was my job to uncover it. In the process layer after layer of my own psyche became uncovered, although an awareness of what was going on remained mostly hidden from me until after the process was all over.

To Be or Not to Be

I began the writing of *Ludwig* the way I have begun every other project – with a reasonable sense of organization and the intention that I would produce 2,000 words a day until the book was finished. My naïvety in assuming I would be able to do this still stuns me. When I look back to how I was then I see myself as a callow youth with little understanding of the processes involved in creation. I was pig-ignorant – ignorant enough not even to have an inkling of how truly ignorant I really was. I found the writing very difficult. I would have to stop for weeks at a time. At one point I discovered that I could not work at all in the light. I would pull down all the blinds in my studio and sit for hours on end in front of my computer screen in the dark. Every day I would get up and run for an hour along the cliffs where I live in West Wales, then I would swim in the sea as I had been doing for years. Afterwards I would return to my darkened room to write.

Before long the whole process had brought me to my knees. Everything I had learned before about writing simply did not apply. I could not, as I had rather arrogantly assumed, write this book from the same practical, matter-of-fact framework that had worked for all my other books. This novel demanded something different. In short, it demanded *everything*. Then one morning as I ran into the sea at dawn I realized that I was so filled with despair and frustration at what I perceived to be the impossibility of the task I had taken on that I wanted to swim out into the Irish Sea and never return. What was happening to me? I knew only one thing: that I had a choice: Do I live or do I die? There in the white foam as the sun rose over the sea that morning I made my choice. I cried out defiantly to whoever or whatever might be listening, 'Okay, if you want to destroy me that is your business but I am not going to help you do it!'

Back on Home Ground

I could not understand what was happening to me. Where was all this anger and despair coming from? I wondered if I was ill. I went to have my endocrine system checked out only to find that most of it – the pituitary, the adrenals, the thyroid, the ovaries – were badly out of order. Instead of worrying me, this news delighted me. Now at least I was on familiar territory, I could fall back on what I knew from my many years of working in health. I knew what to do to help my body. The knowing brought me the only feelings of security I had felt ever since I had entered this new world. So I went on a seven-week juice fast. The practitioner who had examined me and voiced deep concern over how imbalanced my hormone system had become was amazed. He had never seen anyone recover so quickly. Yet, despite my rapid recovery, the book had to be laid aside for almost six months. I felt as though I had fallen into a great luminous sea – a sea in which all things were possible and anything could be brought into being – which so completely dissolved the boundaries of who I thought I was that I felt I could not function.

The years of my crone's retreat were spent in learning patience and humility – that I was nothing, am nothing, and can do nothing of myself, yet that in my nothingness and out of it all things may be born. So many internal events occurred that it would be impossible to speak of them all. So deeply did my research into Beethoven's life and music take me, and so immersed did I become in the spirit of the book, that in time I began to experience his symptoms. I had the same deafness in the ears, the same pain in the liver and upsets in the colon that are described in his medical reports. My research for the novel took me into two other areas outside Beethoven's life which, although I did not know at the time, were to change my view of the human psyche and of worlds – both seen and unseen – beyond all recognition. The first was the phenomenon of the multiple personality. The second area was the whole question of the nature of human freedom and the political and economic forces that stifle it. Before my retreat began I had voiced only the vaguest interest in either subject.

Some of what I experienced during those years went into the novel itself. In the process of creating it I was forced to make my own descent. I learned first hand about the archetypal nature of the hero's journey, about the vast nature of the human psyche and about the quality of the wasteland. Until then these were nothing more than ideas which I had read about with detached curiosity. I was to learn that a woman's experience of the descent is very different indeed from the rather facile description of it you can find in many books on psychology. I learned that myth is the only language one can legitimately use to speak of it. I discovered, too, that a woman's inner world and outer one are but reflections of one another – as within, so without. And, in a messy piece-meal way, I made my passages. They were not passages of my own choosing; from some deep inner place within they had been chosen for me. My teacher and guide was the task I had chosen. My challenge was to use my crone's retreat to complete it. I followed this imperative, never knowing from one day to the next if that would happen.

The first two-thirds of the book took me three and a half

years to write. During most of that time making words was like squeezing blood from a stone. Like many women I was riddled with self-criticism and hardly dared to think that I might succeed. Even to contemplate such an action went against all my conditioning. I discovered that I had all my life been carrying around a notion that a woman should sacrifice her needs for others. It is an idea which now seems ancient history. During the last three months I wrote the final third of the novel – mostly in a frenzy. Suddenly words began to spill forth in such profusion and intensity that I could hardly get them down. I would get up at three in the morning to begin work, my body stiff with pain. For, although most days I still ran along my cliffs, I had become so completely immersed in the mythic world out of which the novel grew that I badly neglected the needs of my body. I would say to it, 'Just support me for a few weeks more then I will take care of you.'

Caterpillars and Butterflies

One day the novel was finished. Six hours later I left for New Zealand to do a series of lectures and workshops for International Green Month. When I arrived there I felt like someone who had come back from the dead – a caterpillar who, bound inside its cocoon, had watched while its body dissolved into a white gel in the hopes that one day it might be re-formed as a butterfly. Now, three years later, it feels as though I may be just beginning to emerge from that cocoon. My wings are very stiff and very wet. My menopausal passage is over. The world is different. I have had to learn all sorts of brand new languages to live in it. What did I gain from all of this? Only the absolute knowing that there is an incredible natural order which regulates our lives even when we perceive ourselves to be in total chaos. Within this order is to be found a quality of love and a compassion which goes far beyond anything I could ever have imagined. It continually asks that we venture deep into the realm of wisdom and it knows exactly what is right and necessary from one moment to the next in our lives. Now I am in the process of having to learn to trust it with all of my being. This is all I know. Except perhaps for

Chapter Twenty-one
The Return

After any hero's journey has been completed there are certain issues which arise. One of them is the issue of boundaries – where you end and others begin. Being fosterers of life, women often give their souls away to those they love or those who are in need of care, believing that this is the best way to help. One of the important awarenesses which begins to develop during the return part of the journey is the awareness of how important it is to decide that you will not allow other people to live off your energy, nor will you live off theirs.

Sealing the Self

There are several things that can help one to do this. First, allow yourself to become aware of energetic shifts that take place and, without passing any judgement, become conscious of situations in which either you feel yourself giving away your energy or being drained of energy by others. Once a woman is aware of this, it is a relatively easy matter to stop it from happening. This is very important on a physical level too: for energy boundaries work very closely together with the immune system and if you allow your boundaries to be breached on an energetic level you are also opening the immune system to compromise, increasing your susceptibility to illness and to degeneration.

Another thing that can be helpful when you sense an energy drain is happening is something I learned from Sandra Ingerman. Ingerman suggests that women in any situation in which we feel vulnerable to energy loss or leakage envisage themselves – their whole body – surrounded by a translucent blue egg, and then say silently, 'I will not give up my soul to you.' It takes a bit of practice to get the hang of it but this little exercise can bring a remarkable sense of wholeness and integration, and help break through years of habitual energy loss.

Something else we usually need to learn on the return – something which many women who lead busy dedicated lives forget to do – is to continually set aside enough time to restore yourself. Go into the garden and sit, go for walks by yourself, and take time to listen to music, learn to honour yourself and care for yourself, and take your needs seriously. It can also be helpful to learn the practice of transmuting negative emotion, both your own and those of others. Anger, grief, sorrow, resentment – all these are nothing more than energy, whether they are feelings that are being felt by you or feelings of others that have been directed towards you. Once you become aware of them, without making any judgements about them, you can choose to transmute them into healing energy for yourself and for the planet, by simply asking internally that this be done.

Living Now

A woman returns from her journey with a new understanding of who she is and what she needs. Week by week this becomes clearer as an awareness of one's own identity begins to emerge. When you begin to experience the freedom that comes after, some conscious decisions need to be made. You might decide, for instance, no longer to put your energy into worrying about what is going to happen next and how you are going to survive, choosing instead to use your new-found freedom as creatively as possible in your life. This usually involves searching to find out what brings you the greatest joy and the greatest sense of meaning, then immersing yourself more and more in doing it as the days go on. The more you do, the more physical energy is likely to be available to you. Following one's passion and feeling one's joy releases all sorts of energy which before may have been wrapped up in worry, frustration and negative feelings towards yourself or others. Women who in earlier years have suffered chronic fatigue are often surprised how it is replaced by a new vitality, for so much of our energy gets locked up. I think this must be what anthropologist Margaret Mead was talking about when she spoke of 'post-menopausal zest'.

For all energy is neutral and, unless it is directed towards the positive, we are always in danger of finding it creates even more entanglements, frustration and negativity. It becomes important to ask the question, 'How can I express my core energy in my life?' You don't have to be an artist to do this, neither do you have to have big ambitions. Quite the contrary. In fact it is best to take things one step at a time. Think of one single thing that you enjoy doing and then promise yourself that you will do it, whether it be dancing, tapestry, taking long walks, doing some sort of public service, or learning about a subject that intrigues you for the sake of learning itself. Then the more you direct your creative energy the more energy there seems to be to direct. Once it starts to flow steadily you will find that other outlets suggest themselves. When these impulses arise, follow them until gradually the flow of energy, rather like the flow of water in a river, grows larger and larger and can be directed into any number of activities or concentrated to be experienced in whatever you choose.

Joseph Campbell used to urge people to 'follow your bliss', and 'participate joyously in the sorrows of the world'. It is good advice. By following your bliss he does not mean going out of your way to have a good time or chasing rainbows. Far from it. He means coming in touch with whatever is your particular individual passion and then pursuing it for its own sake, simply because it brings you joy. For women this may be gardening or going back to university or travelling. The whole point about following one's bliss and honouring one's passions is that doing so leads step by step down a road towards the kind of fulfilment that has nothing to do with striving for success or the approval of society. It is rather like rediscovering the joy of being a child when for hours one could sit and perform a particular act or work with a particular skill, all the while experiencing the joy of living in the moment.

Not long ago I discovered what brings me bliss. What I like doing best in the world is making beautiful things – anything beautiful – from a salad to a piece of sculpture or a painting, although I have no training and no particular gifts for either.

Nine months ago a close friend gave me a dreamcatcher – a circular mandala-type of wall hanging that comes out of the

Native American tradition. Dreamcatchers are made from leather thong, chamois, beads and feathers. They consist of a circle inside which is woven a web-like structure, from which is hung long pieces of beaded chamois and feathers. A dreamcatcher is hung above the bed. It is designed to catch your dreams. It is said to eat the bad dreams, the way the spider eats the fly. Your good dreams get caught by the web and, when the web grows fat enough with them, they will spill over it making their way down the beaded chamois, leather, beads and feathers, intensified the way that water flows faster as it spills over a waterfall. So the good dreams are given back to you in abundance.

I had seen one or two dreamcatchers, found them interesting, and had evidently mentioned this to my friend. She decided to gather together what was necessary and make me one. I was fascinated by the gift, I hung it above my bed and a few nights later became aware that what I wanted most to do was to make a dreamcatcher of my own. I asked her to show me how to weave the beautiful web which forms the net. It turned out to be very easy, and I began to make dreamcatcher after dreamcatcher. To my surprise I rediscovered a sense of joy and excitement in what I was doing that I had not experienced since childhood. This is something I have rarely experienced as a writer. I am a woman who, after I have created something, no longer has any interest in it. I have always tended to feel little satisfaction from anything that I have made. I found that working with dreamcatchers was completely different. I would sit in the middle of my studio surrounded by a total chaos of beads and stones, shells and chamois, small pieces of wood and dried flowers, and spend hours at a time twisting things and building upon the webs to create dreamcatchers of great diversity. Each one seemed a universe in itself.

To Catch a Dream

My experience of making dreamcatchers was so intense for me that at times I would feel I was running a fever while working on one. For the first time in my life I was able to work without thinking, that is to say without making any rational judgements or having to control what I was doing. I would begin by weaving a web, a repetitive process which I found stilling to my mind and satisfying. Once the web was woven then I would allow my instincts to direct me towards putting together whatever objects, beads or forms I wanted to add next. At first I experienced some of the same fear I often do when I am beginning a writing project – a fear that I don't know how to do anything, and that I need to see the overall picture to make it work. But in my dreamcatcher making, I was conscious that there *was* no way I could see the overall picture. So I would just begin anywhere, putting together different forms and objects. I found out that I don't have to know where I am going with each dreamcatcher to get there. Each dreamcatcher has a soul of its own and all I have to do is work in a dedicated, intuitive way, letting myself put together one thing after another to discover it. If something didn't work I simply ripped it apart and began again. The delight I felt working with very ordinary physical objects like stones and feathers and beads was such that for the time I was working on a dreamcatcher it could totally absorb me.

Each time I finished a dreamcatcher I would stand back to look at it and feel a sense of awe at the richness of the form that had somehow come through me into this object. It was for me very much an experience of following my bliss. From it I have learned that one does not have to know exactly where one is going when one begins a task or takes up a challenge. You need only work with clear intention from one step to the next. And there is great joy in this because it means that you are living in the moment and most important of all you love what you do. Meanwhile, somehow, the dreamcatchers made themselves simply by my carrying out my intention and trusting that it would happen.

Rituals of Intention

Freeing ourselves from beliefs and attitudes that have been blocking us creates a great open space ahead. What we need to fill it is just two things – intention and trust. This trust is not only in life to support your intentions and help you fulfil them, but trust in yourself. At some point near the end of the journey a woman is being asked to stretch her visions beyond what she used to be capable of doing and to let go of any roles or attitudes that may be in her way. In directing creative energies and living a life that has meaning, it is enormously helpful to be clear about what you intend. Rituals can help a lot here. One ritual which I like very much is to sit and write down three, four, even half a dozen things that are important to me which I want to be, or feel, or accomplish. They can be internal things, such as 'I want to feel at peace' or external things such as 'I want to create a home for myself at such and such a place'. Write each of them down on a separate piece of paper, writing before each one the words, 'I intend', followed by the things that you want. Each morning sit quietly during a time of meditation or recollection and, holding it in your hand, read through each intention three times before going on to the next. Let your mind play on the words. Then give thanks for its fulfilment even before it is fulfilled. In the non-ordinary world there is no such thing as time or space and the sense of gratitude that is created out of experiencing a fulfilled intention is a powerful ally in bringing it about. Then go on to the next intention. Such intentions repeated every morning and every evening can be a useful way to gather one's energy, and also draw upon our unseen helpers, allies, spirits and ancestors, who can help us fulfil them.

Powers of the Circle

When one has made a journey to the core and retrieved pieces of one's own soul that have not previously been lived out, and discovered other treasures from the underworld, these treasures have to be brought back and lived out within the community. Community, a sense of connectedness with others, begins to take on a new meaning. Many women find that during menopause and afterwards their relationships with other women deepen dramatically, especially women who have followed the pathway of daughters of the father and have sometimes experienced a considerable sense of loneliness in doing so. There is something remarkable about relationships between women. Unlike male relationships which tend to be hierarchical – between a dominant and subordinate male – relationships between women tend to be egalitarian, circular rather than linear. There is no hierarchy, only a sense that each woman brings to the circle or community what she has to bring and takes away what she needs. The circle is the simplest and the most profound shape in all of life. It has no top and no bottom, no start and no finish. It excludes nothing and embraces all.

I discovered this for myself many years ago when I decided to have a large circular table made for our home while my children were growing up. I had some vague idea, although I couldn't explain it, that a circular table might create an atmosphere of unity and equality between everyone in the family and enable each person to express more easily and more fully eye-to-eye whatever it was that he or she thought or felt. When the table was finished we brought it to the house and had a bit of a celebration sitting round at dinner that night. I was amazed at the effect the shape seemed to exert on all of us. There was much livelier conversation than there had been before, a closer sense of connection between us and lots more laughter. I figured that Arthur must have known what he was doing in creating the round table for his knights. Because a circle has no beginning and no end, everyone who sits within it feels himself or herself to be an equal part of the whole.

Like women's menstrual cycles and the cycles of the moon, all transformation takes place in a circle. The interconnectedness that women experience in a circle or community – most especially one of other women – can bring us much closer to an understanding of our own individual nature and how we fit in with life around us. To a woman who has never experienced real community it can be a revelation around the time of menopause – beginning to share dreams, hopes, disappointments and experiences with other women in an open and unguarded way. It can also bring a sense of self-acceptance which is hard to come by via any other means. Such community both encourages and inspires. It fires women with a desire to walk, talk and live from their soul. One of the wonderful things about egalitarian female energy is the way it helps women celebrate the successes of other women rather than feeling threatened as men so often do. After menopause many women find that they come together to celebrate the cycles of life and to give thanks for their connections with each other, to help each other overcome their personal fears, and to encourage each other in the expression of individual creative energies, whatever form they take. Such community helps a woman develop courage, compassion, humility and patience. It can also help her accept the parts of her which have remained unloved or which have exercised tyrannical influences over her.

Such community does not have to be experienced only through people, of course. It can also come through animal friends – dogs, cats, horses, birds. It can even be experienced through objects, when you create a special place in your home to keep the things you find or have been given which have particular meaning for you. They, too, remind you of your power and restore your centre when periodically you seem to lose it.

My own experience of menopause and new community continue to make me clear about what I think and what my values are. I believe:

- that each woman is born unique and gifted with great creativity of soul. This, which I call her *seedpower*, is wrapped in the cloak of her soul. A woman's purpose on the earth is to live out that seedpower fully – in effect, to live out the truth of her own being.
- that creativity is wild and free and female in nature even when found in a man.
- that too often a woman's creativity is stillborn. Her seedpower has been crushed and her soul has been silenced by her culture or by her own lack of self-belief. Unless she takes action herself it tends to remain imprisoned.
- that every woman has a right to walk her own path and speak with her own voice. More than a right, it is essential that she does so if her creativity is to come to fruition.
- that all life, art, sexuality, wishes and dreams move in cycles as do the flow and ebb of a woman's hormones and the changes of the seasons on the earth.

- that as women we have tended to allow our own imprisonment and to treat it as normal. It is as though we seem to volunteer to remain caged even though from a logical point of view we should be able to break free. Imprisoned creatures, women among them, who have been held captive for too long, suffer deep injuries to their instinctual nature so that they no longer feel able to defend themselves. I believe it is important that this damage to instinct be brought to light and healed.
- that making a hero's journey at some time in a woman's life is essential for her to find her freedom.
- that a woman must above all honour her instincts.
- that a woman's wild spirit, energy and creativity is best fed when she surrounds herself with what she loves and does the things she likes doing best.

Our cultural conditioning has taught us to undervalue the wild feminine within us – that part which is instinctual, irrational, non-moral and full of passion. The male-dominated linear society in which we live is so frightened of these things that we ourselves have been taught to fear the feminine within us and judge it harshly. Too often we swallow our anger even when it is righteous, we put our needs and wants below those of others. We crush our wild nature. We judge ourselves wrongly and we see ourselves as ugly. Doing so dissipates our power and fragments our soul. Only when we learn to embrace the irrational feminine and honour her can any of us – man or woman – fully complete the hero's journey and return in wholeness. The most difficult task any woman comes up against is that of accepting the part of herself which she finds most ugly and loathsome. Yet, locked within what we most hate and fear lies the greatest power for our transformation. Let the tale be told in myth.

*   *   *

One Christmastide Arthur rode out with his knights to hunt. By chance he became separated from his companions and found himself at the edge of a great brackish pond. There a knight in black armour emerged from the shadows and challenged him to a fight. Arthur reached to draw his sword Excalibur and call on its power to protect him from all harm. Alas, he had come away from court without it. He could feel every ounce of strength drain away from his body in the presence of the dark and evil stranger who raised his sword and threatened to kill him. Being a responsible king, of course, Arthur told the dark knight he didn't think that killing him was a good idea – he had a country to rule, after all, and knights to look after. Where would *they* be without him? The stranger, bored at the thought of such an easy kill, relented and replied, 'I won't kill you so long as you return to this place in three days with the answer to a riddle I shall give you. If you fail I shall remove your head in one full sweep.'

Arthur agreed. He reckoned that, given half a chance and a mug or two of fancy mead, his pals back at the castle would be sure to come up with something. The riddle the stranger posed was this: 'What does every woman want?' So Arthur headed home to ask all his knights and wise men to give him the answer. Everyone from Merlin to a goose girl he met along the road had a go. Each gave him a different answer. 'A woman wants beauty,' said one. 'A woman wants power,' said another, or fame, or jewels, or sanctity. None could agree.

Time was running out. Finally, although he had done his best to hide from his beloved Guinevere the seriousness of the situation, the third morning arrived. Bound by his word of honour to the Black Knight, Arthur had to return as promised. Along the road to the meeting at the brackish waters Arthur came upon an old woman. She sat on a tree stump by the side of the road calling his name. Arthur dismounted and approached her with all the courtesy he could muster. The closer he came the more ghastly this old hag appeared. Although she was dressed in fine silk and wore magnificent jewels on her gnarled and twisted hands, she was unquestionably the most hideous thing he had ever seen, or dreamed of for that matter. Her nose was like a pig's, her mouth was huge, toothless and dribbling. What hair remained on her head was greasy, and the skin all over her misshapen and bloated body was covered in oozing sores.

Arthur swallowed hard, forcing himself not to have to look away. 'My lord,' she said in a surprisingly gentle voice, 'why look you so dismayed?' Summoning up all his chivalrous training, Arthur apologized for his manner, trying to explain it away by telling her he was most unsettled at the prospect of returning to meet his death at the hand of an evil knight because he could not tell him the answer to the riddle, 'What does every woman want?' 'Ah,' said the hag. 'I can tell you that. But such knowledge cannot be given without payment.' Arthur, hoping once again for a reprieve from death, replied, 'Of course, madam, anything you desire shall be yours for the answer – even half my kingdom.'

The Loathly Lady made Arthur bend down while she whispered a few words in his ear. The moment Arthur heard them, he knew his life and his kingdom had been saved. He was about to leap on his horse again and ride off to meet the stranger when she tugged on his cloak and said, 'Now I want my reward.' 'Of course, madam, what is it that you want?' he asked. 'I want to be the wife of your bravest knight and live at your court.' Arthur, who only a moment before had felt his spirits soar, was plunged into the deepest despair. How could he possibly expect any knight to consent to marry such a hideous hag. And what would it be like to have to endure such ugliness every day at court? 'But, madam, that is impossible!' he said. The words slipped through his lips before he could catch them. Aghast at his own lack of courtesy and agonized by having to ask any of his knights, Arthur said, 'I beg your pardon, madam. You are quite right. Come to court tomorrow. There waiting for you will be your future husband.' So saying, he mounted his horse and rode off to meet the Black Knight to convey to him the answer to the riddle.

When he got back to the castle, Arthur was distraught. The knights questioned him. He confessed that he had won his life from the Black Knight but then told them at what cost and reported his promise to the Loathly Lady. 'My very honour is at stake,' said Arthur, wringing his hands, 'unless one of you will agree to wed her.' His knights were horrified at the prospect and tried to avoid his gaze. But one, the youngest knight of all, Sir Gawain, the most courageous and purest of heart stood up. 'Worry not, my liege,' Gawain said, 'I shall save you. I will marry the woman no matter what her mien.'

Gawain did not have long to rue his offer. The marriage was planned for the following morning and the hag arrived at court. When he looked upon her, even Gawain, with all his chivalry, did not know how he could go through with the ceremony. It demanded every ounce of his courage. Somehow he managed it. But things got worse. When the festivities were over, the couple were obliged to retire to their chamber for the night. Gawain, unable to face the hideousness of his wife, sat for long hours in their bedchamber with his back to the lady, writing at his desk and praying she would go to sleep without him. Was he to spend the rest of his life shackled to such a hideous monster?

Long past midnight, as the candle burned low, he felt a hand come to rest upon his shoulder. 'Will you not come to bed now, my lord?' a voice whispered from behind him. Shuddering with horror, Gawain mustered his courage to look at her. To his astonishment there stood not the ugly hag he had married but the most beautiful woman he had ever seen. She had golden hair and ivory skin. 'Why do you seem so surprised, my lord?' she said to him. 'I am indeed your wife. I was enchanted by a wicked magician. But now the enchantment is half broken by your having consented to marry me and so you see I stand before you now in my true form.' Gawain could not believe his luck.

'Half broken?' he asked. 'Yes, my lord,' was the reply. 'Sadly I am only allowed to spend half the time in my true form. For the rest I must return to the shape of the same hag which this afternoon you married. And now you must choose, my lord. Would you have me be my true self at night when we are alone together and the hag during daylight hours?' Gawain, whose mind was flooded with passion at the thought of her beauty in his bed each night, replied eagerly, 'Yes, that is certainly how it must be.'

In the eye of his beautiful lady appeared a tear. 'But Sir,' she said, 'would you then have me suffer the humiliation of the court who cannot conceal their horror at my ugliness?' Now Gawain, if he was nothing else, was compassionate. He could not bear to cause this beautiful woman a tear of sorrow. 'No, of course not,' he replied. 'It shall be the other way round, of course. You shall be my beautiful wife for the court during daylight hours and the hag at night.' But this only made the lady weep the more. 'Oh, sir, would you then deny me forever the joy and pleasure of your embrace?' she asked.

Poor Gawain, who after all was but a man (and man has never found it easy to deal with woman's grief), did not know what to do. After much thought he replied, 'My lady, whatever choice I make will be the wrong one. It is therefore for *you* to choose which you prefer.' At the sound of his words the lady threw herself into his arms in glorious laughter. 'In so saying, my lord, you have given the right answer. You have bestowed upon me what every woman wants – *her own way*. The spell at last is broken. You will never have to look upon the hideous hag again. I am my true self and it belongs to you forever.'

* * *

Such is the power of accepting that which to ourselves is most loathsome. And such is the power of myth in reminding us of it.

RITES AND RITUALS

Chapter Twenty-two

Angels in the Architecture

Osteoporosis is characterized by a decrease in bone mass and a deterioration in bone tissue which makes bones fragile and creates a high risk of fracture. Osteoporotic fractures create disability and can lead to death. In the UK alone the total cost of osteoporotic fractures is estimated at £640 million each year. However, osteoporosis is not a normal part of menopause, is in no way inevitable and, as a growing number of doctors working with natural methods have discovered, can be healed even in women long past menopausal age.

How do you know if you have osteoporosis? The simple answer is that you don't, because of its insidious nature. A woman often does not know that she has it until a bone breaks. Osteoporosis used to be called *menopausal* osteoporosis since nobody ever thought of it occurring before menopause. A woman may have lost a quarter of her bone by the time menopause arrives and be totally unaware of it until a fracture appears two years later.

There is a simple test that you can carry out for yourself to give you some idea of what your bone status is. Have your husband or a friend mark your height against a wall every couple of months. If your height drops as much as 3 millimetres in a year you have osteoporosis and need to take action. Bone shrinkage cannot be reversed by anything except serious changes in eating and lifestyle habits including regular weight-bearing exercise as well as natural progesterone and nutritional supplements.

Common Tests

There are various medical techniques used to measure bone density. The original way was by taking X-rays. Although still used in many places it is a relatively useless method of measurement since X-rays cannot reliably measure bone mass loss or gain until there has been a change of about 30 per cent.

Even if you were to have an X-ray taken at 40 years of age and then another at 45 the radiologist – no matter how good – cannot tell you whether you have gained or lost bone until the change has exceeded the 30 per cent mark.

Now, with the advent of better methods, some tests are so good they can measure bone density at 96 to 98 per cent accuracy. This means they can detect a change of anything over 2 per cent. That change is real – you can count on it. One of these methods is dual-energy X-ray absorptiometry (DXA), where low-dose X-rays are used. This is the most widely practised method. Measurements can be made of the spine, femoral neck, forearm and total body skeleton. Recently measurements have also been made of the lateral lumbar spine by DXA. DXA is accurate, as is computerized tomography (CT), but both involve radiation (especially high doses in the case of CT) which many doctors concerned with natural menopause would rather not subject a woman to. Other methods, such as single photon absorptiometry (SPA) and dual photon absorptiometry (DPA), are safer, since they do not rely on radiation but rather on passing light through the skin. They work rather the way a flashlight held against the palm of the hand in a darkened room enables you to see the shape of bones as the light shines through. Photons are passed through the skin of the body. They bounce off the minerals of the bones, instead of passing straight through, and therefore cast a shadow. The energy that is lost when photon beams are sent through the body is then calculated by a machine to give an accurate reading of bone density.

Drug Treatments

There are a number of common drug interventions officially touted to be useful in slowing bone loss and preventing fractures. Most have little to offer. They include calcitonin, the biphosphonates, anabolic steroids and, the most commonly prescribed of all, sodium fluoride. All can have serious side-effects and none are truly effective. Be wary.

Fluoride supplements are frequently touted as a treatment

for osteoporosis since initial research showed that fluoride does increase bone mass. But follow-up studies have shown that, although bone mass does increase slightly when fluoride is given, the new bone has a very poor structural quality, is highly brittle and actually makes bones *more* prone to breakage. Stay away from fluoride.

Risk Factors

- Poor calcium metabolism as a result of inadequate vitamins and minerals, including vitamin C, vitamin D, zinc and magnesium during the menstruating years, often from years of living on a diet of processed foods.

- Excessive phosphorus intake from colas or processed meats which leaches calcium from bones.

- Excess alcohol which renders your blood acidic. Acidosis destroys bones because the body has to steal alkalizing minerals (calcium) from them to keep blood pH from dropping into the acid range where it can damage cells.

- Physical inactivity and lack of weight-bearing exercise.

- Smoking.

- High-protein diet. Excess protein also creates a negative calcium balance, leaching calcium from bones and causing more to be lost in the urine than is taken in through food.

- Malabsorption of nutrients either from low levels of hydrochloric acid in the stomach or as a result of using antibiotics.

- Antacids which contain aluminium. They disrupt normal calcium/phosphorus interactions on which the maintenance of good bone depends.

- The regular use of drugs such as cortisone, thyroid hormones, barbiturate anticonvulsants and heparin.

- Progesterone deficiency. Inadequate bone building results from anovulatory menstruation, especially in the 5 to 8 years before menopause where, although periods appear normal, inadequate progesterone is being produced. This reduces the activity of osteoblast cells so that more resorption of old bone is taking place than building of new bone.

- In a *few* women there is a risk of inadequate oestrogen after menopause. This results in increased osteoclast bone resorption. Oestrogen supplementation can slow resorption but its use carries serious potential health risks (unless you use oestriol E3). It will only help as long as you continue to take it. Oestrogen can do nothing to *reverse* bone loss.

Wise Woman Ways

Horsetail Drink horsetail tea regularly. Steep 1 teaspoon of the dried herb in a cup of boiling water. It is rich in silicon. Other herbs that go well with horsetail are sage, alfalfa, uva ursi leaves and nettle which you can mix together and use as a tea.

Exercise

Probably the most neglected of all the actions a woman can take to prevent and to treat osteoporosis is exercise. It needs to be *weight-bearing* exercise. But it has taken until very recently for official bodies such as the United States Academy of Sciences to come out with the statement that weight-bearing exercise is essential to build and maintain bone strength. A lot of the 'official line' booklets such as those sent out by the National Osteoporosis Society in Britain make only vague references to it saying that women should not be inactive or suggest that 'walking, dancing, playing tennis and keep-fit are ideal' as though any old exercise will do. The fact is that although walking, running, cycling and aerobics might be great for your heart and lungs, they will not get the job done when it comes to strengthening your bones because they stress only the long bones of the legs and don't supply enough load. You need weight training – whether the weights be tins of beans held in each hand, dumb bells or bar bells. The simpler they are, the better. Moving weights around in a way that stresses the muscles and bones all over the body is what builds strong bones. Weight training also builds muscle tissue and enhances your Lean Body Mass to fat ratio (see Body Heat, p. 178). This is particularly important for women as they get older since a shrinkage in lean tissue depletes the body of hormones and energy and makes the body and the face look older. So important is weight training for overall wellbeing that the American College of Sports Medicine recently altered its standard advice on using exercise to retain fitness and health to include exercise with weights. Thirty to 45 minutes of this kind of regime three times a week will have your bones brimming with the piezoelectric energy that builds them beautifully.

Diet

For the prevention and treatment of osteoporosis, diet is the first order of the day – low in fat and moderate in protein with plenty of green leafy vegetables, no colas or processed soft drinks, and little meat and alcohol. Official World Health Organization figures calculate that we need no more than half a gram of good-quality protein for each kilo of body weight. So if you weigh 70 kilos (11 stone) that means about 35 g of protein a day. The average western diet serves up between 60 and 150 g of protein a day – far more than we need.

The countries with the highest consumption of protein per capita and the highest consumption of dairy products are where you find the highest incidence of hip fractures and osteoporosis. To prevent acidosis of the blood which is not only a major factor in osteoporosis but also in chronic fatigue, depression and many other negative conditions that women are frequently faced with, it can be useful to be aware of the foods that tend to be acid-forming, those that are relatively neutral and those which are alkaline-forming. Then you can choose your menus leaning heavily on the neutral and alkaline-forming foods.

Acid-forming	Neutral Foods	Alkaline-forming
alcohol	apples	bicarbonate of
artifical sweeteners	apricots	soda
beef	aubergines	blackberries
butter	bananas	broccoli
carob	beans – fresh and	celery
casein	dried	chicory
cheese	blueberries	cinnamon
chicken	buckwheat	diakon radish
chick pea	cauliflower	garlic
chocolate	carrots	ginseng
cocoa	cherries	grapefruit
coffee	courgettes	kohlrabi
corn	dates	lentils
fried foods	eggs – chicken,	limes
jam	duck	mangoes
ice-cream	figs	melon
lard	fish	mineral water
lobster	goats' cheese	miso
most medication	grapes	molasses
nuts	honey	mushrooms
oat bran	lemons	mustard greens
oils – hydrogenated	lettuce	nectarines
pasta	maple syrup	onions
peas	milk – cows, goat	papayas
pork	oatmeal	peppers
rye	organic flaxseed oil	potatoes
soy beans	organic olive oil	raspberries
soya milk	oranges	sea salt
sugar	peaches	sea vegetables
veal	pears	shitaki mushrooms
vinegar	pineapple	soy suace
	plums	sweet potatoes
	pumpkin	tangerines
	raisins	turnips
	rice – wild, brown	watermelon
	strawberries	yams
	turkey	yannoh

Eat More

- Fresh fruits eaten raw.

- Fresh green leafy vegetables, at least 50 per cent of which are eaten raw: broccoli, collards, kale, cabbage, mustard greens, Swiss chard, lambs' lettuce, rocket.

- Fresh green herbs.

- Legumes such as beans, peas, lentils, chick peas, etc.

- Whole grain breads, cereals, pasta and noodles – preferably two different varieties of grain a day, together with one pulse, which will give you all the essential amino acids you need even without meat. Steer clear of wheat if you suspect any sensitivity to it.

- Nuts, tofu, soya milk and other soya products including soy beans, free-range eggs, fish, free-range chicken and game, and seeds in moderation. Remember that it is not necessary to eat any animal products if you don't want to.

Eat Less

- Dairy products, except for butter in small quantities, including milk, cheese, cream and anything containing them. Natural live yogurt is something everyone needs to experiment with to find out if they are better off without it. Cut it out for a fortnight along with all other dairy products or anything containing them and examine how you feel.

- Refined foods such as white bread, white rice, white pasta and most breakfast cereals which are not only refined but riddled with sugar.

- Sugar

- Soy-based ersatz meat substitutes.

- Margarines, golden oils.

- Fried foods. Use only cold-pressed extra virgin olive oil or soya oil.

- Drink less coffee, tea or colas – and avoid cigarettes.

Bone Makers	Bone Breakers
Adequate magnesium	Processed convenience
Alfalfa and barley high in	foods, junk fats
minerals and trace	diuretics and antibiotics
elements	Crash dieting
Boron	Deficiencies in minerals and
Calcium in moderation	trace elements
(best from food sources)	Smoking
Leafy green vegetables	Soft drinks including diet
Moderate protein diet	colas
Organically grown wholefoods	Salt
Progesterone	High protein diet
Sea plants and green	High-fat diet
supplements – spirulina,	Sedentary lifestyle
green algae and chlorella	Coffee
Silicon	Antacids which contain
Soya-based foods	aluminium
Sunlight and vitamin D	Sugar
Vegetarian diet	Fluoride and chlorine in
Vitamin C which improves	drinking water
calcium absorption	Weight training
Whole grains	Too many dairy products
Zinc	Alcohol

Nutritional Support

Calcium The best source of calcium is not in supplements but in foods. Rarely is it necessary to take calcium supplements and you should never take calcium on its own. Instead change your diet so that you are getting calcium in foods, preferably not milk products. The ratio of calcium to magnesium is 8 to 1 in milk – far too high. When magnesium isn't absorbed in proper relation to calcium then the calcium does not end up in your bones. It is more likely to end up in inflammatory areas, causing tendonitis, carpel tunnel syndrome, arthritic spurs and extra calcium deposits around tendons. Doctors will be likely to call it arthritis or rheumatism and – because they have not been trained in nutrition – will not have the slightest clue that it is a calcium/magnesium imbalance.

Get your calcium instead from plants -- whole grains and vegetables, especially sea vegetables. Calcium is not in the roots; it is in the structure of a plant – the leaves, the stems and the stalks – and it is not at all difficult to get 600–800 milligrams of calcium a day from plant sources. Research suggests that the megadoses of calcium supplements which many women take may actually decrease bone strength and in animal studies has been shown to induce internal bleeding. A vegetarian or someone on a good moderate-in-protein diet needs only 500–600 mg of calcium a day. Eating good unprocessed foods makes it easy to get this amount, especially if you include sea plants in your menus. Calcium is found in good quantities in whole grains such as rye, wheat, millet, brown rice and quinoa, as well as pulses or legumes. These foods are also rich in magnesium. The thing to remember about calcium is that once you get it out of the stomach into the bloodstream you have to get it into the bones. This is where exercise comes in as well as adequate progesterone (or testosterone in the case of men). I have given a list of common foods and the amount of calcium each contains.

CALCIUM CONTENT OF FOOD AND DRINK

Vegetables	Calcium Per Cupful (Cooked)
beet greens	165 mg
broccoli	175 mg
Chinese leaves	125 mg
kale	180 mg
mustard greens	100 mg
pak choy	200 mg
parsley	122 mg
spinach	300 mg
turnip greens	250 mg
wild greens	350 mg

Pulses and Legumes	Calcium Per Cupful (Cooked)
black beans	135 mg
chick peas	150 mg
pinto beans	130 mg
soy beans	130 mg

Sea Vegetables	Calcium Per Cupful (Cooked)
agar agar (dry flakes)	400 mg
dulse	570 mg
hiziki	610 mg
kelp (kombu)	300 mg
wakame	520 mg

Mineral Water	Calcium Per Litre
Contrexéville	450 mg
Perrier	140 mg
San Pellegrine	200 mg

Nuts	Calcium Per Cup
almonds	300 mg
brazil nuts	260 mg
hazelnuts	282 mg

Soya Products	Calcium in 112 grams (4 oz)
tempeh	170 mg
tofu precipitated with calcium salts	300 mg
tofu soy-bean curd	100 mg

Other Foods	Calcium
blackstrap molasses	140 mg per tablespoon
spirulina	30 mg
tahini	120 mg per 14 g ($^1/_2$ oz)

In comparison:

Dairy Products	Calcium
cheese	200 mg per 25 grams (1 oz)
low-fat cheese	150 mg per cup
milk	300 mg per cup
non-fat yogurt	295 mg per cup
skimmed milk	285 mg per cup

While spinach also contains a good quantity of calcium, it is also high in oxalic acid which decreases calcium absorption and should not be relied on as a calcium source. If, for any reason, you decide to take some form of calcium supplement, choose a food-state calcium, chelated calcium or calcium citrate rather than the usual calcium carbonate or one of the other cheap versions which are not well absorbed. Also consider using betaine hydrochloride.

Hydrochloric Acid One of the major factors in ensuring you get enough calcium is adequate hydrochloric acid in the stomach. The plants containing calcium go into the stomach; to get the mineral from there into the bloodstream you need two things – plenty of hydrochloric acid and adequate B vitamins. If either is missing then this will stop the absorption of calcium, making it pass on through the colon and out of your body. This is important to know because many women as they get older don't produce enough hydrochloric acid in their stomachs to absorb calcium. An important question to ask yourself is, 'Are there foods that I used to be able to eat but now I can't?' If there is even the slightest indication that this may apply to you, it can be useful to take a supplement of hydrochloric acid – usually in the form of betaine hydrochloride. What many women don't realize is that a lot of indigestion comes not, as the advertisements would have us believe, from 'over-acidity' but rather from the lack of hydrochloric acid. John Lee tells an interesting story which illustrates this situation.

> One of the first patients I had with osteoporosis was in her seventies. She had come from a clinic and she wanted to be treated for osteoporosis because it was bad. They wanted to give her fluoride and she didn't want that. I tried the progesterone cream and the diet but in six months' time I could see no improvement. Then she said, 'I don't think I am absorbing the calcium.' I said, 'Why do you think that?' She said 'I've been taking those calcium pills and when I go to the bathroom I can see them in the toilet.' I said, 'Right, I don't think you're absorbing the calcium.' She said, 'Maybe if I took it as a liquid?' I said, 'No, that doesn't help, your not absorbing it means you are lacking either vitamin D or hydrochloric acid.' She was already taking vitamin B so I said, 'You have to take the hydrochloric acid.' She said, 'Oh, they're treating me for indigestion by giving me Tagamet and antacids.' They said her indigestion was from too much acid. I said, 'How old are you?'

She said, '74'. I said, 'No, your indigestion is from not *enough* acid, and you are not going to absorb the calcium unless you get some.' So I gave her some betaine hydrochloride and lo and behold those calcium flakes did not show up in the toilet any more. Her indigestion went away and her bone mineral density took off. Within three years she had gained 48 per cent new bone. I discovered then that, provided a woman has enough hydrochloric acid and eats a good diet, she will get all the calcium she needs from her foods.

Supplementing main meals with hydrochloric acid also improves the digestion of proteins and helps many people avoid indigestion and food sensitivities by protein foods not being broken down adequately in the stomach. (See Resources, p. 510.)

Magnesium Sixty per cent of the body's magnesium is contained within the bone. Although it makes up only 0.1 per cent of bone (compared to calcium's 20 per cent), magnesium is vital to good bone formation as it both increases the absorption of calcium from the foods we eat and also enhances its role in mineralizing bones. Magnesium helps convert vitamin D into its active form in the body and it also helps fix calcium into the bone tissue. There are over 300 enzymes known to require magnesium.

Foods high in magnesium include black-eyed peas, curry, almonds, whole grains and pulses, eggs, liver and green vegetables.

Vitamin D This vitamin is necessary in good quantity for the transportation of calcium and phosphorus into bone tissue. It also helps prevent too much calcium being lost in the urine. The best sources of vitamin D are natural sunlight which enables the body to synthesize the vitamin from exposure to sunlight and natural vitamin D found in fish oils.

Zinc This mineral is also essential in the formation of new bone and, like magnesium, it is processed out of our foods. Zinc deficiencies have now become so widespread that supplementing the diet with zinc appears to be important for many people. Zinc tends to be low in women with osteoporosis and in women who take calcium supplements. A co-catalyst for enzymes that change beta-carotene into vitamin A in the body's cells, zinc is essential for the formation of the collagen matrix on which both strong bones and healthy skin depend.

Vitamin C Another important player in the bone formation game, vitamin C is essential since the matrix to build bone with calcium cannot be made without vitamin C being present. Vitamin C levels decline as women age. They are also drastically reduced by exposure to pollutants in the air including cigarette smoke. A couple of extra grams of vitamin C each day can protect bones.

Silicon An important trace element in the formation of connective tissue, bone, cartilage, hair and nails, silicon also helps protect the body from some of the damage caused by aluminium in the system. Concentrated in sites of active calcification in the bones of the young, silicon is an unusual element. It is the second most widespread element in nature after oxygen. Silicon is enormously hard and has the ability to bind into tissues other minerals which are needed there. Silica is readily available in unprocessed vegetables, but hard to come by when eating processed foods or foods grown chemically. This is why supplements of silicon can be useful. It can also be taken in the form of horsetail tea (the plant which has the highest content of the trace element) and can do wonders for improving the state of nails, hair and skin.

Boron Only recently has boron, another trace element, been thought to be important as a nutrient. During the 1980s a number of studies indicated that boron may affect calcium, markedly reducing its urinary excretion (as well as that of magnesium). The presence of boron reduces calcium loss and increases the level of some of the oestrogens in the body. In one study of 12 postmenopausal women on a low-boron diet for 119 days, 3 mg of boron daily reduced their calcium excretion by an average 44 per cent and also increased their production of oestrogen. Boron also affects hormone levels in women and appears to help normalize them. Boron has been shown to improve the metabolism of calcium, phosphorus and magnesium, and aid the manufacture of vitamin D by the body. Alfalfa and kelp are good sources of boron as are some of the other seaweed foods.

Vitamin B6 Working together with magnesium, this member of the B complex vitamins is a co-catalyst for such a variety of enzymes in the body that it would be tedious to list them all. It supports the production of progesterone and helps minimize inflammatory reactions in connective tissue as well as encouraging the formation of important new collagen. A number of studies indicate that women with osteoporosis have low levels of this vitamin.

Dr John Lee's Typical Osteoporosis Treatment Programme

Diet	Leafy green and other vegetables emphasized. Avoid all 'sodas' and limit red meat to 3 or fewer times per week. Limit alcohol use.
Vitamin D	350–400 iu daily.
Vitamin C	2,000 mg per day in divided doses.
Beta-carotene	15 mg per day (equivalent to 25,000 iu of vitamin A).
Zinc	15–30 mg per day.
Calcium	800–1,000 mg per day by diet and/or supplements.
Magnesium	300 mg per day.
Oestrogen	Use in minimum doses 3 weeks/months only if needed for vaginal dryness. Do not use if contra-indicated for any reason.
Progesterone	Natural progesterone cream applied daily during the last two weeks of oestrogen use or 3 weeks/months if oestrogen not used. Use one jar per month initially for 3 months. Later half the amount per month may suffice, as determined by serial BMD tests.
Exercise	12–20 minutes daily, or $1/2$ hour 3 times a week.
No cigarettes	
Report any occurrence of vaginal bleeding	

From *Natural Progesterone* by John R. Lee, MD, BLL Publishing, Sebastapol, CA, USA, 1993

Typical Supplementation for Osteoporosis

- **Magnesium** 300–600 mg a day in divided doses as magnesium citrate or chelated magnesium.
- **Vitamin D** 350–400 iu a day.
- **Zinc** 15–20 mg a day as zinc citrate or picolinate.
- **Vitamin C** 2,000–4,000 mg a day in divided doses.
- **Silicon** Take as horsetail tea.
- **Boron** Take 2–8 mg a day.
- **Vitamin B6** 50 mg a day before bed.

In addition to Dr Lee's programme other experts in natural menopause suggest using 50 mg of B6 once or twice a day, spirulina either taken in tablet form (see Resources, p. 511) or in powder form stirred into a glass of juice or a cup of vegetable broth, and a cup of horsetail tea each day. Also eat plenty of seaweeds in salads, in soups and in vegetable dishes, since sea plants are rich in boron and trace elements and other micronutrients vital for flexibility and strength of bones. So are organically grown grains and vegetables and many sprouts including alfalfa.

Progesterone

Progesterone helps spur the osteoblasts to make new bone. The message which progesterone carries is 'make new bone'. Some pretty remarkable results have been reported from doctors who in the last 15 years have used progesterone creams. It has brought clinical relief of osteoporotic pain, stabilization of height loss, reduction in fracture incidence and improved density *regardless of age*, even in women who already have osteoporosis – in both women who have used progesterone cream alone and in those who have used small doses of oestrogen as well. When height has been lost as a result of crush fractures in the vertebrae, the pressure on the nerves is often alleviated with the use of progesterone cream and exercise. When you put a woman into a warm swimming pool up to her chest and let her walk, the buoyancy of the water takes the weight off the spine. Exercise like this can help the bones relocate themselves the micro-millimetre distance it takes to relieve pain. The nerves in the spine are very tough and hard to kill and space created where they arise can compensate for the pressure that has occurred. John Lee reports having seen women, with what looked on X-ray like total obliteration of the parameter where nerves emerge from the spine, who in time have been restored to pain-free normal states.

Because natural progesterone applied in cream form has so many other benefits and virtually no side-effects, it would seem unwise for a woman who has any indication of bone loss or who is concerned about preventing osteoporosis not to use it. (See Magnum Force, p. 425 for protocols.) The nutrients listed in this section are important for progesterone to be efficiently used by the body. It generally takes about three months for women who begin progesterone treatment to begin to experience the sense of wellbeing which generally accompanies it. If you have been diagnosed as osteoporotic then it is wise to have serial vertebral bone density studies done at intervals of six months to a year to monitor progress.

Bad Blood

Mounting xenoestrogenic pollution in our environment and widespread use of artificial hormones for birth control and HRT have produced an epidemic of female problems which develop out of a state of oestrogen dominance in a woman's body. It is this that is creating a need for progesterone supplementation. They have set the stage for the development of the *bad blood* plague of the late twentieth century we are experiencing. Here are some of the most common bad blood conditions now appearing in ever greater numbers.

Endometriosis

A mysterious and rapidly increasing condition of modern times in the westernized world, endometriosis is where the normal endometrium or uterine lining which develops each month during the follicle phase of the menstrual cycle, instead of breaking down and being shed fully with menstruation, proliferates inside the uterine cavity. Tiny islets of endometrial tissue can arise in or migrate to other areas of the pelvis, the fallopian tubes, the surface of the ovaries – even beyond occasionally – to the sides of the pelvic wall and occasionally on to the bowel. Endometriosis can be accompanied by pelvic pain, cramps, infertility and disturbed menstrual cycles. Pain is often worse at ovulation and during menstruation or just before a period begins. Although many women can experience endometrial build up without apparent symptoms, in others it results in painful intercourse because of the pressure, or pain when moving your bowels. The only sure way to diagnose the condition is via laparoscopy, although sometimes endometrial lesions can be seen during a pelvic examination on the vagina, vulva or cervix. Often endometriosis and fibroids are found together.

Because these endometrial islets are of the same endometrial tissue as found in the womb they swell and diminish with the ebb and flow of monthly hormones, then are shed at menstrual time, bringing pain in their wake. The incidence of endometriosis has increased dramatically in recent years, perhaps partly because women are giving birth later and having fewer children, and most probably because of widespread oestrogen dominance. For oestrogen is the hormone of proliferation – responsible for the build up of endometrial tissue. When it gets out of hand, endometriosis can be one of the results.

Common Treatment

The standard medical treatments for endometriosis include giving birth control pills in an attempt to artificially cycle the build up and sloughing of the womb lining, using a progestogen to suppress menstruation, prescribing analgesics and narcotics to kill the pain, or giving a GnRH agonist drug which acts directly on the pituitary to stop its cyclic hormonal secretions altogether – in effect rendering a woman menopausal so long as the drug continues to be given. Although they can relieve pain so long as you take them, GnRH agonists in common use do carry a number of potentially unpleasant side-effects, including the thinning of vaginal walls, hot flushes and osteoporosis. Other drugs such as danocrine sulphate, which is also commonly used for the treatment of endometriosis, can bring masculinization such as facial hair growth. None of these treatments have been shown to be very successful. Surgery is another standard treatment for endometriosis – either for the removal of the endometrial lesions themselves or, more radically, a complete hysterectomy as well as ovary removal. Since adequate progesterone inhibits the secretion of LH and FSH and therefore the proliferation of endometrial tissue, it is not surprising that a growing number of doctors, nutritionists and naturopaths prefer to recommend the cyclic use of natural progesterone so that the pain and menstrual flow are adequately reduced and the need for surgery eliminated.

Soul Searching

There are always complex interactions and imbalances between thoughts and feelings that affect a woman's immune system when endometriosis is present. Many women with the condition also show auto-immune characteristics such as having developed antibodies towards their own tissues which in turn disrupts reproduction.

Endometriosis is often called the 'career woman's' ailment. It is a way in which a woman's female power can be demanding her attention through pain or abnormal menstrual cycles – asking her to turn back from total absorption in the externals of her life and become more self-nurturing, self-examining, self-honouring. Listening to the symptoms you are experiencing is important, as is writing down whatever comes to you as you do so. This works best if it is done without paying much attention to what you are writing – just letting the words pour out of you. You may be surprised to find some of the impulses that get expressed and some of the desires. Honour what comes. Do you need more time alone? Do you need to allow yourself more freedom of self-expression in your work? Your relationships? Are you in need of self-care? Time off? Are you resting enough? What changes would you like to see in your life if anything were possible? Are you in any way living somebody else's values – your parents, your boss's, your family's – rather than your own? Do you feel helpless – a victim of your condition and your pain or do you conceive of the possibility that you can change your life?

Castor Oil Packs

Castor oil packs are an age-old remedy traditionally used to treat everything from colitis and peptic ulcers to arthritis and female problems – from back pains to fibroids, PMS and endometriosis. They work. Preliminary research at the George Washington School of Medicine in the United States has shown that they are likely to improve the functioning of the immune system. They are an excellent helper for endometriosis not only to alleviate discomfort but also to help speed recovery. Use at least three times a week, preferably every day.

What You Need

- Cotton or wool flannel cloth (can be a piece of an old sheet if necessary, but make sure there are no synthetics in the fabric).
- Plastic freezer bag or plastic sheet.
- Hot water bottle or electric heat pad.
- 2 safety pins.
- 150 g (6 oz) castor oil.
- Bath towel.

Prepare the flannel cloth by tearing and folding so that it is 2 to 4 thicknesses and, when folded, turns out to be about 25 cm (10 inches) wide and 30 cm (12 inches) long. Pour castor oil into the cloth so that it is saturated with the oil but not dripping. Whilst lying down, apply to the abdomen then lay the plastic bag or sheet over the soaked flannel. Put the hot water bottle or heating pad on top of that as warm as you can manage, then cover with the towel folded lengthwise over the whole area. You can leave a castor oil pack on all night if you can manage it. One hour is a minimum. While using the pack let your mind gently wander over questions such as those above and see what comes to you. Afterwards cleanse the skin using water to which a teaspoon of baking soda has been added. Provided it is kept clean, the soaked flannel can be used many times.

Wise Woman Ways

Two herbs are traditionally used with success in the treatment of endometriosis by wise women: raspberry leaves and Chastetree or *Vitex agnus castus* (Chinese variation is Man Jing Zi – *Vitex rotundifolia* or *Vitex trifolia*). They work well together.

Raspberry leaves Raspberry leaf tea is easy to make. Simply steep a tablespoon of the dried herb in a pint of hot (not quite boiling) water for five minutes and drink hot or cold throughout the day with a little honey if you like.

Chastetree *Vitex agnus castus* can be taken in the form of fresh powdered berries (3-4 capsules a day with food), made in tea form from the powdered berries or, easiest of all, taken in tincture form (15 drops in a little water two to three times a day).

Vitex, which has been used for two millennia, has a reputation for being virtually free of side-effects. It is rich in flavonoids and micronutrients. Although it contains no phytosterols itself, it is an enormously useful natural remedy for severe hot flushes that occur as a result of low levels of oestrogen. It can help eliminate flooding, spotting, irregular cycles, fibroids and endometriosis while balancing emotions, making skin clearer and improving vaginal dryness. It is also a great remedy for relieving hormonally related digestive distress from constipation to poor digestion. It also counters most of the usual PMS problems from headaches and depression to water retention and breast tenderness. *Agnus castus* is slow acting but profound in its effects, thanks to its ability to enhance certain hormones such as progesterone and leutotropic hormone and inhibit others such as follicle-stimulating hormone and prolactin. It can also increase your sense of emotional wellbeing as it has been shown to increase the production of the brain hormone dopamine. I first learned the virtues of *agnus castus* from Dr Dagmar Leichti von Brasch (see p. 142).

Important to remember *Agnus castus* is slow acting. Results begin to show in two or three months of daily use and can become permanent after a year – a botanic well worth persevering with.

Diet

Throw out the coffee, sugar, colas and dairy products. Cut out all milk and milk products. Throw out anything containing hydrogenated oils such as margarines, junk fats, cooking oils and convenience foods. Eliminate shellfish. Eat 50 per cent of your foods raw (see *The New Raw Energy* by Susannah and Leslie Kenton), especially fruits and vegetables, as well as making sure you eat plenty of high-fibre whole grains, lentils and beans. Avoid red meat; use organic tofu as a protein food. Use a green drink of chlorella, spirulina, green barley or wheatgrass in water or fresh vegetable juice daily.

Nutritional Support

- **Natural iron tonic** such as Floradix.
- **Good B complex vitamin**.
- **Vitamin B6** 50 mg three times a day for three to six weeks then 50 mg a day taken in the evening.
- **Pantothenic acid** 100 mg three times a day.
- **Vitamin C** in buffered form (calcium ascorbate) 2,000 mg three times a day.
- **Bioflavonoid complex** once a day.
- **GLA** (gamma linolenic acid) 2 x 500 mg capsules three times a day.
- **Magnesium Citrate or Chelated Magnesium** at least 200 mg, three times a day.

Progesterone

Used in the form of a cream rubbed on the skin twice a day or in oil or pellet form either sub-lingually or intra-vaginally from day 10 or 12 to day 26 of your menstrual cycle (see p. 425 for additional information). Says John Lee, 'I recommend that a woman increase the dose of the cream until she is satisfied her pelvic pains are decreasing. Once that dose is reached, a woman can continue for three to five years before gradually lowering it.' Lee finds that this regime decreases menstrual flow and gives the body time to heal the endometrial lesions. If the pains recur he advises women to continue the treatment until menopause. Lee has treated patients with mild to moderate endometriosis in this manner for the past thirteen years and none of them has ever had to resort to surgery.

Vary the sites to which you apply the cream – breasts, back, belly, face, neck, thighs. Progesterone oil can be useful when symptoms are severe since it contains more progesterone. To use the oil put 4 or 5 drops under the tongue and keep it in the mouth for at least five minutes without swallowing (this takes a bit of practice). Vaginally, you can drop the oil on your finger and then apply it to the walls of the vagina from where it is readily absorbed. Vaginal absorption is more efficient than sub-lingual. Increase or decrease the dosage of the oil or cream depending upon the severity of the symptoms and on how rapidly the cream is absorbed. Oral progesterone can also be prescribed by your doctor, usually in doses of between 50 and 200 mg a day. However, much of the hormone is wasted when taken orally because of first pass liver actions.

Fibroid Tumours

Fibroids are benign (non-cancerous) tumours of the uterus. They are whorls of tissue, very much like the tissue of the womb itself, that grow into unusual shapes which either lace the lining of the womb or are attached by a stump to its outer walls. Probably 50 per cent of women in the West have fibroids although most never know they are there. They are more common in black women than in white and if you are going to get them they usually develop in the 8 to 10 years before menopause when anovulatory menstruation and lowered progesterone levels occur most commonly. Fibroids can be tiny or can weigh as much as a newborn baby or more. (The biggest reported in medical history weighed 80 pounds!)

Only if fibroids cause trouble do doctors usually consider that they need to be removed. Many women with fibroids have no symptoms at all. Others experience menstrual cramps, pelvic pains, pressure on the bladder or rectum, a swollen belly, or extremely heavy periods, which can result in long-term fatigue and anaemia. When a woman's hormones are fluctuating wildly, as they can do in the years just before menopause or when she is under a lot of stress, fibroids can grow quickly, sometimes even causing haemorrhaging. Fibroids are responsible for a third of women's gynaecological problems and are the most common reason that hysterectomies are performed for they can often be hard to remove without taking out the womb. Occasionally fibroids are removed without taking out the uterus through an operation called a myomectomy, but this is generally only done when there is a single large fibroid present or when a woman is wanting to become pregnant, since the operation is difficult. Fibroids are *very* rarely cancerous.

Fibroids have a tendency to grow and shrink in size as a woman's hormone levels shift during monthly cycles. They are highly oestrogen dependent so are most prevalent in oestrogen-dominant women, particularly women who have not had children early on in life and are in their late thirties or forties. The good news is that once menopause arrives and oestrogen levels diminish sharply, fibroids shrink so small that often they can no longer be detected by pelvic examination. The presence of fibroids in a woman is usually confirmed by a sonogram or ultrasound since it can be difficult for a doctor to distinguish between an ovarian growth and a fibroid through pelvic examination alone.

Common Treatment

Until recently the best treatment for most fibroids – provided they are not creating too much discomfort in a woman – has been to watch and wait for menopause when they would go away, provided, of course, that a woman was not given oestrogen replacement. Now, doctors at the forefront of the natural menopause revolution urge women to make dietary changes and recommend the use of progesterone cream or oil. Sadly, the majority of doctors and surgeons, even those considered to be 'experts' in the gynaecological fields, continue, unnecessarily, to remove women's wombs.

Soul Searching

Many transpersonal psychologists and clairvoyant healers insist that fibroids are directly related to frustrated creative energy. In some women they almost seem a physical manifestation of plans, projects or dreams that have either outlived their usefulness or have not yet been brought to birth. Fibroids tend to develop when powerful creative energies have been truncated in some way or have been dissipated. Sometimes fibroids are linked with conflicts over whether or not to have a child or an intimate relationship. Sometimes they can appear to be the physical manifestation of hard, immovable anger or deep frustration.

Energy Medicine

Don't use an electric blanket. Help pelvic energy to flow via meditation for ten minutes twice a day. Visualize drawing life force down from the head and chest into the pelvis and vagina and flooding it with warmth and gentle light. Some women report benefit from spiritual healing, the laying on of hands healing or Reiki. Investigate energy medicine treatments from scalar wave generators or magnetic field therapy (see Alchemy of Energy, p. 185).

Take long Epsom salts baths regularly. Take 2 cups of household grade Epsom salts (available from the chemist), pour it into the bath and fill the bath with blood-heat water. Then immerse yourself for 20 to 30 minutes, topping up with warm water when necessary to maintain a comfortable temperature. Afterwards, lie down for 15 minutes or, better still, have an Epsom salts bath just before you go to bed.

Castor Oil Packs

Use three times a week or more when there is any discomfort, heavy bleeding, abdominal pressure or other symptoms (see p. 315–316).

Wise Woman Ways

Lady's mantle (*Alchemilla vulgaris*) tincture has long been used as a natural treatment for fibroids among herbalists. Also called lion's foot, this is one of the sacred plants among wise women. *Agnus castus* is also useful, as is a combination of mistletoe and butterbur.

Lady's Mantle Lady's mantle is said to carry magical properties offering support to any woman either entering the role of motherhood or leaving it. It is also good for excessive menstrual flow and flooding taken as a tea – 28 g (1 oz) of the herb to 570 ml (1 pint) of boiling water or, in tincture form, 10 to 25 drops several times a day. Lady's mantle is excellent for relieving headaches too.

Agnus Castus (*Vitex agnus castus*) Chastetree berries (see p. 316) are also good in tincture form: 10 to 20 drops 2 to 3 times a day. Both of these herbs are anti-oestrogenic in their actions. They can be profitably used together.

Mistletoe and Butterbur A combination of mistletoe (*Viscus album*) and butter bur (*Petesites hybridus*) is also one of the best herbal remedies for shrinking fibroids. It was developed by the Swiss physician Dr A. Vogel. When American pharmacist Lynne Walker gave it to six women with fibroid tumours in 1991 she found that within a week all the women reported that bleeding and other painful symptoms had decreased significantly. Before long two of the women found that their fibroids had reduced from the size of a grapefruit to that of a walnut. Soon after, the combination which Walker was using was taken off the market in the United States. The FDA refused to let it be sold because it apparently was not listed among the 'accepted' herbs there. Other doctors, naturopaths and wise women who have tried the combination are delighted with the results. It is available in most countries in the form of Petasan tincture made by Bioforce. Normal dosage is 10 to 20 drops, three times a day.

Diet

Whole grains are full of lignins (compounds which are anti-oestrogenic in their effects on the body). Eat plenty of rye, millet, soya products, oats, buckwheat, barley, corn and brown rice. Sprinkle 2 tablespoons of fresh flaxseed ground in a coffee grinder and sprinkled over porridge in the morning or over a salad. Reduce your fat intake to 15 to 20 per cent of your calories. Try to take 50 per cent of your foods raw (see *The New Raw Energy* by Susannah and Leslie Kenton). Avoid coffee, cocoa, chocolate or sugar and stay away from junk fats, from margarines to golden cooking oils, and from anything which contains trans-fatty acids. No junk foods or fried foods (see Order Out of Chaos, p. 161).

Nutritional Support

- **High potency B complex**.
- **Beta-carotene** 50,000 to 300,000 iu a day.
- **Zinc Picolinate or Zinc Citrate** 22–25 mg a day.
- **Vitamin C** 2,000 mg a day minimum.
- **Flaxseed oil** 3 capsules a day.
- **Vitamin E** 600 iu of d-alpha tocopherol a day.
- **Vitamin B6** 50 mg three times a day for a month, then twice a day for two weeks, then once a day.

Caution The Chinese herb Dong Quai or Tang Kuei (*Angelica sinensis*) which in general is excellent for many female problems should not be used if you have fibroids since it has been shown to increase their size in some women. Avoid oestrogen replacement since this, too, increases their growth.

Progesterone

Provided dietary changes are also made, when enough progesterone is supplied fibroid growth is arrested and frequently reversed. Good herbal support (see above) works well with both. Progesterone cream should be rubbed on different areas of the skin twice a day. It can also be used in oil form either sub-lingually or intra-vaginally from day 12 to day 26 of your menstrual cycle. Use enough cream so that you get through a jar during this two-week period, varying the sites to which you apply the cream – breasts, back, belly, face, neck and thighs. Progesterone oil can be particularly useful when symptoms are severe since it contains more progesterone (see p. 425).

Progesterone plays an important psychological-cum-spiritual role in women with fibroids by helping to soften the frustration or anger often associated with them so that these feelings can then be examined and life change more easily instigated. This is thanks to progesterone's role as a precursor to important brain chemicals and stress hormones.

My sister, Christi, is 41 years old. She suffered from fibroids and heavy bleeding for several years, and spent a fortune in New York going from doctor to doctor and test to test in an attempt to do something about them. She started using progesterone cream and then, after a month, added the oil too. She discovered that her fibroids shrank progressively so that in two months she was completely free of the pain which she had had for two years, as well as of the heavy bleeding. Delighted though she was to be free of both, in many ways the psychological and energetic effects of the natural progesterone meant even more to her. Not only did she experience a return of energy and enthusiasm for life that had been missing for years, she reported: 'For five years I have felt oppressed by the universe. Now I feel as though the universe is supporting me. At least I am no longer a victim. I feel I can do whatever I want.' Her experience is a good example of how physical change through diet, herbal supplements and natural progesterone can help shift long-standing psychological or spiritual blockages as well. It is always worthwhile to have your doctor monitor the results of such natural treatment by way of regular ultrasound scans or sonogram tests three or four times a year to verify shrinkage.

Vaginal Irritation, Dryness and Thinning

Some women at menopause experience a thinning of the vaginal tissues which can lead to irritation and in a few cases to repeated urinary infections. The lining of the vagina is a cornified epithelium which makes it strong and resilient. After menopause some women shed the outer layers of this cornified epithelium so that their vagina walls become thinner, have less protection and can more easily become irritated, causing dryness, itching and pain during intercourse. In some women an increase in the normally low pH of the vagina makes it more susceptible to bacterial infection. This thinning of the walls of the vagina and the things which can accompany it – referred to by the medical experts as *atrophic vaginitis* or *vulval dystrophy* – is by no means inevitable. Many women, especially those who are physically active and have active sex lives of any sort which brings regular stimulation to genital tissues, never experience it at all. Others have had to handle a tendency to dryness since their twenties.

Soul Searching

Forget the feeling that you are somehow odd or incapable of enjoying intercourse or that this is the inevitable consequence of growing old. Vaginal thinning, which is a natural part of lowered oestrogen levels in menopausal women, can be simple to counter without ever having to resort to potentially dangerous hormone drugs. So just in case you have been feeling bad about yourself or timid, lay those feelings aside and do something about it. Your body will thank you for the renewed sense of comfort. If you have been leading a celibate life and suddenly find yourself in the embrace of a lover, it is important to be gentle with your body. It has been in a kind of sexual hibernation so give it time to thaw out. Also make sure that you never force intercourse before your vagina is ready for it – and this means before your soul is ready for it. Vaginal moistness and receptivity depend on arousal and, despite what all those Hollywood movies with people continually surrendering themselves to passionate embraces would have us believe, arousal is a soul-centred activity not a mechanical response to external stimuli. Regular sex itself keeps the vagina plump and healthy.

Wise Woman Ways

Stay away from soaps, bubble baths, shower gels, and nylon tights or underwear, since all of these things can make this condition worse. There are several botanicals which are great to treat it: motherwort, chastetree taken internally, and calendula, aloe vera and comfrey used externally. They can also help prevent recurrent vaginal and bladder infections.

Motherwort Taken as a tincture, 15 to 20 drops in a glass of water several times a day, motherwort is an excellent way of restoring thickness to vaginal tissues when it has been lost and of remoisturizing the vagina (see also p. 353).

Chastetree A tincture of this berry enhances many hormones in a woman's body including progesterone and luteinizing hormone. Although it was used in the Middle Ages to calm the lascivious thoughts of celibate monks (hence its name), it has a powerful stimulating effect on women's libido taken over a few months. It is also excellent for bringing moisture and circulation to vaginal tissues when they are hungry for them (see also p. 359).

Calendula This herb in a good cream base (see Resources, p. 508) can help soften yet toughen vaginal tissues and tissues of the vulva. It can also relieve itching when applied three times a day and helps protect against infection.

Comfrey In a cream base (see Resources, p. 508) comfrey is the best soother of all for itchy vaginal tissue. It can be applied both externally and internally to foster the growth of healthy new epithelial cells in the vagina. It can also be used as a lubricant instead of the usual Vaseline or KY jelly during intercourse. Use it three times a day for three months and you may never need to use it again.

Aloe Vera Pure aloe vera juice is useful when vaginal tissues have become hot, dry and uncomfortable. Simply wipe it on several times a day.

Cesium Gel This is the *pièce de résistance* when it comes to rejuvenating vaginal tissues. When Dr Zhen Lin at Jishuitan Hospital in Beijing in 1975 made an important discovery about acupuncture, little did he know it would have powerful implications for regenerating tissue. This esteemed Chinese surgeon discovered that stimulation of acupuncture points by needle, finger pressure, magnetic fields or the burning of a traditional herb (moxabustion) had a positive effect on the body because they triggered activity of one particular enzyme at the point treated – acetylcholinesterase. This enzyme acts on the neurotransmitter acetylcholine creating a stimulation through the nervous system, in effect heightening 'aliveness' in that area at a molecular level. A year later Zhen began his hunt for a completely safe-to-use substance which would have a strong acetylcholinesterase-releasing effect that could be put directly on skin. He found it in cesium salts. He began treating various diseases with solutions, creams and plasters soaked in these mineral salts and found that many were either cured or dramatically improved – everything from sprains and stuffy noses to primary hypertension, asthmatic bronchitis and trigeminal neuralgia. He even used cesium plasters to prevent the pain of cervical dilatation during abortion. A light colourless gel containing cesium salts was developed by Beth Jacobs. You can apply it to encourage the healing of cuts, acne, sores, burns and other skin problems (as well as banishing the pain of injuries and muscles in spasm) and it has remarkable skin-rejuvenating properties when you put it on clean skin twice a day before applying moisturizers or treatment creams. It is also excellent rubbed on the vulva and in the vagina three times a day as an energy treatment for vaginal thinning. It affects not only superficial tissue on which it is applied but at a much deeper level as well. Cesium gel is also useful during intercourse when extra lubrication is needed or to heighten pleasure.

Natural Oestrogen Cream

There is a very good natural oestrogen cream which can be ordered from the United States (see Resources, p. 506). High in the safe natural oestrogen oestriol (E3), it can be used sparingly on vaginal tissues and tissues of the vulva. Usually an application of as little as a $^1/4$ of a teaspoon two times a week is enough to remoisturize and thicken vaginal walls.

Pre-Menstrual Syndrome

PMS is a very big problem. Today somewhere between 40 and 60 per cent of menstruating women in the western world suffer to some degree from premenstrual syndrome. There are no specific laboratory tests for PMS. Neither are there specific clinical signs for the condition, which is why it is called a *syndrome* – a symptom complex appear to have one specific cause. Each month PMS usually comes on after ovulation and before menses. Women with PMS can experience symptoms (from bloating and depression to mood swings, headaches, weight gain, irritability, fatigue and lack of interest in sex) which begin a week or more before a period starts and usually decline dramatically within 24 hours of menstrual onset. The common symptoms associated with PMS are included in the chart on page 328.

COMMON SYMPTOMS ASSOCIATED WITH PMS

Psycho-Energetic	Neurological-Digestive	Respiratory-Skin	Oedema-Reproductive
chronic fatigue	migraine	sinusitis	weight gain
irritability	epilepsy	chest infections	swollen extremities
mood swings	dizziness	runny/blocked nose	tender breasts
weeping	diarrhoea	bronchitis	abdominal bloating
sudden anger	fainting spells	asthma	period pains
depression	headaches	skin rashes	lowered libido
drug abuse	flatulence	acne	joint/muscle pain
alcohol abuse	poor digestion	conjunctivitis	
attempted suicide	constipation	thinning hair	
lethargy	backache	soft/brittle nails	
insomnia	palpitations	tonsillitis	
cravings	herpes	dry skin	
food binges			

Dr Guy Abraham, former Clinical Professor of Obstetrics and Gynaecology at the University of California in Los Angeles, has done more to study the physical causes and treatments for premenstrual syndrome than anyone else in the English-speaking world. He categorizes premenstrual syndrome into four types. Type A, he says, is accompanied by anxiety, mood swings and irritability. Type C is accompanied by sugar cravings, headaches and fatigue; Type H by bloating, breast tenderness and weight gain; Type D by depression, memory loss and confusion. Other experts such as Dr Susan Lark, author of *Premenstrual Syndrome Self-Help Book*, have identified two other common sub-groups: the first in which women experience acne, pimples and oily skin and hair; and the second in which women experience dysmenorrhoea with cramps, low back pain and nausea.

Soul Searching

The causes of PMS are many: some nutritional, some psychological or stress-related. Even a woman's attitude towards menstruation has a part to play in the development of PMS. In our culture menstruation has long been associated with the work of the devil. It is often called the curse. The whole cycling in a woman's body involving the build-up and flow of blood has been treated as humiliating rather than inspiring a sense of awe at the magnificence of its complexity and power for bringing to birth new life. This has created a situation where literally millions of women have never experienced the miracle of inheriting a female body with its finely balanced hormonal system. They grow up fearing that there is something diseased and unclean about their body or even that somehow they are being punished by God. Instead of the period of menstruation itself being an exciting time of heightened emotion, creativity and personal drive, it turns into a period of suffering. In the last 50 years women have been stuffed with thyroid supplements, prescribed tranquillizers and given psychiatric counselling, all in an attempt to help them handle PMS.

Exercise is important for PMS not only because of the biochemical and physiological benefits that regular exercise bring a woman's body but also because regular exercise can enhance self-esteem and help a woman experience a sense of *living in her body*, thereby erasing the old patterns of feeling a victim who goes through monthly suffering. Menstruation is a woman's time to celebrate mysterious female power – the dark moon phase of a woman's monthly life during which she is said to be able to touch the greatest mystery of all. Nothing should be allowed to interfere with that.

Wise Woman Ways

There are a number of botanicals and herbs which bring potent medicine to a woman wrestling with PMS. Some of the best botanicals are motherwort, wild yam (either *Dioscorea villosa* or *Dioscorea mexicana*), black cohosh and Dong Quai (see also pp. 349–364).

Motherwort My favourite plant of all for PMS – particularly for the emotional ups and downs – is motherwort. Ten to 25 drops of tincture of motherwort works wonders when you are feeling unsettled. Alternatively you can take 5 to 15 drops of the tincture every day for a month or two to stabilize emotions long-term. Motherwort is the most comforting herb I have ever come across. It brings a sense of inner security and calm strength. It is also strengthening to the heart and tends to enhance courage and self-esteem.

Wild Yam The most effective single botanical for PMS for most women is wild yam, from which so many hormones are derived. Taking 3 grams of powdered wild yam a day, split into two doses, works so well on many women that, unless they are seriously oestrogen dominant and anovulatory, this course of action – together with changes in diet and lifestyle – is often enough to banish the condition permanently. And the nice thing about using wild yam is that after taking it for three to six months, many women find they can stop using it altogether without a return of symptoms (see also p. 362).

Dandelion Root Ten to 20 drops of tincture of dandelion root three times a day with meals usually works for eliminating water retention.

St John's Wort Oil of St John's Wort rubbed on to sore breasts relieves pain thanks to its action on nerve endings.

Yellow Dock Root Tincture of yellow dock root – 5 to 10 drops two or three times a day – can help counter indigestion, constipation and intestinal gas.

Sage Drinking sage tea or taking tincture of sage (10–20 drops three times a day) which is rich in phyto-sterols can help counteract PMS.

The Light Factor

Full-spectrum lighting, such as that which you get in broad sunlight, is important in the treatment and avoidance of PMS, as it is in a woman's hormonal health after menopause. Some experts in light therapy suggest that sleeping with a 100 watt bulb in a bedside lamp from day 14 to day 17 of a woman's menstrual cycle for six months can help regulate periods. Many studies show that exposure to lighting in the form of overhead lights or light boxes which emit full-spectrum light can vastly improve PMS, as well as lift depression and aid a woman's hormonal functions in menopause and beyond. I have used full-spectrum lights and light boxes for the past two years with excellent results. I find I can work far longer without fatigue than I could before and find I no longer suffer from 'February Blues' as a result of long dark winter nights. It works through the stimulating effect which full-spectrum light has on the pineal gland, stimulating the production of melatonin during the hours of darkness which follow. This kind of lighting equipment, which was originally developed to counteract Seasonal Affective Disorder or SAD, needs to be used for only an hour or two a day to work its magic.

Diet

Excessive consumption of animal fat, which triggers an increase in the hormone prostaglandin, also increases oestrogen levels and decreases progesterone levels, thus contributing to PMS. Vegetarians who live on a low-fat and high-fibre diet excrete two or three times more oestrogen in their faeces than meat eaters. They also have 50 per cent less unconjugated oestrogens in their blood than non-vegetarians and much less PMS as a consequence. Studies show that PMS patients consume on average 62 per cent more refined carbohydrates, 275 per cent more refined sugar, 78 per cent more salt, 79 per cent more dairy products, 53 per cent less iron, 77 per cent less manganese and 52 per cent less zinc than do women without PMS. They are also lower in B complex vitamins than normal women. When it comes to eliminating PMS, initiating the dietary changes suggested in previous chapters is instrumental in making deep shifts in metabolism and energy that help make it a thing of the past. Dr Tori Hudson, Academic Dean at the Natural College of Naturopathic Medicine in Portland, Oregon, in the United States, recommends that a diet to protect women from PMS should include fresh vegetables and fruit, whole grains, legumes, nuts, seeds and fish, and avoid all refined sugars, large quantities of protein, all dairy products, free fats, salt, caffeine and tobacco. Another major item to avoid at all costs is junk fats – salad oils, margarines and convenience foods filled with processed trans-fatty acids. These, more than any other single dietary item, interfere with hormonal functions (see Order Out of Chaos).

Causes of PMS

- Poor nutrition.
- High-fat diet.
- Too much calcium and too little magnesium.
- Deficiency of some vitamins such as B6.
- Low levels of progesterone.
- High levels of oestrogen.
- Poor thyroid function.
- Poor adrenal functions.
- Diet high in junk fats.

Using a simple detoxification programme based on fresh foods every four to six months, such as my *10 Day Clean-Up Plan*, or the Miso Detox and Rebuild (see Resurrection, p. 365), can clear away the accumulation of wastes that builds up to interfere with enzyme actions and metabolic processes which are responsible for the proper functioning of the reproductive system. Even a day or two a month on miso broth and seaweed in the premenstrual period helps to cleanse the system and remineralize the body.

Nutritional Support

No nutritional supplement is going to replace a proper diet and lifestyle. However, certain supplements, especially magnesium, zinc, vitamin B6 and the other B vitamins which play important parts in enzyme reactions related to the production, metabolism and elimination of hormones, can be instrumental in clearing PMS and need to be looked at. In an uncontrolled study where women with PMS were given a multivitamin and mineral supplement containing high doses of magnesium and B6, 70 per cent of them showed a reduction in symptoms (see also The Professionals, p. 404).

Magnesium Magnesium is an essential catalyst in many enzyme reactions, particularly those involved in energy production and sugar metabolism. A deficiency in magnesium appears to be a strong causative factor in the development of PMS. Low magnesium often produces symptoms of aches and pains as well as nervousness, lowered immunity, breast pain and weight gain.

Vitamin B6 The liver needs B complex vitamins, especially B6, to break down and deactivate oestrogen in the body. Many studies have shown that vitamin B6 supplements are useful in treating PMS. In one double blind cross-over study 84 per cent of women reported a lowering of symptoms during the period of treatment with B6. In another study, the incidence of acne was reduced by 72 per cent when women were given a supplement of 50 mg of B6 daily for a week before and during the menstrual period. Vitamin B6 is best taken with a high B complex supplement.

Zinc Zinc is another important co-factor in many enzyme reactions related to reproduction, foetal development, sexual functions, fertility and mental alertness. Zinc deficiencies are common in women who have taken synthetic hormones in oral contraceptives and HRT. Coffee and tea drinking interfere with zinc absorption.

Vitamin E The fat-soluble vitamin E oxygenates tissue and protects unsaturated fatty acids, sex hormones and other fat-soluble vitamins from oxidation. Most of the research into the beneficial effects of vitamin E on PMS has centred around mastalgia. However, double-blind studies show that women given vitamin E supplements experience significant improvement in other PMS symptoms as well, including headaches, tiredness, depression, insomnia and nervous tension.

Beta-carotene Precursor to vitamin A, beta-carotene is a safe alternative to vitamin A. But it is best not to take common synthetic supplements. Look for naturally derived beta-carotene. In doses of 100,000 to 300,000 iu per day it has been shown to reduce PMS symptoms in the luteal phase of the menstrual cycle. In animal studies vitamin A has been shown to support the activities of the corpus luteum which produces progesterone. Beta-carotene is believed to be converted into vitamin A when needed by the corpus luteum.

Vitamin B Complex B complex deficiencies result in depressed liver functions. Much PMS develops out of an excess of oestrogens in the blood that results from the liver's inability to clear oestrogens from the system. As far back as the 1940s researchers remarked that there is a relationship between B complex deficiency and menorrhagia, cystic mastitis and menorrhagia as well as PMS. Supplements of B complex vitamins have been shown to help clear these problems.

Bioflavonoids Substances such as quercetin and apigenin act in the body to inhibit oestrogen synthesis and have been shown to be useful in eliminating many symptoms of PMS.

Essential Fatty Acids To manufacture and metabolize hormones properly essential fatty acids – especially linoleic acid and gamma linolenic acid (GLA) – are necessary. The proper metabolism of essential fatty acids demands adequate magnesium, vitamin C, zinc, vitamin B6 and vitamin B3. This is a major reason why all of these nutrients are so important in the treatment of PMS. When the body's enzymes are working properly and the diet is not full of trans-fatty acids from junk fats, it can convert linolenic acid into GLA. In many women with PMS, because of poor diet usually over many years, this conversion is difficult if not impossible for their bodies to carry out. Using borage oil or starflower oil, blackcurrant oil or evening primrose oil supplements which are all high in GLA will bypass this conversion and can be very helpful for PMS in many women.

Typical Supplementation for PMS

- **Vitamin B complex** 25–50 mg of major B complex vitamins a day.
- **Vitamin C** 1–2 grams a day.
- **Vitamin E** 200–400 iu a day.
- **Bioflavonoids** Mixed flavonoids – 1,000 mg a day.
- **Beta-carotene** Equivalent of 50,000 iu a day.
- **Magnesium** 400–800 mg chelated magnesium a day in split doses.
- **Zinc** 18–22 mg chelated zinc or zinc picolinate a day, preferably at night.

- **Linseed or Flaxseed Oil** 1–2 tablespoons of cold pressed refrigerated oil a day on salads or 4 capsules (see Resources, p. 508).
- **GLA, borage oil, starflower oil, blackcurrant oil or evening primrose oil**: 500 mg, 3 to 4 times a day.

Progesterone

Underlying all PMS, whether primarily nutritional, emotional or stress-related in origin, is an imbalance in hormones. In most PMS the imbalance in hormones is a simple one – too much oestrogen and too little progesterone. While this is not the case for *every* woman, it is certainly what happens in the vast majority of cases regardless of which PMS 'group' her symptoms place her. Many of the common treatments for PMS, from the use of extra vitamin B6 to changes in diet, actually work because through one action or another they are able to influence hormone balance. Levels of progesterone lower than they should be in the second half of the menstrual cycle – the luteal phase – can cause the hypothalamic centre to become hyperactive increasing the production of LH and FSH and create many symptoms associated with PMS.

The swelling which occurs near a menstrual period is not simple extracellular oedema. It is *intracellular* where water actually gets blocked within cells. This can mean as much as a six or eight pound weight gain over the course of ten days just before menstruation. In women who experience such weight gain the use of a progesterone cream for three months from day 12 to day 26 or day 27 of their menstrual cycle will almost invariably clear this up. After several weeks of using the cream, John Lee suggests that women weigh themselves during the time of the month that the oedema was always there. 'When a woman sees that the oedema that has always been there is now gone,' says Lee, 'it proves to her that the progesterone is working.' After using progesterone cream Lee's patients reported that they felt much better, that they felt they had a handle on their life again, and that they could get on with things without the disturbing effects of their PMS. 'Not all PMS is due to progesterone deficiency or oestrogen dominance,' says Lee, 'but a large proportion of PMS women have oestrogen dominance and are helped by progesterone.'

Biochemist Ray Peat used transdermal progesterone therapy on 200 women who were suffering from a wide range of PMS symptoms from migraine, depression and acne to lethargy, mastalgia and oedema. He discovered that almost all the women treated were able to determine for themselves the appropriate dose to control their symptoms. He also found that a few women needed thyroid supplementation to shed excess fat from their bodies as well as using progesterone cream. British physician Barry Durrant-Peatfield frequently combines progesterone with thyroid treatment when appropriate with good results. One of the interesting things Peat reported was that many women have difficulty at first grasping how a condition such as PMS which is hormonal in nature can be cleared using a hormone.

Another expert in PMS is Joel Hargrove MD, Director of the PMS and Menopause Clinic at Vanderbilt University in the United States. Hargrove, too, is an advocate of natural progesterone. Unlike Lee, he uses it orally, prescribing much higher doses of the steroid since progesterone taken by mouth is largely destroyed in the liver before it can reach the bloodstream. Hargrove gave progesterone in doses of 500–800–1,000 mg a day orally to several thousand women whom he studied for twelve years. He reported a 94 per cent success rate. A jar of progesterone cream contains only about 900 mg of progesterone. If that is used over the course of the month you are most likely to take in 30–60 mg a day and probably only absorb 15–25 mg. However, that's usually sufficient to establish balance. If you are packing the use of the cream into a 10- to 12-day timetable, then you will be receiving some pretty good levels. 'This is magic stuff for PMS,' says Lee, 'I don't say 94 per cent, maybe 80 or 90 per cent. That is pretty darned good for PMS. And you don't have to use diuretics and tranquillizers and pep pills – which neither I nor my patients were ever happy with.' Lee suggests that women using a progesterone cream can best monitor themselves. 'If they feel the PMS getting worse on a certain day they should just apply more,' he says. 'It is unnecessary to pick the dose exactly. It usually picks itself through the woman using it. It is also usually best rising progressively in the ten days before a period.'

Here are some of John Lee's protocols for PMS.

Use a jar of cream in a ten-day period, ending just before expected menses. With experience many women discover that the progesterone dose can be applied in a manner to produce a *crescendo* effect in the 4 to 5 days just before menstruation begins. In fact some women prefer to add the use of sub-lingual drops during the last 4 to 5 days in addition to the transdermal progesterone in the cream. Others find that additional cream can be applied several times a day close to a period, depending on their symptoms. 'The important thing to remember about dose', says Lee, 'is that the right dose of progesterone for any particular woman is the dose that works.' The way Lee achieves the crescendo dose is for a woman to use a full jar in 10 or 12 days from days 14 to 26, or days 12 to 28, aiming to have finished the jar two days before the period. In the last five days Lee adds four drops of progesterone oil sub-lingually to create the crescendo effect. You can also use progesterone in the form of sub-lingual pellets or granules which most women find easier to manage. Taking progesterone sub-lingually is a little tricky to get used to as the oil has to be held under the tongue for three to five minutes to allow it to be properly absorbed through the mucous membranes of the mouth. It often takes practice to hold the oil there for long enough without swallowing.

Never Come Morning

Insomnia is one of women's greatest fears. Eight times more women report sleep difficulties to their doctors throughout their lives than do men. Apart from the motherhood-induced insomnia which comes from having to feed a baby, if ever you are going to have trouble sleeping it is most likely to be during the perimenopausal years, just before your periods stop, or much later on in your seventies and eighties. People sleep less as they get older for a number of reasons not the least of which is a decrease in the production of a substance called melatonin which regulates the body's circadian rhythms (see p. 343). Hot flushes and night sweats can interfere with sleep, too, and taking action to ease them (see Field and Forest p. 346) is often enough to make you sleep blissfully through the night.

Sleep patterns vary tremendously from person to person. Some women need only four or five hours a night while others need eight or nine. Short sleepers are often more outgoing, contented and lively than their long-sleeping sisters who may get as much as 10 hours a night. Studies show that long sleepers tend to worry more, be more introverted and anxious. How much sleep you need can change depending on your life circumstances. When you are pregnant, eat less wholesome foods, or are under stress or ill you may need more sleep. You need more sleep when you gain weight. When losing weight or during a detoxification regime you will often sleep less.

The sleeplessness that occurs in women around the time of menopause and in the few years just before is most usually not a difficulty in going to sleep but a tendency to awaken regularly at the same time each night (usually 2 or 3 in the morning) and to lie in bed wide awake. Because we are accustomed to sleeping through the night, we assume that there must be something wrong. Yet sleeplessness can sometimes bring new insights, if you are ready to receive them. Many artists, writers and composers will tell you that they receive inspiration for new projects and discover ways of overcoming creative challenges on awakening in the night.

Common Treatment

That being said, when sleeplessness becomes chronic it can leave you feeling exhausted, hopeless and washed out. Sleeping pills are not the answer. Their side-effects include digestive problems, poor concentration, disorders of the blood and respiration, high blood pressure, liver and kidney troubles, problems with vision, depression, dizziness, confusion and damage to the central nervous system. Using them can even lead to worse insomnia. There are better ways.

Soul Searching

Native Americans refer to the unseen world of inspiration, myth, spirit helpers, animal helpers and magic as *dreamtime*. They insist that once a woman claims her own right to the transformation of menopause by embracing her power and learning to hold her wise blood within her body, then the magic implicit in dreamtime becomes present to do her bidding and sleep comes at her command. But this, they say, does not happen until she has passed through the energetic chaos which is part of the transformative journey – chaos which can manifest as flushes of hot and cold, surges of energy, waves of fatigue and powerful emotions. These are all part of the transition from the ordinary world of the childbearing woman to the extraordinary realm of the young crone.

One of the most wonderful experiences for a menopausal woman is that of letting go of all time constraints and freewheeling. If you can manage it, take a weekend or even a week away from all responsibility either by staying at home alone or by going on a retreat (see Resources, p. 503–504) so you can sleep whenever you like. Freed from the bonds of time you can nap at any time of the day or night and heed any creative impulses that arise. Forget your watch, don't watch television or listen to the radio. See what it is like to move away from the restrictions of outward time and to align yourself with the times of the earth, the sun and the moon as well as your own internal rhythms. It can have a remarkable effect both on your creativity and also on eliminating once and for all the feeling of being trapped in time and full of anxiety if you don't sleep as much as you think you should.

A Breath of Medicine

When sleeplessness arises out of anxiety or brings worries in its wake it can be useful to shift the focus of your energy towards the breath using one of the most simple yet powerful techniques I know from yogic breathing. Practise it first when you are relaxed so you know it well. Call on it during sleepless nights to transform your anxious energy into calm and at any time during the day when you may feel worried or a sense of panic comes on about anything.

Sitting straight in a chair or with your legs crossed on a cushion on the floor – once you get the hang of it you can do this exercise lying down as well – place the tip of your tongue on the ridge on your pallet just behind your front teeth. Keep it there during the whole of the exercise. Breathe out completely through your mouth, pursing your lips a bit if necessary, and letting the air move out around your tongue (it makes a soft whooshing sound). Now you are ready to begin.

- Close your mouth and silently inhale through the nose to a count of four.
- Hold your breath to a count of seven.
- Now exhale fully through your mouth again, making a whoosh sound as you do so to a count of eight.
- Repeat the whole of the above four times.

The inbreath is taken silently through the nose with the mouth closed and the outbreath, which takes twice as long, is made through the slightly opened mouth. How much time you spend on each phase of the breath is up to you. In the beginning it is likely to be faster and later on, when you have used the exercise a lot, it is likely to slow down a great deal. This really does not matter. What is important is that you maintain the same 4:7:8 ratio during the whole exercise and that your tongue remains on the ridge just behind your upper teeth. The reason for the tongue placement is that according to yogic theory there are two kinds of energy in the human body – positive and negative nerve currents – one being solar and the other lunar. They begin and end at this spot behind the upper front teeth and at the tip of the tongue. By putting the two together you are completing a circuit that enables you to hold the power of breath energy within your body rather than letting it dissipate, thus restoring balance and serene wellbeing.

This is a marvellous exercise which brings about an instantaneous shift of consciousness after only four breaths. After you have learned it and used it for a few weeks, extend from four to eight breaths for even deeper calming effects. This is not a good idea until you know it well since it might make you slightly light-headed. Use it whenever anything disturbing happens in your life.

Wise Woman Ways

There are some excellent helpers from the 'plant people' which various wise women have taught me to use. Each has its own spirit and character. Some will work better for you than others.

Valerian This is the root of the plant *Valeriana officinalis* which was the primary herbal sedative used on both sides of the Atlantic before the advent of barbiturate sleeping pills. It is a safe and well-tested herbal remedy with a smell like dirty old socks (the smell drives some people's cats wild). Don't let that put you off since valerian is a powerful and useful tool for inducing safe sleep – more potent than most of the other natural tranquillizers such as hops or skullcap or chamomile.

You can taken valerian in two ways but I like the tincture best: 10 to 20 drops in a little water before bedtime or in the middle of the night when you awaken. Alternatively, you can use a couple of capsules of the dried root. Valerian in lower doses is also useful when your nerves feel 'shot' during the day. Very occasionally valerian will be too strong for a particular woman so that she awakens with the sense of a slight hangover in the morning. If this applies to you, either cut down on the dose or try another milder remedy. In any case it is a good idea to change remedies every so often so your body doesn't become accustomed to one, rendering it ineffectual.

Passion Flower (*Passiflora incarnata*), also known as Maypops, is a climbing plant that boasts magnificent white flowers with a purple centre. It has a wonderful sedative and mildly narcotic effect on the body. Passion flower is most useful for women who wrestle frequently with nervous tension and particularly helpful when nerves seem to be edgy before and around the time of menopause. It is also useful for relieving pain, thanks to its mild analgesic and anti-spasmodic qualities, all of which have been well demonstrated in laboratory and clinical tests. Passion flower can also be useful for a woman troubled with PMS. It is not as strong as valerian in its actions, is more calming than sedating and as such is a great alternative to tranquillizer drugs. Use 10 to 20 drops of the tincture or the same amount of the liquid extract in water. Alternatively, take two capsules of the dried extract up to four times a day as needed. Where you might take valerian at night just before going to bed, the best results from passion flower often come from taking it during the day to calm nerves and make everything easier and less stressful.

Chamomile Tea (*Matricaria chamomilla*) was one of the nine herbs sacred to the Anglo-Saxon god Wotan. Chamomile was also much loved by the Romans. Its name *Matricaria* is derived either from the Latin word *mater* meaning mother or from *matrix* meaning womb. For thousands of years it has been used as a woman's herb to help painful menstruation, to calm anxiety and aid sleep – even to help build strong bones, since it contains a form of readily absorbed calcium. Chamomile is also a uterine tonic – something else which has been scientifically evaluated. It boasts many other therapeutic properties such as being anti-bacterial in its actions and good for skin. The easiest way to take chamomile is in the form of a tisane or tea. Infuse 5 to 10 grams of the dried flowers in hot water before bedtime or whenever you need to relax. Chamomile works particularly well when taken together with passion flower.

Hops (*Humulus lupulus*) The flowers from this British herb are often used together with other remedies to treat everything from indigestion to calming nerves. Like valerian, hops have a pronounced sedative effect but are milder. Unlike valerian, hops smell sweet and can be used without concern for side-effects. You can use hops in the form of a tincture but, particularly for women who are awakened in the middle of the night and have trouble going back to sleep, it is good to drink hop tea which you make before going to bed by steeping the flowers for 10 minutes in hot water then straining and allowing to cool. Put the tea, sweetened with honey if you like, by the side of your bed so you can drink it when you awaken in the night. Also wonderful is a little pillow stuffed with dried hops' blossoms which you put under your neck when you go to bed or if you awaken.

Oatstraw (*Avena sativa*) The straw from oats has an ability to restore energy when nerves have been frayed and is useful for counteracting insomnia. It can help ease night sweats, calm anxiety and even relieve headaches. Stuff a little pillow with oat husks or infuse them in hot water as a drink (see hops above).

Hormone Magic: Melatonin

Melatonin, a hormone from the pineal gland, decreases the time that a woman is awake before falling asleep again as well as reducing the number of times she awakens. It also increases daytime alertness and energy levels. The dose generally recommended is between 3 and 15 mg, preferably taken on an empty stomach an hour before going to bed, although some people seem to need more. Melatonin is one of those compounds which, although it has often been given in much higher doses (between 40 and 80 mg), appears to be more effective for many women in low doses (see also p. 414).

Sleep Rituals

When it comes to getting ready for sleep each night the body loves routines. They foster relaxation and let it know what to expect.

Routines Make bedtime and rising time as regular as possible and go through the same routine each evening of putting the cat out, opening the window, reading a book, or whatever suits you.

Movement Take plenty of aerobic exercise each week, preferably out of doors. Experiment with exercising at different times of the day to see which time works better for you in terms of relaxing you and making you ready for sleep at night.

Stay Awake Don't take on any new activities late in the day and don't take a nap in the evening or late afternoon.

Eat Early Don't eat dinner late in the evening – the earlier the better. Make it the smallest meal of the day and avoid snacks after dinner since they can interfere with sleep. Everybody sleeps better on an empty stomach despite what the hot-drink manufacturers would have you believe.

Midnight Soak Soak in a lukewarm (not hot) bath for 30 minutes, topping up with hot water to maintain the temperature at just blood heat. Blot your skin dry without friction and go straight to bed moving slowly. This can be a great thing to do in the middle of the night if you awaken. Use a candle instead of turning on the light and let yourself relax as you probably never can during the day when a telephone could ring or someone might demand something from you.

Sleep Alone Insist that you sleep in a room by yourself if you want to be alone. Many women stay in the same bed with their mate night after night, year after year, out of habit, insecurity, or a fear of upsetting the boat should they voice a need for solitude at night. It is every woman's right to sleep alone when she wishes. In fact it is sometimes not so much a question of right but of necessity if you are to make your own passage to power and come to know your emerging self.

The Water Margin Drink plenty of water during the day. Sleep is induced by the brain and brain cells need adequate hydration both to stay awake during the daylight hours and to trigger the dreamy relaxation that brings on sleep. Hardly anyone drinks as much water as they profitably could. I discovered this a couple of years ago and regularly consume at least 3½ pints (2 litres) of mineral water a day now, in addition to whatever other drinks I may have.

Cut out Stimulants Eliminate all stimulants from your life – coffee, tea, colas and chocolate as well as some of the stimulating plants such as guarana (a caffeine source from South America), yerba mate (another one) and ma huang or Chinese ephedra which is a natural source of ephedra. All of these stimulants work against a good night's sleep when they are in your system even if you have taken them many hours before bedtime.

Give Thanks Count your blessings and say your prayers. It is an old-fashioned idea but it is a true key to deep relaxation and blissful sleep. Each night as you turn out the light think of six things during the day which you have to be thankful for, regardless of your physical or emotional state or how difficult your life may be at any time. Give thanks for them and surrender your body to the bed asking that the love of sleep wash over you cleansing and renewing you for tomorrow. It gradually trains the mind to dwell on pleasurable themes even when you are awake. It can even improve the quality of your dreams.

Chapter Twenty-five
Field and Forest

Using plants and herbs for health and healing offers many advantages. First their powers for balancing an organism and restoring or enhancing health go far beyond their ability to alleviate symptoms. As living things they are *supraphysical* in their ability to affect a woman's vital force. Besides all their chemical properties botanicals carry to the body their own brand of the ineffable life energy. Wise women often like to use the whole of a plant, rejecting the principles of allopathic medicine which chooses to give isolated active ingredients or drugs. In medicinal plants there are two kinds of compounds, each of which has an important part to play in treatment. The first are the active ingredients. These are what capture the imagination of chemists and drug producers who often isolate them from a plant and then go on to chemically modify them and make molecular analogues which can be patented and sold as drugs. The second are the compounds and substances which drug manufacturers ignore altogether and seek to eliminate but which wise women and good herbalists insist play a supportive role in the healing which a particular herb can bring to the body. These compounds work synergistically with the actives making them more easily assimilable or buffering the action what are otherwise potent plant chemicals – helping to protect the body from side-effects. Some even help protect from taking too much of a particular active ingredient by causing nausea if the body's safe level of tolerance is passed. It is the synergy of these primary active ingredients and their secondary helpers that makes herbs work so well.

There are many different substances and compounds in plants and herbs which offer health-supporting abilities – the volatile oils, the mucilages, the tannins, alkaloids, bitters, glycosides, flavonoids, anthraquinones and saponins. For the purposes of treating female problems and enhancing women's health the most important are the steroidal saponins. The steroidal saponins fall into various categories.

Some resemble cholesterol from which the body makes its own steroid hormones or cortisol, i.e. the oestrogens, progesterone, the androgens or vitamin D. Others (the tri-terpenoid saponins) give to the body a unique ability to regulate its own hormonal balance and activities probably because they provide the raw materials out of which the body can make whatever hormones are needed to enhance health. These plants are known as adaptogens. They include many of the herbs long used by wise women to help menstrual and menopausal problems. Because of this balancing ability, unlike drugs or isolated ingredients, they are often used to treat two apparently completely opposite conditions. Ginseng, for instance, can be used to treat both high and low blood pressure. Wild yam is useful for progesterone insufficiency as well as low oestrogen. Some of the adaptogens – wild yam and liquorice for instance – also act as anti-inflammatories.

PREPARATIONS

Herbs can be taken in many different ways – as infusions, decoctions, syrups, tinctures, suppositories, and in baths, as ointments and creams as well as in capsules to bypass the taste buds on the tongue. You can even grow your own herbs and then, using these or herbs you have bought in bulk, make up your own infusions. The dried plant is by far the cheapest way to use herbs since you can buy 500 grams of most powdered herbs from a good supplier very cheaply and even encapsulate them yourself in capsules that you fill by hand. It is often easiest if you are a complete beginner, however, to rely on good-quality ready-made herbal products – whole herbs, herbs in capsules and herbal extracts. Tinctures are quite concentrated extracts which employ both water and alcohol to draw out a plant's chemical constituents and preserve them. They are taken in a little water. They are best either bought ready made from a reputable supplier or left until you have mastered the use of herbs in other ways, as each herb demands a specific ratio of water and alcohol to plant material. This ratio can be found in a pharmacopoeia.

It is worth remembering that, just as plants have different personalities, so do people. One plant might work better than another for different individuals.

Infusions

These are made the way you would make a cup of tea using the leaves, stems or flowers of a plant, whichever is appropriate. Take a couple of teaspoons or 25 g (1 oz) of the dried herb or 50 g (2 oz) of the fresh herb and put into a large teapot. Fill with boiling water (or water just off the boil for fresh herbs) cover immediately and steep for 10 to 15 minutes. Strain and drink immediately or store for up to two days in a refrigerator and use as needed. Sometimes infusions are taken by the cupful, sometimes by the spoonful, depending upon the plant.

Tinctures

The part of the plant you are using can be fresh or dried, finely chopped or powdered. I prefer to use fresh plants in a ratio of 1:2 or one part of the plant to two parts of the fluid. If the plants are dried the ratio becomes 1:5 as a general rule. In the case of chamomile, for instance, use 200 g (1/2 lb) of the dried flowers and pour over it 1 litre (1³/₄ pints) of the alcohol, the correct ratio of alcohol for this flower being 45 per cent. The best alcohol is vodka but you can also use brandy, remembering that 60 to 70 proof is equal to 45 per cent alcohol. Put the mixture in an airtight container and allow it to macerate in a dark place away from direct sunlight for two to four weeks, shaking the jar thoroughly twice each day. Now the mixture is ready for pressing. Using a muslin bag or clean cloth press as much of the fluid as you can from the herb so you waste as little as possible. You can use a cheese or a wine press for this if you like. Then throw away the waste from the herb (it is great for making compost) and, placing the tincture in a dark bottle, store in a cool place. Tinctures will keep almost indefinitely although I would never use one more than two years old.

Herbal Vinegars

Take a bottle of organic cider vinegar. Fill a jar with the part of the fresh plant you are using – root, rhizome, leaves, berries or flowers – then cover with the vinegar and allow it to sit for six weeks. Vinegar must never be allowed to come into contact with metal for it will corrode it, so cap the jar with plastic or protect the top with a piece of cellophane before closing. Vinegars are particularly good for plants which have a high content of alkaloids since they dissolve well in the medium. Vinegars can be taken by the spoonful mixed into a glass of spring water.

THE PLANTS

Here is a small and simple repertoire of herbs for women. Get to know them. They are like making new friends. Each has its own personality and characteristics. All have been used for centuries for menstrual and menopausal treatments. The therapeutic actions of many have been scientifically validated.

Black Cohosh *Cimicifuga racemosa*

Also known as squaw root, black snake root, or Sheng Ma in Chinese herbal repertory, this pungent root comes from the hardwood forests of the New World. It has been used for hundreds of years by Native Americans for its ability to treat disorders of the womb, promote and restore healthy menstruation, sooth irritation and congestion in the cervix, womb and vagina, relieve pains and promote a trouble-free delivery in childbirth – hence the name they gave it, squaw root. It is one of the great plants for managing menopause well. Black cohosh contains phyto-oestrogens and, as an adaptogen, has the ability to balance hormones in a woman's body. It can be particularly useful when a woman has aches and pains to deal with as well as anxiety, rheumatic problems, arthritis or mental stress. In a German study carried out in 1988 it was shown to relieve hot flushes, sleep disturbances and irritability as effectively as HRT but without dangerous side-effects.

How to Use

By infusion: 1 teaspoon of the dried root in a cup of boiling water for 12 minutes then allowed to cool and taken by the spoonful every few hours during the day. Tincture of the fresh root: 10 to 30 drops in a little water spread throughout the day.

What It Can Do

- **Calm hot flushes and decrease their frequency** Rich in phyto-sterols and micronutrients, black cohosh helps the body to produce the hormones it needs to rebalance itself while reducing LH when you use it regularly over a few months.

- **Ease aches and pains** The root contains natural salicylates which help relieve pain in the body.

- **Heighten energy and calm nerves** As an adaptogen the root can raise the body's vital energies and improve one's ability to handle stress; it is traditionally used to treat hysteria. It also alleviates water build-up in the tissues.

- **Help prevent prolapses** The root has long been used in Oriental medicine to correct prolapses of the womb and bladder.

Caution Black cohosh is never used to treat pregnant women or when there is menstrual flooding.

Sage *Salvia officinalis*

Also called garden sage, red sage or Shu Wei T'aso in the Chinese pharmacopoeia, to Native Americans as well as the ancient Romans sage was a sacred plant burnt to clear negative energy from places and people. I use sage in its many forms all the time. I often burn dried sage to cleanse the atmosphere of a room, calm stress and heighten awareness. The name sage means 'to save'. Sage is a plant with an affinity for female energy, which has a powerful force for deep cleansing and for drying out that which is too wet. This is one of the reasons it can be so helpful in the treatment of night sweats and the kind of hot flushes that produce copious perspiration. Sage is a plant rich in phyto-sterols and flavonoids. Like black cohosh, it can be as effective as the synthetic oestrogens of HRT in banishing hot flushes. It is also used to treat infertility, is the best gargle for a sore throat you will find anywhere, and makes a great mouthwash. Sage is one of the easiest herbs to grow – it will grow just about anywhere. As the Latin saying goes, *cur moriatur homo cui salvia crescit in horto* – no man should die while sage grows in his garden.

How to Use

Make an infusion of 1 teaspoon of the dried leaves in a cup of water, let it sit for 10 minutes, then drink 1 tablespoon of the cooled mixture 1 to 8 times a day. Alternatively, use 10 to 25 drops of a tincture made from the fresh leaves every day. Also use sage in cooking sprinkled on steamed or wok-fried vegetables and salads, in cooked grains, soups and casseroles.

What It Can Do

- **Calm anxiety, banish depression and balance mood** A natural tranquillizer, sage helps calm the nerves and create peaceful sleep since it is rich in the calming minerals – magnesium, calcium and zinc. It also helps balance emotions and banish emotional swings, in no small part because it helps replenish lost minerals from your system.

- **Reduce infection** Sage is one of the best herbs in the world for helping the body overcome infections. Its essential oils concentrate in the urine countering bacterial growth and helping to clear infections there; used as a mouthwash or a gargle it counters a sore throat and drunk as tea or taken as a tincture it helps banish infections in the body as a whole.

- **Relieve headaches** The herb supports the actions of the liver and encourages good circulation while many of the saponins it contains help ease pain in the head.

- **Banish night sweats and hot flushes** Often acting quickly to bring relief, sage can calm sweats day or night; half a cup of sage tea taken at bedtime can make all the difference to women who awaken drenched in sweat.

- **Balance hormones in the midst of change** Sage has been used for thousands of years by wise women to help women at major times of change – to ease menarche, to increase fertility in childbearing years, to make menopause a smooth transition, thanks to its ability to balance hormones regardless of whatever imbalances are present in a woman's body.

- **Improve digestion and strengthen the liver** The volatile essential oil of sage which contains both alpha and beta thujone with cineole, borneol and other chemicals helps both the stomach and the liver produce more enzymes making digestion work better and eliminating nausea and gas.

- **Relieve flooding and menstrual cramps** Sage's tannins and volatile oil relieve pain in the womb and help dry up menstrual excess.

- **De-age the body** A natural anti-ager, sage is full of anti-oxidants, antiseptics which protect against bacteria, and minerals to act as co-factors for enzymic processes which decline with age; it has been used for generations by wise women to protect hair from greying and skin from wrinkling, and helps prevent cancer and other degenerative conditions.

- **Eases inflammation and clears joint pains** Its phytohormones help oil the joints, dissolve mineral deposits in the joints and ease aches and pains.

Caution Sage is a drying herb and, as such, should not be used by a woman who is experiencing vaginal dryness or a dry mouth. It is a herb to use frequently when needed but not continuously over long periods of time without a break or it may lose its effectiveness.

Motherwort *Leonurus cardiaca*

Also called lion's tail or Yi Mu Cao in the Chinese pharmacopoeia, motherwort grows in waste places. It has gained its name from the ancient practice of using it to reduce anxiety during pregnancy. The plant has good sedative properties which have been well validated by scientific experiments and is able to calm the nervous system while at the same time acting as a tonic to the body as a whole. Culpepper, who believed that motherwort belonged to the goddess Venus and to the astrological sign of Leo, wrote, 'There is no better herb to drive melancholy vapours from the heart, to strengthen it and make the mind cheerful, blithe and merry.' I think this sums up the virtues of motherwort very well. Its leaves are full of mind-altering natural chemicals which studies in China have shown to decrease the levels of blood lipids and exert a regulating action on muscles such as the womb and the heart, bringing calm in its wake. This is one of the reasons why, in addition to being used by women to ease hot flushes, banish insomnia, and even restore elasticity to the walls of the vagina, it is an excellent herb for the treatment of many heart conditions. I find it is the most physically and psychologically comforting plant I know.

How to Use

Motherwort is rich in alkaloids and bitter as an infusion. It is easier to take as a tincture or made into a herbal vinegar. Take 10 to 25 drops of the tincture made from the fresh plant every 2 to 6 hours or 1 to 2 teaspoons of the herb vinegar as desired.

What It Can Do

- **Calm the nerves** There is something so calming and balancing about motherwort that it is hard to describe to someone who has never used it; used frequently it can relieve anxiety, nourish the nervous system and relax tensions, while at the same time act as a tonic for energy; it is wonderful used just before confronting stressors of any kind.

- **Minimize hot flushes** The herb can reduce the intensity, length and frequency of hot flushes, even helping to calm the dizziness or faintness that can accompany them, thanks to its ability to oxygenate the blood, detoxify thyroid, liver, heart and womb, and invigorate circulation. For best results you need to use it regularly for 12 weeks or longer but sometimes 10 drops or so of the tincture in a little spring water can ease a hot flush while it is happening.

- **Promote undisturbed sleep** This herb is a wonderful help when you awaken in the night with sweats and have trouble dropping off again. Take 10 to 20 drops of the tincture (kept at the side of your bed with a glass of spring water) and swallow some each time you wake up. It will even help banish anxiety and bad dreams.

- **Eliminate waterlogging** Take a little motherwort every few hours and it acts as a natural diuretic, reducing water retention; this is useful after a flight when legs and feet can become swollen.

- **Tonify and elasticize womb and vagina** Improving circulation and thickening tissues which have lost their elasticity and tone, the herb can rejuvenate the tissues of the bladder, womb and vagina when you take it several times a day for two to four weeks (see p. 325).

- **Relieve cramps** Simply the best for clearing up menstrual and uterine cramps when the menstrual flow is absent or light to moderate. Use 5 to 10 drops of the tincture or 1/2 to 1 teaspoon of the vinegar every few minutes until they have gone and repeat as necessary; prolonged use strengthens the muscles of the womb and makes it resistant to cramping in the future.

Caution Motherwort is not a herb to use when a woman is experiencing menstrual flooding since it can aggravate this tendency.

Ginseng *Panax ginseng*

Oriental ginseng which is widely cultivated in China, Korea, Japan and Russia is probably the most studied plant in modern times. It is more potent and effective than its American cousin *Panax quinquefolium* and best chosen carefully as there is a lot of relatively worthless ginseng on the market. It has been praised for centuries for its rejuvenating properties, its ability to protect against illness, to enhance the body's ability to handle stress – even to prolong life. The herb is a great ally – the most potent of all the plants for handling very severe symptoms in menopausal women. You should be aware that many of ginseng's benefits will be lost if you take more than 2 grams a day of vitamin C, while taking vitamin E will enhance ginseng's actions. The most effective ginseng is the dried root which you chew or a good tincture made from it. Extensive research has shown that for ginseng to work it has to be replete with ginsenosides – the active compounds from the plant. Ginseng can heighten immunity, improve the functions of the heart and lungs, counter fatigue and balance female hormones, thanks to its oestrogenic effects.

How to Use

Always buy the best ginseng you can afford and take it either as a fresh root tincture (5 to 20 drops 1 to 3 times a day), as an infusion or as a tea in which 1 oz (25 g) of the dried root is taken in a cup of water each day, or by chewing on a piece of the root the size of the tip of your baby finger every day. The effects of ginseng are cumulative so you need 6 to 8 weeks of taking the plant to feel its full benefits.

What It Can Do

- **Regulate hormones and banish menstrual flooding** Rich in phyto-sterols, ginseng encourages the body to produce the quantities of oestrogen and progesterone it needs along with other steroid hormones, gradually making it possible for the body's endocrine system to completely rebalance itself; this can be particularly helpful in the years just before menopause when it can balance menstrual flow and prevent flooding up to menopause.

- **Enhance the ability to handle stress** Nothing compares with ginseng's adaptogenic abilities to strengthen the body's adrenals and support the functions of glands such as the thyroid, pituitary and hypothalamus involved in stress protection; ginseng banishes fatigue and slowly rebuilds stamina and energy.

Echinacea *Echinacea purpurea*

Purple cone flower or Black Sampson is a plant native to the prairies of North America with unequalled properties to stimulate the immune system, heal wounds, enhance skin, counter infection and calm inflammation. The Sioux used it for snake bites, blood poisoning and wound healing. Until the twentieth century its roots and rhizomes were primary agents for the treatment of fever and infections from 'flu and colds to serious conditions such as typhoid, meningitis, malaria, diphtheria, boils and abscesses. When drugs came into being in a big way the beautiful echinacea plant was almost forgotten – except in Germany. There researchers began to quantify its effects on the body discovering that it has properties equal to and often greater than most antibiotics to prevent and heal infection. It offers cortisone-like anti-inflammatory activity, interferon-like activity to heighten immunity, an ability to stimulate T-cells – important mediators in the body's immune system – and can even help slow down the rate at which the body and skin ages. This later property comes as a result of its ability to prevent the breakdown of one of the body's primary defence mechanisms – the so-called H-system of hyaluronic acid which cements cells together and acts as an effective barrier against infection. Echinacea is a plant product I would never want to be without. I use it to protect from infection through the long dark winters and to treat illness in myself and my family.

How to Use

By capsule of the ground herb: 1 to 4 capsules 3 to 4 times a day, depending on whether it is being used as a prophylactic or treatment for illness. In the form of fresh plant tincture it can be taken in a little water: 15 to 50 drops at a time once or twice a day for prevention; several times a day as treatment; up to 2 teaspoons an hour for a day or two at the onset of illness.

What It Can Do

- **Bring health insurance against illness and premature age-ing** Used throughout periods of stress, echinacea contains two polysaccharides – inulin and echinacea – which reinforce the body's defence mechanisms and heighten immunity, making it easy to ward off colds and 'flu as well as fungal infections by continually detoxifying the body and strengthening its vital powers to resist illness and degeneration.

- **Boost immunity when illness strikes** The immunostimulatory activities of echinacea make it a bold ally in fighting off viral or bacterial infections including boils, abscesses and carbuncles as well as to heal wounds; the plant's polysaccharide fractions activate macrophages and trigger an increase in interleukin I to enhance immune functions and help the body heal itself.

- **Protect skin and body from degeneration** Hyaluronic acid is the intercellular cement that forms a barrier against infection and helps keep skin strong, resilient and youthful. As the body ages an enzyme attacks the hyaluronic acid so it loses its viscosity and changes from a firm jelly to a thin watery fluid. Echinacea prevents the enzyme from dissolving so inhibiting the spread of infection and maintaining good collagen and elastin in the skin.

Caution Like many plants, echinacea should not be used continuously since the body can become accustomed to it and this may negate some of its potent health-enhancing abilities.

Golden Seal *Hydrastis canadensis*

Favourite cure-all of the Cherokee Indians, golden seal has in recent years won praise from scientists for its widespread benefits which include banishing morning sickness and nausea, calming digestive disturbances, banishing skin diseases and haemorrhoids. A potent nerve and endocrine gland tonic, it includes among its active principles berberine and hydrastine which are both potent antibiotics. It can be used as a douche in the treatment of vaginal infections, as a mouthwash in the treatment of gum problems and to fight off the infections of 'flu and fevers. One of the most generally effective of all remedies, this is another remedy I would never want to be without.

How to Use

Use the powdered root in capsule form rather than as an infusion since golden seal is very unpleasant tasting (1 to 4 capsules three times a day). Tincture of fresh herb: 10 to 30 drops 3 to 4 times a day.

What It Can Do

- **Soothe digestion and ease liver problems** A bitter tonic, golden seal was much used in the nineteenth century to soothe disorders of the stomach and heal the liver – good for gastritis, dyspepsia, peptic ulcerations, colitis and a liverish feeling. The berberine alkaloids which the root contains stimulate bile production and secretion, destroy unhelpful bacteria in the gut and increase the tone and movement of the gastrointestinal tract. The root has overall tonic actions on the nervous system, and is excellent applied topically (on the skin) in strong infusion or tincture against eczema and many other skin problems.

- **Counter infection** Excellent for the treatment of all kinds of infection including mucous membranes and body tissues, golden seal can banish catarrh in the head, throat and bronchial passages, and clear up infections of the teeth and gums when used as a mouthwash.

- **Calm uterine contractions** Gently strengthening to muscle tone and circulation, it has a mildly sedative and muscle-relaxing effect on the body and helps stabilize blood sugar. It can be used for menstrual disorders especially menorrhagia.

Caution Do not use when pregnant.

Chastetree *Vitex agnus castus*

Also called Monks' Pepper, the equivalent in the Chinese pharmacopoeia is Man Jing Zi, *Vitex rotundifolia* or *Vitex trifolia*. This plant gets its name because of its ability to calm the lascivious desires of men. For most women however it has the exact opposite effect – stimulating libido and energizing the whole system while balancing emotions. Chastetree is the most helpful and far-reaching in its effects of all plants for perimenopausal, menopausal and postmenopausal women. It works superbly whether hormones are deficient or in excess by acting on the pituitary to harmonize imbalances. What is wonderful about the berries is that it is hard to get too much of them since the herb never forces the body to make more of any particular hormone than it needs. It is far better known in Continental Europe and the Orient than in Britain and the Americas. There, its berries have been used for centuries to protect against and even to help cure cancers of the breast and womb, to reduce breast lumps and tenderness, banish oedema, clear skin problems, moisten vaginal tissues that have dried, and banish hot flushes, as well as eliminating menstrual cramps and restoring emotional calm. Research shows that these remarkable berries used daily increase the production of the brain hormone dopamine. They also tend to enhance progesterone and LH while they inhibit FSH and prolactin. Vitex is not a phyto-sterol rich plant, it relies on its glycosides, micronutrients and flavonoids to work its wonders so be patient. Chastetree goes deep in its effects on the body and psyche but this takes time. Look for good results after daily use for 8 to 12 weeks. In about a year to 18 months you will probably be able to stop using the plant and find that improvement has become permanent.

How to Use

As an infusion: one cup of tea made from freshly ground berries each day. As fresh powdered berries in capsule form: 1 capsule 3 to 4 times a day. Fifteen drops to 1 teaspoon of the tincture 1 to 3 times a day.

What It Can Do

- **Eliminate hot flushes** German research shows that the chaste berry can increase LH, stimulating progesterone synthesis and secretion and balancing high FSH and excess oestrogen which can cause flushes in some women.

- **Regulate periods and banish cramping, endometriosis and fibroids** Whether the problem is spotting, flooding or irregular periods this plant can help, due to its action on the pituitary. Its anti-inflammatory properties can also help soothe the endometrium and shrink fibroids when used regularly for 12 to 36 months.

- **Keep vagina moist** Thanks to its oestrogen-balancing abilities, chastetree helps regulate vaginal secretions while offering protection from oestrogen-dominant illnesses such as cancer.

- **Strengthen bones** Due to its ability to increase progesterone production, it is an important ally against osteoporosis and may even help reverse bone loss.

- **Ease constipation and digestive problems** Sluggish digestion is no match for the chaste berry which helps restore digestion easily and permanently, provided you take it for long enough. It can also clear skin troubles that develop as a result of hormonal change and banish waterlogging from the tissues with regular use.

- **Eliminate depression and balance mood** Typical PMS problems from migraines and depression to ordinary headaches and anxiety can yield slowly but permanently to *Vitex* which helps ground women. This usually takes about 6 months and it is wise to continue with the plant for another 6 months at least to make the benefits permanent.

Caution None.

Dong Quai/Tang Kuei *Angelica sinensis*

This is the most prized of all the Oriental plant treatments for women's hormonal problems. Studies have shown that this root, which acts like a sister to ginseng in its actions, quickly clears the kind of hot flushes which are the result of too little or the wrong kinds of oestrogen in your body and performs many other useful tasks as well. It will lower blood pressure, fight bacteria and viruses, get rid of water retention, improve the body's use of oxygen at a cellular level, calm menopausal anxiety, stimulate a sluggish metabolism, protect the cardiovascular system, and eliminate insomnia, nervousness and depression. This remedy works fast – usually in a week or two. It is best used together with ginseng since it is yin in nature to ginseng's yang and they perfectly balance each other. Ginseng's yang chi or energy is toxifying while dong quai's yin energy nourishes the blood deeply. Chinese teaching about menopause is that it is the yang or active expression of yin or wise blood. The Chinese often use dong quai together with other herbs such as peony root. Western wise women sometimes suggest taking dong quai for a fortnight then ginseng for the next fortnight to reap the highest benefits from both.

How to Use

Like ginseng, a thin slice of dried root can be chewed 3 times a day. As an infusion, $1/2$ to 1 cup a day. Fifteen to 30 drops of the fresh root tincture 1 to 3 times a day.

What It Can Do

- **Improve sleep** Rich in calming minerals like magnesium, trace elements such as cobalt and in phyto-sterols, dong quai can be a blessing when trying to handle the sleeplessness of menopause; it calms nerves and soothes mood swings in the daytime too.

- **Moisten vagina** Known for its ability to moisten a vagina which has become dry, dong quai soothes the whole of the pelvis, relieving cramps and aches and restoring warmth and vitality to the tissues.

- **Ease hot flushes** Fast working, this root is excellent for treating hot flushes particularly if by nature you tend to be cold; it is not the plant of choice for a woman who tends to be naturally very warm since taking it can make you warmer.

- **De-age skin** This plant's ability to nourish the energy – which in Chinese medicine is known as wise blood – improves circulation to the skin and brings a glow to the face, smoothing out fine lines and thickening skin that has thinned from age. It also thickens the walls of the vagina and bladder which have thinned and relieves many rheumatic aches and pains.

Caution Dong quai is not a remedy to use if bloating, menstrual flooding or diarrhoea regularly occur nor if you have fibroids. Neither should it ever be used if you are on blood-thinning herbs or take aspirin. Any tenderness or discomfort in the breasts while using it is a sign that it should be discontinued.

Wild Yam *Dioscorea villosa*

There are many related species of the dioscoriaceae family which have similar properties to *villosa*, including *Dioscorea Mexicana*. Root and rhizome found commonly in the United States and some tropical countries may hold the secret to natural birth control although you will not find this attribute listed among its virtues in any herbal pharmacopoeia (see p. 146). Wild yam was traditionally used to prevent miscarriage, as a natural tonic and for natural birth control without side-effects as it does not interfere with normal periods. Then in 1936 Japanese scientists found that the glycoside saponins of a number of Mexican wild yam species yielded steroid saponins such as diosgenin from which progesterone itself could be easily converted. Progesterone is an intermediate compound in the production of cortisone. Since then wild yam has been used to produce steroid drugs derived from diosgenin including oral contraceptives, androgens, oestrogens and corticosteroids through a series of chemical steps. That is why it is now grown and used widely by pharmaceutical manufacturers. The whole plant which supplies the raw materials for the body to make hormones has much to offer perimenopausal, menopausal and postmenopausal women. It is also useful for its anti-inflammatory properties in calming joint and muscle aches and pains, it soothes the nerves, eases menstrual pains and encourages the production of progesterone in a woman's body to counter oestrogen dominance and the many conditions associated with it. It is useful to counter intestinal gas, colic, nausea and calm nerves. It stimulates libido in many women. The root has also been shown to lower blood cholesterol and blood pressure which is too high.

How to Use

As an infusion of the dried root: $1/2$ to 1 cup once or twice a day; or as a tincture of the dried root 10 to 30 drops 3 or 4 times a day. You can also take the ground root in capsules. According to midwife Willa Shaffer, wild yam can be used as a means of natural birth control provided it is taken for three months along with some barrier form of birth control before relying on it alone. A maximum of 1,500 mg of the plant must be taken in capsule form *absolutely* regularly morning and night. In practice this usually means 4 to 5 capsules morning and night daily (depending on the size of the capsules). Shaffer insists that high doses of vitamin C – above 3 or 4 a day – invalidate its actions. You can also use wild yam on the body in the form of a cream which contains converted natural progesterone as an antidote to osteoporosis and helps to reverse bone loss after it has occurred (see p. 425 for protocol).

What It Can Do

- **Ease joint and muscle pains and headaches** The root is one of the best anti-inflammatory plants known to man.

- **Reverse osteoporosis** Progesterone cream increases the rate of bone formation; as John Lee writes in *The Lancet* (24 November 1990), 'the signs and symptoms of osteoporosis cleared in every patient [using the wild yam cream] and the incidence of fractures dropped to zero'.

- **Moisten vagina** Due to its hormone-balancing capacities, when taken internally, wild yam helps calm itching and burning in the genitals of menopausal and post-menopausal women; wild yam cream with natural progesterone is also effective in doing this when applied directly to the vagina, labia and whole genital area.

- **Banishing PMS and menstrual pain** Because of its ability to stimulate the production of progesterone in a woman's body wild yam is enormously helpful in soothing the nerves, easing menstrual pain, preventing flooding and countering PMS in most women; some who also use it as natural birth control claim that it has changed their lives completely, making them feel content, balanced and in control of their own destiny.

Big Note of Caution Remember that all of the information on wild yam used for birth control is anecdotal. There have been no controlled studies done on it and probably never will since no pharmaceutical company is likely to fund them. If you decide to use wild yam as natural birth control, be absolutely sure of the purity of the plant you are using and of the exact amount. Steer clear of prescription drugs and high doses of vitamin C (above 2 a day) or Willa Shaffer warns that it will not work. Use some barrier form of birth control for three months before relying on it completely.

Chapter Twenty-six

Resurrection

A time of death and rebirth, menopause offers a woman approaching it or passing through it an unequalled opportunity to regenerate and rejuvenate her body and, in the process, to transform her life both physically and spiritually. It is as though the energies involved in the changes her body is experiencing at this time – energies which may have been dormant for years – are now rising to the surface and becoming accessible. Take advantage of them. Menopause is also a time to take stock of what works in your body and what does not; a time to begin listening to the rhythm of your body and your soul even if you, like many of us, seem to have forgotten how or wonder if there is any soul there to be heard. There are many techniques and compounds that can help a woman do this – from immune stimulants and green medicines, to nutritional supplements and brain enhancers (see The Professionals p. 404). Now is the time to explore what they can offer. But, first, for any woman to make the most of them her body needs to be as clear and pollution-free as possible. For most of us this calls for carrying out a simple programme of detoxification which can eliminate body pollution that may have built up over the months and years, while at the same time helping to supply the body with a good quantity of minerals, vitamins and micronutrients to support enzyme reactions and hormonal balance.

Such a programme can be as useful to a menstruating woman who wants to minimize PMS as it can to a menopausal or postmenopausal woman wanting to regenerate her body. Deep cleansing the body can be done in a number of ways: by spending time at a clinic where the principles of nature-cure are put into practice with deep cleansing regimes, by carrying out a spring clean such as the one in my *10 Day Clean-Up Plan*, or – and this is my favourite in mid-life – by making periodic use of a Miso Detox and Rebuild. It is a programme which is best used for at least a week at a time but can be carried out for several weeks to great advantage. During the first week of the programme it is best to stop all supplements you may be taking except for a high-quality vitamin C supplement which can actually help in the detoxification process. After that it can be useful to add specific supplements either recommended by your health practitioner or following the general guidelines in The Professionals (see p. 404). Most important of all you need to increase your intake of pure water to 1-2 litres ($1^3/4$–$3^1/2$ pints) a day.

Let Food Be Your Medicine

Miso – pronounced MEE-so – is also known as fermented soy bean paste. It is a savoury paste made from soy beans and grain which has been cultured with *Aspergillus oryzae* – a micro-organism highly beneficial to the human body due to its ability to help set up virtually ideal conditions in the colon so that intestinal flora support digestion in the best possible way. This in turn facilitates the body's manufacture of B vitamins important for energy and for protecting the body from excess stress; enabling a continuous effective elimination of toxic waste build-up.

For generations Japanese folklore has insisted that miso broth is beneficial to health and longevity. As a result, it still forms the basis of breakfast for over 70 per cent of the population of Japan. Recently, a number of scientific studies have been carried out to quantify the effects of taking miso regularly. Scientists have been able to identify some of the specific ways in which it benefits health. The daily use of miso has been shown to lower cholesterol, to alkalinize blood made acid by too much sugar, refined foods and meat, and to neutralize many of the negative effects of environmental pollution on our bodies including cigarette smoke. In many ways, most fascinating of all is miso's apparent ability to neutralize many of the effects of radiation, helping to prevent the free radical damage which underlies early ageing and the development of degenerative diseases from cancer to coronary heart disease. The first inkling of miso's ability to do this came from the work of Dr Shinchiro Akizuki. As Director of Saint Francis Hospital in Nagasaki, Akizuki spend his life treating atomic bomb victims a few miles from ground zero and investigating the use of foods as preventative medicine. Although his team spent years close to the place in which the atomic bomb had been dropped neither he nor his colleagues experienced the effects of radiation poisoning which devastated the lives of the patients whom they were treating. Akizuki wondered if this may have been because he and his staff drank miso soup regularly through each day. Then, in 1972, his hypothesis was confirmed when scientists discovered that miso is rich in an alkaloid called dipicolonic acid which is able to link up with molecules of heavy metals in the body such as lead, mercury, aluminium and radioactive strontium and, by chelating them, carry them out of the body. A few years later at Japan's Cancer Research Centre, other researchers discovered that people who regularly use miso soup have significantly lower levels of many forms of cancer and heart disease. And, recently, scientists at Tohoku University in Hokkaido have been able to isolate compounds in miso which appear to wipe out the carcinogenic or cancer-causing effects of many chemicals on the body. Scientists at Hiroshima University's Atomic Radioactivity Medical Lab under the direction of Professor Akihiro Ito have confirmed with animal experiments the free radical protection against radiation which the regular use of miso can infer. The liver cancer rate of animals not fed miso and then exposed to radiation is 100 to 200 per cent higher than those of animals that are fed miso.

Miso Detox and Rebuild

Miso comes in many flavours, and ranges in colour from the sweet pale tan varieties to the dark rich brown and red misos. Some misos are made from barley, others from rice or chickpeas. In texture they resemble a soft nut butter which can be spread on bread, added to soups, grain dishes and casseroles, and used in salad dressings. The cornerstone of the miso diet for detoxification is the use of miso broth. The kind of miso which is best for this is organic *genmai* miso made from soya and brown rice. It is dark, rich in flavour and has a thick texture. Although the preparation of miso soup in Japan is an art in itself and makes use of their famous dashi broth and superbly cut vegetables, it is simple to put together an instant broth by placing a heaped teaspoon to a tablespoon of the miso in the bottom of a large cup or bowl and pouring boiling water over it. Then you can add sea vegetables such as flaked nori or other sea plants, spirulina flakes or other green powerhouses like green barley or wheatgrass to taste. I like to add a splash of good soya milk and sometimes a crushed clove of garlic or two. Once you break through old habit patterns that force us all to look upon breakfast as a time for packaged cereals and coffee, you find that such a breakfast is not only satisfying, it also helps keep your energy levels steady all through the morning and beyond. After a couple of weeks of miso broth taken once or twice a day all of the body's elimination processes move into top gear enabling it gently yet inexorably to cast off all kinds of stored wastes.

The basic principles of the Miso Detox and Rebuild are simple. Remove all foods that can interfere with the body's natural abilities to cleanse itself. These include heavy proteins like meat, dairy products, wheat, sugar, junk fats and other highly processed items. Cut out stimulants such as coffee and tea, and depressants such as alcohol, which tend to distort body energies and build up toxicity. Then you take in foods with deep-cleansing abilities such as raw fruits and vegetables and miso to encourage the elimination of stored wastes from the cells. Finally, you supply a high level of easily available nutrients from power foods such as sea plants, sprouted seeds and grains and the green foods as well as low-fat easily absorbed protein foods rich in phyto-hormones such as the soy products tofu, tempeh, soya milk and miso itself. While carrying out a Miso Detox and Rebuild, the foods to use and those not to use are given below.

Choose From	Avoid
sprouted seeds and grains	coffee
organic miso	tea
fresh fruits	alcohol
fresh vegetables	sugar or anything containing
seaweeds	sugar

green foods (spirulina, chlorella, green barley, wheat grass)
buckwheat and buckwheat noodles
organic brown rice
fresh seeds
fresh nuts
soya milk
fresh herbs
low-salt vegetable bouillon powder
soya seasonings (e.g. organic tamari)
raw honey
tofu
tempeh or soya cheese
legumes
extra virgin olive oil
herb teas
spring water

artificial colourings and flavourings
convenience foods
wheat and wheat products
meat
fish
game
cigarettes
drugs
chocolate
colas
milk and milk products

Here is what a fortnight of the Miso Detox and Rebuild looks like. Breakfast is simple: a bowl of miso broth every day (see p. 368). It is important to experiment with miso broth in the beginning. You will probably find that some of the green foods I have suggested you add to it will appeal to you while others will not. You will also discover by trial and error the amounts of these various foods your body needs and wants. This is likely to vary from time to time as well. You may find at the beginning that you want only the miso broth with a little soya milk by itself. It doesn't matter. But do try to add the green foods bit by bit as you get used to this new kind of breakfast.

The other two meals of the day are interchangeable and can be adjusted to fit what is available on the menu of a restaurant when you need to eat out.

SAMPLE WEEK'S MENU FOR MISO DETOX AND REBUILD

	Main Meal	Light Meal
Monday	Grilled tofu spread with tamari. A fresh salad of raw beetroot and apple dressed with fresh orange juice and curry powder. A fresh peach.	Vegetable soup made with root vegetables, green vegetables, garlic, onions and low-salt vegetable bouillon. Melon.
Tuesday	Risotto of organic brown rice, vegetables. A salad of fresh sprouted seeds or grains topped with mixed three seeds: pumpkin, sesame and sunflower. Half a grapefruit or tangerines.	Crudités with a dip made by blending organic tofu with garlic, lemon juice, seasoning and Worcester sauce. Miso broth with soba (100% buckwheat noodles).
Wednesday	Sweet potatoes or baked yams topped with grated fresh ginger and extra virgin olive oil. Salad of grated celeriac, carrots, red pepper and black olives with olive oil and lemon dressing. Baked apple with raisins and cinnamon.	Fresh spinach, mushroom and garlic salad with dressing made by blending tofu with brown rice vinegar, garlic, vegetable bouillon powder and herbs. Fresh fruit salad.

Thursday	Baked carrots and parsnips with almonds or cashews spread with miso. A cooked buckwheat and raw vegetable salad including whatever fresh vegetables and sprouts are available. Slices of orange topped with raisins which have been plumped by soaking in spring water overnight.	Dairy-free muesli (for recipe, see p. 402). Bowl of miso broth if desired.
Friday	Leek, parsnip and yellow split-pea soup made with garlic, seaweeds and vegetable bouillon. Fresh cucumber slices topped with a dressing of olive oil, finely chopped onions, grated fresh ginger, slivered mushrooms and miso.	Sliced tomato and sesame seed salad with fresh basil if available, cubes of organic tofu and crushed cloves of garlic. Dress with cider vinegar, olive oil, miso and honey.
Saturday	Tofu slices spread with miso then grilled served with wok-fried fresh vegetables. A bunch of grapes.	Brown rice salad with chopped carrots, green onions, olives, tomatoes, parsley, celery and garlic, dressed with olive oil, lemon, sesame seeds and sprinkled with sea salad vegetables.

Sunday	Scrambled tofu with green salad made from Chinese leaves, herbs, celery, green pepper, spring onions and rocket. Half a melon filled with blueberries or strawberries.	Barley pilaff salad with miso sauce. Cook and cool the barley and mix with finely chopped raw vegetables. For miso sauce: $1\frac{1}{2}$ cups water, 2 tablespoons arrowroot, $\frac{1}{2}$ cup miso, juice of 1 lemon, 6 tablespoons apple concentrate. Mix half the water with the fruit concentrate and the miso in a food processor until thoroughly blended. Mix arrowroot into a small amount of the remaining water and blend, adding more and more water until all the water is used. Heat on a medium heat, stirring briskly, until the starch gels. Remove from the heat and stir in the miso mixture. Squeeze in the lemon juice at the last minute. Mix thoroughly. Almond milk made in a blender from $\frac{1}{2}$ cup of blanched almonds, raw honey, spring water and pure vanilla essence.

Secrets of Water

Water is the principal constituent from which your blood, your cells, your muscles – even your bones – are mostly made. A healthy person who weighs just over 65 kilos (10 stone) carries about 40 litres of water around – 25 litres inside the cells, 15 litres outside, including 5 litres in the blood. Let yourself become dehydrated and the chemical reactions in the cells involved in fat burning become sluggish. Your cells cannot build new tissue, toxic products build up in your bloodstream, your blood volume decreases so that you have less oxygen and nutrients transported to your cells – all of which are essential to fat burning. Dehydration also results in your feeling weak and tired and can lead to overeating as it disturbs appetite mechanisms so you think you are hungry even when you are not. The role of water in weight control and health in general is almost completely ignored. The brain too is 75 per cent water. This is why the quantity and quality of water you drink also affects how you think and feel. If the water you drink is polluted by heavy metals or chemicals then the biochemical reactions on which clear thought and emotional balance depend will become polluted as well.

Liquid Energy

Drinking enough brings dynamic energy. Yet few of us drink enough. When Sir Edmund Hillary set out to conquer Everest he had a shrewd doctor named George Hunt on his ascent team. Hunt knew this precept well. He had studied the records of the recent failed attempt by the Swiss team and discovered that their climbers had drunk less than two glasses of water per day per man. So he ordered special battery-operated snow-melting equipment for the kit and urged the British climbers to take a minimum of twelve glasses of water each day of the climb to reduce their fatigue as they scaled the peaks.

Since then, research with athletes at Harvard University and Loma Linda University in the United States carried out to explore the relationship between water drinking and energy has demonstrated that drinking extra water reduces fatigue and stress and increases stamina and energy to a remarkable degree. During one of the Harvard studies, researcher G. C. Pitts set athletes walking at $3^{1}/_{2}$ miles an hour, allowing them to rest regularly but not allowing them to drink extra water. They reached exhaustion after $3^{1}/_{2}$ hours with temperatures of 102° Fahrenheit. Under the same conditions, he allowed them to drink as much as they wanted. The same athletes lasted 6 hours before collapsing. On the third occasion the athletes were forced to drink more water than thirst dictated – in quantities calculated by researchers to replace what was being lost in perspiration. This they were able to continue indefinitely without fatigue or fever until finally, after running out of time, the researchers were forced to bring the experiment to a close. Few of us drink as much water as we need to remain in top form. Even if you pay attention to your thirst and quench it regularly you are likely to replace only about a half to two-thirds of the water your body needs for optimal health.

Water Power

Water plays a major part in digesting your foods and absorbing nutrients thanks to enzymes which are themselves mostly water. If you fail to drink enough water between meals your mouth becomes low in saliva and digestion suffers. Water is also the medium through which wastes are eliminated from your body. Each time you exhale you release highly humidified air – about two big glasses worth a day. Your kidneys and intestines eliminate another 6 or so glasses every 24 hours, while another 2 glasses' worth are released through the pores of your skin. That makes 8 glasses a day – and this is on a *cool* day. When it gets hot, when you are exercising or when you are working hard, the usual 10 glasses lost in this way can triple. On average, in a temperate climate – not sweating from exertion or heat – we need about 6 pints a day for optimal health although few of us consume as much as 2 pints. The important thing to remember is that how thirsty you are is *not* a reliable indication of how much water you need to drink. If you want to grow lean and stay that way you need to do as French women have done for decades. Keep a large bottle or two of pure, fresh mineral water on your desk and make sure you consume your quota of this clear, delicious health-giving drink. Here's how to work it out.

Divide your *current* weight in kilos by 8. If you weigh 58 kilos then 58 divided by 8 equals 7.25 big glasses. Then round the figure upwards to the next glass and there you have it: 8 glasses a day. But remember that is only a base calculation for a cool day. *You will need a lot more during exercise or on a hot day.*

Provided you do not suffer from a kidney or liver disease, drinking 8 big glasses or more of water a day not only helps you to lose weight and keep it off permanently but also improves the functioning of your whole body.

There is another way in which drinking optimal quantities of water plays a central role in detoxifying the body. It has to do with your kidneys. The kidneys are responsible for recycling all the water in your body – some 800 glasses of it a day – and for filtering out any wastes present. The filtering mechanism responsible for all this in the kidneys is made up of millions of microscopic bodies known as glomeruli. They identify waste products such as urea which need to be removed as well as screening out other chemicals and unwanted metals and minerals. At the same time they pour back into the bloodstream the minerals you do need and regulate your body's acid-akaline balance. When some part of you needs more water, your kidneys make sure it arrives. For instance, when you are hot and sweating a message is sent to the pituitary gland in the head telling it to release the anti-diuretic hormone which in turn tells your kidneys to let more water be resorbed into the blood. Your urine at such times can become highly concentrated and a dark colour. Provided you replenish the water you are losing in sweat by drinking more your kidneys remain happy and well-functioning and the appetite/thirst messages from your brain do not become confused. When your body's water level gets too low, however, your kidneys cannot carry out their cleansing efficiently and the liver's role in detoxification becomes overburdened. Water is also the world's best natural diuretic. If your body tends to retain water this is often because you don't drink *enough* so it tries its best to hold on to the water there is. Once you do begin to drink enough this tendency to waterlogging decreases and usually disappears completely.

And, by the way, if you are worried about puckered thighs, the best way to help eliminate them easily is simply to *drink more water*. During a Miso Detox and Rebuild you need to drink plenty of water. Keep a litre bottle on your desk or in your room and see that you drain it every day regardless of whatever else you drink.

Only the Best

The quality of water you drink matters a lot too. If you can afford the best spring waters buy them. If not, at least get yourself a good water filter and use it, always changing it regularly. Bottled waters differ tremendously from one to another. Some are nothing more than tap water which has been run through conditioning filters to remove the taste while doing nothing to improve the quality. Just because they say 'spring' on the label, that doesn't mean a thing. The word may be nothing more than the brand name used to sell the product. Other bottled waters are excellent in taste and quality. Few countries do much to regulate standards for bottled water and what regulations there are, are generally even poorer than those applied to tap water. Except in France.

There are some 1,200 springs in France. Several dozen of them supply bottled waters the quality of which has long been monitored and controlled by official government bodies. A few have been granted the title *eau minerale naturelle*. This means that they maintain a constant mineral content. It also means that they have a reputation for specific therapeutic properties. These waters should be safe from bacterial or chemical contamination and you can be sure they have not been mixed with any foreign substance when they are bottled. Two of the best mineral waters are Volvic, an exceptionally pure still water from the Auvergne mountains in central France, and the sparkling Perrier, which arrives in a carbonated form from a spring in Vergèze in southern France. The Volvic spring is surrounded by seventeen square miles of countryside free from industry, intensive farming and other nearby sources of pollution. Volvic is lightly mineralized with a lot of character and a vibrant quality. Vittel is also good as is Evian.

It takes a bit of practice at first to make sure you get your water quota each day but soon it will become second nature. Start by drinking two glasses of water first thing in the morning when you get up, either neat or with a twist of lemon or lime. You can heat the water if you like. This helps with elimination. Then drink two or three glasses between breakfast and lunch and another two or three between lunch and dinner. When you exercise or when it is hot remember to drink more. Getting the water habit will quench your appetite, improve your body's ability to eliminate wastes, heighten your energy levels, improve the look of your skin and help your metabolic processes function at their peak. You will be amazed to discover just how potent are its gifts.

During a Miso Detox and Rebuild it is also important to get plenty of rest – you will need more than usual for much of the body's energy will be involved in deep cleansing itself. Take a nap in the middle of the day whenever you can and spend more time in bed at night reading or listening to music, or doing anything else that brings you pleasure. It can be helpful to take long walks and get plenty of gentle exercise.

Brush your skin before a bath or shower using a natural bristle dry brush which encourages good lymphatic drainage and cleansing.

The Detox is also an excellent time to explore what meditation or a deep relaxation exercise practised once or twice a day can do for you or to begin recording your dreams or writing spontaneously in a journal whatever happens to come into your mind without censoring any of it. The whole process of deep cleansing the body – breaking out of living habits which do not support health and energy – is but one part of cleansing the whole being. It can open up new vistas and help you to see your whole life in new ways.

When you stop eating the foods you are accustomed to eating and substitute the cleansing and regenerating foods, your body begins to throw off its stored wastes at an incredible rate. This can sometimes lead to a coating of the tongue and teeth with a most unpleasant-tasting stuff, headaches, a feeling of being unwell for a few hours or, in the case of those who have been heavy drinkers or who have long polluted their bodies through poor nutrition, even temporary nausea or diarrhoea. Sometimes one will even run a bit of a fever in the first few days which comes as a result of the toxin-burning processes that have begun. These unpleasant symptoms (and they by no means occur in every case) are simply a sign that the detox is working; they need no special treatment, just patience and rest and they usually pass quickly. Then, as stored wastes are eliminated from your body, your skin takes on a new glow and translucence. Lines on the face are softened and your eyes become clear and bright. In addition, your mind becomes clearer so that thinking is easier. Many writers and artists use detoxification regimes such as this or a high-raw diet before beginning a new project since it can heighten creativity. It is no accident that throughout history saints and philosophers have turned to abstinence as a way of increasing spiritual awareness and improving mental clarity. Following this kind of regime for between one week and several weeks can actually help create a bridge between a woman's previous existence and a new way of living. It is a mid-life ritual which can carry with it not just regeneration on a physical level but, in a very real sense, the resurrection of one's being.

Chapter Twenty-seven

Seeds of Change

The basic principles of balancing a woman's hormonal system are, by and large, the same nutritional principles that keep you vibrant and full of energy. Much of what follows I have already investigated in previous books but it forms the core of using food to enhance health and life energy. Never were these more important to any woman than after she passes the age of 35.

Making changes in the way you eat means making changes in how you cook. Not only are the methods of food preparation and the equipment you need in preparing life-generating foods special, so is the shopping. You may find your larder stocked with a whole new set of ingredients – particularly if until now you have been living on convenience foods or meat and two veg. The foods which you will use for most of these recipes are not only good for you, they are delicious – grains and legumes, nuts and seeds, fruits, vegetables and herbs. These can either be bought at great cost, or, if you shop around, very cheaply. I buy many of my fruits in crates from a wholesaler at less than half the price I would pay at the greengrocer. You can pay dearly for nuts and seeds, grains and pulses in some health-food stores where they come in tiny packages (and are often not very fresh). But beans and legumes, nuts and seeds, can also be bought cheaply in good supermarkets or in bulk at reasonable cost from many of the new wholefood emporiums which are beginning to appear everywhere. Obviously the more you buy at one time the cheaper they are. Be sure to refrigerate your nuts after purchase to keep their oils from going rancid. And if ever you buy a package of anything which you find on returning home is not absolutely fresh, take it back and complain. That is the only way to protect yourself while improving the quality of what is being sold. Here is a brief guide to stocking a larder with life-generating foods to give you some idea of just how much variety you have to choose from.

Fruit

Not only are fruits some of the most delicious natural foods available, they also have remarkable properties for spring-cleaning the body and are excellent biochemical antidotes to the stress that ages. Because fruits contain many natural acids such as citric and malic acid, they have an acid pH reaction in digestion. However, since they are also a rich source of alkaline-forming minerals, their reaction in the blood is always alkaline. This reaction helps neutralize the acid by-products of stress as well as the waste products of metabolism which are also acidic. That is why fruits are so highly prized as a means of internally cleansing the body.

Fruit contains very little protein but it is very high in the mineral potassium which needs to be balanced with sodium for perfect health in the body. Because most people in the West eat far too much sodium in the form of table salt and an excess of protein as well (which leaches important minerals from the bones and tissues), eating good quantities of fruit can help re-balance a body, improve its functioning, and make you feel more energetic as well.

Finally, because fruits are naturally sweet and because we are born with an innate liking for sweet things, a dessert of fresh fruit after a meal can be tremendously satisfying to the palate. And there is such a variety of beautiful textures, colours and tastes to choose from – from the sensuous softness of persimmons and the super-sweetness of fresh figs, to the exhilarating crunch of the finest English apple.

Vegetables

The best vegetables are those you grow yourself organically. If you are lucky enough to have a garden – even a small one – save all the leftovers and turn them into compost for fertilizer. Even in winter you can grow some delicious salads and root vegetables in a greenhouse or under cloches. The quality of organic produce is far superior to chemically fertilized fruits and vegetables – not to mention all the vitamins which are lost in foods when they are picked, stored, shipped and sit on shop shelves. In summer I go to the garden to pick my vegetables and fifteen minutes later they are gracing the dinner table. That is the best way to preserve their nutritional value as well as to experience the fullness of their flavour. If you are a flat dweller without a garden you can sprout fresh seeds and grains in jars or trays on your windowsill (see p. 387).

How you treat your vegetables once you cut them or buy them from the shops determines a lot how they taste and how much of their energy-enhancing goodness you preserve. Scrub anything that will stand up to a good scrubbing, using a brush marked *veg only*. Scrubbing vegetables is better than peeling since many of the valuable vitamins and minerals are stored directly beneath their skins. Never soak vegetables for long periods. They are better washed briefly under running water so you don't allow water-soluble vitamins to leach out of them. Always keep vegetables as cool as possible (even carrots and turnips are best kept in the fridge) and use them as soon as you can. When shopping for fresh things be demanding – choose your own cauliflower and make sure it is a good one. Don't be intimidated by pushy greengrocers who want to foist the leftovers on you before they bring in their new stock. Demand the best and you will get it. Your palate and your health will be grateful that you do.

Grains

Thousands of years ago Zarathustra the Persian sage waxed ecstatic about grains. 'When the light of the moon waxeth warmer,' he said, 'golden hued grains grow up from the earth during the spring.' I have always thought his words beautifully captured the richness and delight of the grain foods. When a good portion of what you eat comes from grain foods, because of the effect on the brain of the complex carbohydrates they contain, it tends to improve your disposition, make you feel calm and bring you energy that lasts and lasts. Grains, like legumes, need special handling. They should not be eaten raw. This is why many of the packaged mueslis cause digestive upset in many people. It is only by cooking them (or by sprouting or soaking them) that you break the chemical bonds, turning hard-to-digest starches into more easily digested sugars. All grains can be toasted lightly. This process, which is called dextrinizing, not only helps turn starches into natural sugars but also enhances the flavour of grains used as cereals or cooked in other recipes.

To dextrinize grains, spread them on a baking sheet and pop them into an oven at 150°C (300°F) Gas mark 2 for about 20 minutes, stirring every now and then. This is not necessary if you are going to boil them, but it does enhance the flavour and is particularly good if you want to use grains to make porridge or other hot breakfast cereals. The other important thing to remember about grains is that it is best to get as wide a variety as possible so if you have oat porridge at breakfast, at lunch you might choose whole rye bread or a bulgur wheat salad or brown rice. The more variety the better since each grain boasts a different balance of essential minerals and micronutrients.

GUIDE TO COOKING GRAINS

Grain (1 cup)	Water (cups)	Cooking time	Yield (cups)
Barley (whole)	4–5	2–3 hours	$3^1/2$
Barley (flakes)	3	45–60 minutes	3
Brown rice	2–$2^1/2$	1 hour	3
Buckwheat	2	20 minutes	$2^1/2$
Bulgur wheat	2	15–20 minutes	$2^1/2$
Couscous	1	15 minutes	$2^3/4$
Millet	$2^1/2$–3	45–60 minutes	$3^1/2$
Oats (whole groats)	5	2–3 hours	$2^1/2$
Polenta	5	45–60 minutes	$3^1/2$
Rye	5	2–3 hours	2
Quinoa	2	20 minutes	$2^1/2$
Wild rice	3	1–$1^1/2$ hours	$3^1/2$
Wheat (whole grain)	5	2–3 hours	$2^3/4$
Wheat flakes	2	45–60 minutes	3

Oils

It is wise not to use oils, except for soya oil and cold-pressed extra virgin olive oil. In heat-processed oils usable 'cis' fatty acids have been chemically changed into 'trans' fatty acids – junk fats (see Order Out of Chaos, p. 168) – which can not only be actively harmful, but actually block the use of any 'cis' fatty acids in the rest of your diet. Olive oil adds a distinctive flavour to salad dressings. It is quite heavy though and some people prefer a lighter oil.

The oil found in flaxseed or linseed is an almost perfect balance of linoleic and linolenic acid – both the omega 6 and omega 3 fatty acids. Linoleic acid is prominent in many seeds. Linolenic acid belongs to the omega 3 family. These are the fatty acids which are generally most prevalent in fatty fishes. What makes flaxseed oil so exceptional is that it has such a high degree of the omega 3 fatty acids which are, incidentally, particularly important in fat burning. The way to take flaxseed oil is by eating the seeds themselves – flaxseed oil that has been extracted is too easily made rancid. I grind flaxseed in a coffee grinder and then put it into a tightly covered jar and store it in the refrigerator. I use 2 to 4 dessertspoons a day. It is important to go for the very best German vacuum-packed linseeds, however, in order to make sure that the precious fatty acids which they contain are protected from rancidity. It is as easy as that to make sure you get all the essential fatty acids provided you steer clear of junk fats and processed oils. Your body will do the rest.

Nuts

Fresh nuts are a good source of essential fatty acids when used in small quantities. The rancid oils in old nuts are harmful to the stomach. They retard pancreatic enzymes and destroy vitamins. If nuts are fresh and whole (unbroken) you can buy a kilo or so at a time and, provided they are kept airtight in a cool dry place (best in the fridge), they will keep for a few months. You can even freeze them and keep them longer. It is a good idea to buy a few different kinds, then if you mix them you will get a good balance of essential amino acids. You will also have more variety in your recipes. Choose from: almonds, Brazils, cashews, coconut (fresh or desiccated), hazels, macadamia nuts, pecans, pine kernels, pistachios, tiger nuts and walnuts.

Seeds

Be sure you buy really fresh seeds with no signs of decay. The three seeds which provide a particularly valuable combination of protein and essential fatty acids are sunflower, pumpkin and sesame. They can be ground fresh in a coffee grinder and sprinkled on salads or cereals. Other seeds worth trying, mainly for seasoning, are poppy, celery, caraway, dill, fennel and anise.

Legumes

Nutritious, economical and delicious when well prepared, beans and pulses are rich in complex carbohydrates, protein and fibre as well as minerals and essential fatty acids. It is important to know how to handle them and to cook them well in order to avoid digestive upset. All legumes should be washed and cleared of any small pieces of stone or spoilt food. Then everything except lentils, split peas and mung beans should be soaked for at least six hours, preferably overnight, before cooking. The soak water should then be thrown away and fresh water should be added. There are two ways to minimize digestive upset when cooking legumes. I use both of them. The first is, after soaking and rinsing, put the legume in the freezer overnight and cook the next day. The second is, after soaking, throw the soak water away, boil up the beans for 20 minutes, throw the boil water away, rinse the beans then put them in more water plus whatever vegetables, herbs and seasonings you may be putting in with them, then cook in a covered saucepan by bringing the beans to a boil, reducing the heat and simmering them until they grow tender.

BEANS AND PULSES

Legumes (1 cup)	Soak	Water (cups)	Cooking time (hrs)	Yield (cups)
Adzuki	Yes	4	3	2
Baby lima	Yes	3	2	$1^3/_4$
Black beans	Yes	5	2	2
Cassoulet	Yes	4	$3^1/_2$	2
Chickpeas	Yes	4	$3^1/_2$	$2^1/_2$
Kidney	Yes	3	$1^1/_2$	2
Lentils	No	4	1	$2^1/_4$
Lima	Yes	5	2	$1^1/_4$
Mung	No	$2^1/_2$	$1^1/_2$	2
Navy	Yes	3	$2^1/_2$	2
Pinto	Yes	3	$2^1/_2$	2
Red	Yes	3	$3^1/_2$	2
Split peas	No	3	1	$2^1/_4$

There are so many things that you can make with legumes that you could fill ten cookbooks with wonderful recipes. I like to make thick soups with them and casseroles. They are great cooked and used cold the next day as a base for a whole-meal salad. In either case I add whatever vegetables I intend to cook with the beans plus some low-salt vegetable broth powder, and whatever other seasoning I am going to use. I then bring the beans to the boil and allow them to simmer for the prescribed length of time. Alternatively, I will bring the beans to the boil and put them in a slow cooker or the bottom of the Aga oven and forget about them for six to eight hours. I sometimes cook beans overnight this way. I soak various kinds of beans, such as lima beans, black-eyed beans, kidney beans, or a mixture of them, pour the soak water away and rinse them, then store them frozen in bags so that I can pull them out whenever I need them to make a casserole or a soup.

Many legumes sprout well, particularly lentils, mung and adzuki beans. Legumes contain a trypsin inhibitor, a substance which blocks the action of some of the enzymes which break down protein in your body, and because of this they must never be eaten raw. Trypsin inhibitors are destroyed when legumes are well cooked. Sprouting also neutralizes them. On p. 385 is a chart that will give you some guidelines to the cooking of legumes.

Sprouts

Seeds and grains are latent powerhouses of nutritional goodness and life energy. Add water to germinate them, let them grow for a few days in your kitchen and you will harvest delicious, inexpensive fresh foods of quite phenomenal health-enhancing value. The vitamin content of seeds increases dramatically when they germinate. The vitamin C content in soy beans multiplies five times within three days of germination – a mere tablespoon of soy bean sprouts contains half the recommended daily adult requirement of this vitamin. The vitamin B2 in an oat grain rises by 1,300 per cent almost as soon as the seed sprouts and by the time tiny leaves have formed it has risen by 2,000 per cent. Some sprouted seeds and grains are believed to have anti-cancer properties which is why they form an important part of the natural methods of treating the disease.

When you sprout a seed, enzymes which have been dormant in it spring into action breaking down stored starch and turning it into simple natural sugars and splitting long-chain proteins into amino acids. What this means is that the process of sprouting turns these seeds into foods which are very easily assimilated by your body when you eat them. Sprouts are, in effect, pre-digested. As such they have many times the nutritional efficiency of the seeds from which they have grown. They provide more nutrients gram for gram than any natural food known.

Because of the massive enzyme release which occurs when a seed or grain is sprouted the nutritional quality of a sprout is extremely good. These enzymes not only neutralize such factors as trypsin inhibitors but also destroy other substances which can be harmful such as phytic acid. Phytic acid, which occurs in considerable quantity in grains, particularly wheat, tends to bind minerals so that the digestive system cannot break them down for assimilation. When a grain is sprouted this mineral-binding capacity is virtually eliminated. Another attractive thing about sprouts is their price. The basic seeds and grains are cheap and readily available in supermarkets and health-food stores – chickpeas, brown lentils, mung beans, wheat grains and so forth. And since you sprout them yourself with nothing but clean water, they become an easily accessible source of organically grown fresh vegetables, even for city dwellers. In an age when most vegetables and fruits are grown on artificially fertilized soils and treated with hormones, fungicides, insecticides, preservatives and all manner of other chemicals, the home-grown-in-a-jar sprouts emerge as a pristine blessing – fresh, unpolluted and ready to eat in a minute by popping them into salads or sandwiches. As such, they can be a wonderful health food to any family concerned about the rising cost of food and the falling nutritional value in the average diet. They are the cheapest form of natural food around. Different sprouts mixed together will indeed support life all on their own. While I would never suggest that anybody live on sprouts alone, I think they are an ideal addition to the table – particularly if the budget is tight.

DIY Sprouting

When you discover how economical and easy it is to grow sprouts you will want to have some on the go all the time. Once germinated you can keep sprouts in polythene bags in the fridge for up to a week – just long enough to get a new batch ready for eating. Most people grow sprouts in glass jars covered with nylon mesh held in place with an elastic band around the neck, but I have discovered an even simpler method which allows you to grow many more and avoids the jar-method problem of seeds rotting due to insufficient drainage. You will need the following:

- Seeds (e.g. mung beans).
- Seed trays with drainage holes, available from gardening shops and nurseries.

- A jar or bowl to soak seeds in overnight.
- A plant atomizer – from gardening or hardware shops.
- A sieve.
- Nylon mesh – available from gardening shops.

1. Place two handfuls of seeds or beans in the bottom of a jar or bowl and cover with plenty of water. Leave to soak overnight.
2. Pour the seeds into a sieve and rinse well with water. Be sure to remove any dead or broken seeds or pieces of debris.
3. Line a seedling tray with nylon mesh (this helps the seeds drain better) and pour in the soaked seeds.
4. Place in a warm dark spot for fast growth.
5. Spray the seeds twice a day with fresh water in an atomizer and stir them gently with your hand in order to aerate them.
6. After about three days, place the seeds in sunlight for several hours to develop the chlorophyll (green) in them.
7. Rinse in a sieve, drain well and put in a polythene bag in the fridge to use in salads, wok-frys, etc.

There are many different seeds you can sprout – each with its own particular flavour and texture. Use the chart (on p. 389) as a guide to the variety of sprouts you can try.

Special Foods

Carob (St John's Bread)

Carob powder/flour is a superb chocolate substitute – and good for you too. Unlike chocolate it does not contain caffeine. Instead it is full of minerals – calcium, phosphorus, iron, potassium, magnesium and silicon – as well as vitamins B1, B2, niacin and a little vitamin A plus some protein. Carob powder is often sold toasted, but the best kind is raw. It is lighter in colour than the cooked kind. It can be bought from most health-food stores and used to make chocolate drinks, desserts and treats.

SPROUTING

Seeds and soak time	To yield 1 litre	Ready to eat in	Length of shoot	Growing tips and notes
Alfalfa (6–8 hours)	3–4 tbsp	5–6 days	3.5 cm ($1^{1}/_{2}$")	Rich in organic vitamins and minerals, and natural oestrogens.
Fenugreek	$^{1}/_{2}$ cup	3–4 days	1 cm ($^{1}/_{2}$")	Have quite a strong 'curry' taste. Good for ridding the body of toxins.
Adzuki beans (10–15 hrs)	$1^{1}/_{2}$ cup	3–5 days	2.5–3.5 cm ($1–1^{1}/_{2}$")	Have a nutty flavour. Especially good for the kidneys.
Chickpeas (10–15 hrs)	2 cups	3–4 days	2.5 cm (1")	May need to soak for 18 hrs to swell to their full size. Replace the water during this time.
Lentils (10–15 hrs)	1 cup	3–5 days	0.5–2.5cm ($^{1}/_{4}$–1")	Try all different kinds of lentils. They are good eaten young or up to 6 days old.
Mung beans (10–15 hrs)	1 cup	3–5 days	1–5 cm ($^{1}/_{2}$–$2^{1}/_{2}$")	Soak at least 15 hours. Keep in the dark for a sweet sprout.
Sunflower seeds (10–15 hrs)	4 cups	1–2 days	same length as seed	Soak them and sprout for just a day. Bruise easily so handle carefully.
Wheat (12–15 hrs)	2 cups	2–3 days	same length as grain	An excellent source of the B vitamins. The soak water can be drunk straight or added to soups and vegetable juices.

Agar-Agar

This starch comes from seaweed. You can use it to make vegetarian gelatin-based sweets and salads and to thicken sauces and toppings. It comes in flakes or granules and sometimes in sheets. Soak the agar-agar in a little water to soften it before adding hot liquid to dissolve it. Use about 1 teaspoon to each cup of water or liquid.

Arrowroot

Made from the pulp of the tuberous rootstocks of a tropical American plant, arrowroot is a nutritious easily digested food high in calcium. When you heat it in water it thickens (use 1½ teaspoons per cup of liquid). It is better than cornstarch or corn flour to thicken gravy, fruit sauces, soups and stews.

Sea Vegetables

If you have never used the sea vegetables for cooking, this is an ideal time to begin. Not only are they delicious – imparting a wonderful, spicy flavour to soups and salads – they are the richest source of organic mineral salts in nature, particularly of iodine. Iodine is the mineral needed by the thyroid gland. As your thyroid gland is largely responsible for the body's metabolic rate, iodine is very important to a woman's energy. I like to use powdered kelp as a seasoning. It adds both flavour and minerals to salad dressings, salads and soups. I am also very fond of nori seaweed, which comes in long thin sheets or tiny flakes. It is a delicious snack food which you can eat along with a salad or at the beginning of the meal: it has a beautiful, crisp flavour. I often toast it very, very quickly by putting it under a grill for no more than 10 or 15 seconds. It is also delicious raw.

Get to know some of the sea vegetables and start to make use of them. Your nails and hair and the rest of your body will be strengthened by the full range of minerals and trace elements such as selenium, calcium, iodine, boron, potassium, magnesium, iron and others which are not always found in great quantities in our ordinary garden vegetables. You can use nori to wrap around everything from a sprout salad to cooked grains in order to make little pieces of vegetarian *sushi*. It's often a good idea to soak some of the other sea vegetables such as dulse, arame and hiziki for a few minutes in enough tepid water to cover. This softens them so that they can be easily chopped to be put into salads or added to soups. Sea vegetables are available in health-food stores and in Oriental food shops. Recommended ones are:

- arame
- dulse
- hiziki
- kelp
- mixed sea salad

- combu
- laver bread
- nori
- wakami

Seasonings

Mustard

Mustard can be bought in dry or paste form. The dry powder is sometimes useful in dressings. I think the most delicious mustards are French. They are milder and more aromatic than English mustard. Moutarde de Meaux is particularly delicious and is great in dressings for all sorts of salads. Dijon and Bordeaux are also nice.

Tahini (preferably unroasted)

A paste made from ground sesame seeds which is delicious and very nutritious. It has many uses including tahini mayonnaise, and is delicious as an addition to many seeds and nut dishes.

Low-Salt Vegetable Bouillon Powder

This is something I use a lot to season just about everything. Use it for soup stocks, to flavour pizzas, grains like brown rice and kasha and even salad dressings, stews and casseroles. It is my favourite of all seasonings. The very best is Marigold's Low-Salt Swiss Vegetable Bouillon. I even take it with me when I travel.

Yeast Extract

This can be used as a substitute for 'vegetable bouillon'. It is rich in B complex vitamins but very salty, so it should also be used in moderation.

Food Yeast

This is sometimes called primary yeast or nutritional yeast. It is not brewer's yeast which is a by-product of beer making. Food yeast is grown specifically to be used as a flavouring. It is light yellow-beige and slightly spiky in its texture and is good to add to soups, sauces, cheeses and dips. You can even sprinkle it on popcorn.

Vanilla Essence

Try to find real vanilla essence rather than the more common vanilla flavouring which is synthetic. It gives a delicious warm flavour.

Plant Sterols Helpers

So many fresh foods are rich in plant hormones. Include them often in your meals. The fresher they are the better: yams, peas, papayas, bananas, cucumbers, raw nuts, bee pollen, sprouted seeds and grains, and the herbs liquorice root, alfalfa, red clover, sage, sarsaparilla, and sassafras. The green vegetable juices, particularly figs and garlic, dates, avocados, grapes, apples, seaweed, wheatgerm and chlorella can all be helpful in countering menopausal and menstrual problems. Grapes, cherries, citrus fruits and red clover are excellent sources of the bioflavonoids which also have weak oestrogenic activity and have shown themselves to be useful in countering hot flushes, mood swings and in helping to prevent heavy irregular menstrual flow. Plant foods high in phyto-sterols are good insurance against cancer, too, since they help prevent oestrogen dominance in the body and xenoestrogens in the environment from binding with hormone receptor sites and causing long-term damage.

The anti-oxidants in fresh plant foods also offer protective properties against cancer. These include vitamin C from fresh fruits and vegetables, vitamin E which is rich in fresh whole grains, vitamin A from fish liver and beta-carotene. The fibre found in plants is protective against oestrogen dominance and cancer via another mechanism. Breast cancer is highly related to oestrogen levels as well as to the consumption of high levels of meat and fat. Women on a vegetarian diet high in fibre excrete a much higher level of oestrogen than other women and have much lower blood levels of the hormones. In Britain and the United States the use of milk products has been correlated with breast cancer. Sea plants and green vegetables, spirulina and chlorella are far better sources of calcium than cheese and milk. Some of the best products of all are the soya-based foods from the Orient, together with naturally fermented foods – often of Japanese origin.

Tofu

Its other name is bean curd. This white, bland soft food made from soy beans is easy to digest, high in protein, low in calories and fat, cheap, and you can use it for just about anything. It behaves a bit like a sponge which will absorb whatever flavour you soak it in. When you cook it, it becomes firmer. You can mix it with herbs, make sauces or low-fat mayonnaise from it, dips for vegetables, pizza toppings and stir-fries. You can even substitute it for cheese in some of your favourite recipes, except that it doesn't melt under the grill. Buy it in the supermarket, health-food store or Oriental food shop and keep it sitting in water in the fridge so it doesn't dry out.

Miso

A fermented soy bean paste which is rich in digestive enzymes and high in protein. It can be used for seasoning soups and sauces. It is also a delicious addition to dips for crudités and salad dressings (see Resurrection, p. 365).

Tamari

This is a type of soya sauce made from fermented soy beans, but unlike soya sauce it contains no wheat, although it does contain sea salt so should be used in moderation. It is good for giving a 'Chinese' taste to dishes as well as a rich flavour to bland dressings or sauces.

Soya Flour

Made from cooked, ground soy beans, soya flour is sometimes added to grain-based flours to increase their protein content. It can be used to make soya milk and soya cheese.

Soya Milk

Made from cooked, ground, and strained soy beans this is often used for bottlefed infants who are allergic to cow's milk. I use it as a substitute for milk on cereals and in recipes. You can make your own very cheaply. I prefer this since ready-made varieties are often packed in aluminium-lined cartons and it is best to avoid aluminium (see Resources, p. 512, for the best soya milk).

Herbs

The magicians of life-generating cooking, fresh herbs can transform a humble recipe into a Pasha's delight. I use them constantly, lavishly, and occasionally with utter abandon. I have been known to add as many as seven different leafy herbs to a simple green salad which becomes more of a herb salad than a green salad by the time I have finished. I grow most of my herbs in the garden because there is something about freshness which you can't recapture from the dried varieties. With fresh herbs you needn't worry much about choosing the wrong ones. Some of my favourites for salads include lovage (which I also use to season many salad dressings), basil, dill, the mints, winter savory, fennel, chives and the parsleys. In the summer I cull them from the garden. Some I dry by hanging from beams in the kitchen for a few days and then store them in airtight jars for winter use. Others – the more succulent herbs such as parsley, basil and chives – can be deep-frozen in sprigs then simply chopped and used when needed. If you live in a flat or don't have a garden you can grow herbs in pots in the kitchen window where they lend their own beauty to the room as well as offering a constant supply of culinary delights. Thyme, marjoram and winter savory will grow beautifully in pots indoors over the winter. So will parsley. Once you begin to play about with herb magic you will probably find, as I have, that you never want to be without these lovely plants. Here are some of the most common herbs and what I find them useful for.

Herb Magic

Basil I probably use this herb far too much because it is available only in the summer months and because it is simply so lovely. It has a distinctive flavour which is an ideal garnish for tomatoes or in large amounts mixed in a green salad. Use the leaves whole for the best possible flavour.

Chervil This herb is a cousin to parsley, with a delicate aniseed flavour. We use it lavishly in salads. It mixes particularly well with chives, tarragon and parsley.

Chives More beautiful in looks than in flavour, I think, chives are great for sprinkling on to sunflower wafers or in seed cheeses. I find them not strong enough for most salads and prefer instead spring onions or a little chopped shallots.

Dill It goes wonderfully with dressings, cucumbers, and beetroot and apple salads, and has a gentle delicate flavour which reminds me of quiet afternoons under sun-shaded willows.

Fennel A lacy aniseed-flavoured herb which grows immense in the summer. It goes well with salsify salads and with cucumbers, tomatoes and in vegetable loaves. It is also a lovely decorative herb to place around the edge of a dish of salads.

Lovage Perhaps the most underrated of the common herbs, lovage is wonderful mixed with the mints and yogurt as the base of a herbal salad dressing which is as beautiful in colour as it is in flavour. We use lots of it in our dish salads.

Marjoram This herb comes in many variations – sweet marjoram, pot marjoram, winter marjoram, golden marjoram. Each is a little different. The sweet variety is lovely with plain green salads and goes well with tomatoes and Mediterranean vegetables. Oregano is a wild marjoram akin to our winter variety.

The Mints There are even more varieties than the marjorams – spearmint, peppermint, apple mint, pineapple mint, ginger mint, eau de cologne mint. I use spearmint and apple mint in green salads and many dressings. Pineapple mint, with its splendid variegated leaves, makes a wonderful garnish for fruit salads, drinks and also salad platters. Ginger mint is great in summer drinks, sorbets and punches.

Parsley This common herb comes in two main varieties – fine and broadleaf. For most raw dishes we prefer the broadleaf parsley because it is more delicate and pleasant to munch. Both have a rich 'green' flavour which works well with other herbs. It is great chopped in patties and loaves, in green salads and for dressings, as well as being a lovely garnish for almost any dish.

Sage This herb has a strong individual flavour and a particular affinity for onions. It is good in savoury nut dishes and adds flavour to seed and nut ferments.

Thyme It comes in many varieties, some of which are much richer in flavour than others, but all have a wonderful warming sweet flavour which enhances peppers, courgettes and nut dishes as well as giving a unique flavour to sprout salads.

Seven Days of Supermeals

For energy that lasts, eat breakfast like a king, eat lunch like a prince and supper like a pauper. For example, breakfast would be a bowl of miso broth with green foods (see p. 368) or a grain dish, i.e. porridge, raw muesli or sugar-free granola. In addition you might eat one or two pieces of fruit, wholegrain bread (best wheat-free) or toast with a fruit or nut spread. Lunch would become your main meal, consisting of a main course plus some vegetables – crudités, salads or sprouted seeds and grains, plus a yellow and green vegetable if not already incorporated. You might want to add wholegrain bread (best wheat-free) with a fruit spread. Supper now becomes a light meal consisting of a fruit dish or fresh fruit salad or perhaps a light soup.

Monday

Main meal 100 per cent corn pasta with garlic olive oil and steamed vegetables. Charismatic carrot salad made with shredded fresh raw carrots and tangerine sections dressed with orange juice, curry powder and chopped parsley.

Baked bananas made using organic brown rice syrup, a dash of rum and a squeeze of lemon juice.

Light meal A dish salad where whatever raw vegetables are available have been arranged in segments – grated carrots, red or yellow bell peppers, half an avocado, radish slices, a handful of Chinese bean sprouts, a few slices of cucumber, a grated raw beetroot or white radish, and some mustard and cress dressed with tofu vinaigrette. For this you will need $3/4$ cup of tofu, 3 tablespoons of rice wine vinegar or cider vinegar, the juice of two lemons, a tablespoon of Dijon mustard, 1 clove of crushed garlic, salt and fresh herbs put into a blender and processed. (This dressing will keep for a few days in the fridge.)

Tuesday

Main meal Carrot soup with orange and fresh ginger made with: $1/2$ cup chopped green onions, 1 cup orange juice, 1 cup water, 2 cups diced carrots, 2 teaspoons chopped fresh ginger, 2 tablespoons low-salt vegetable bouillon (to taste), freshly ground pepper and a teaspoon of coriander. Boil the carrots until tender then add the orange juice and bouillon powder, reheat and serve.

Slices of organic tofu which have been spread with miso and grilled along with raw mushrooms.

Serve with a selection of steamed vegetables all cooked in the same pot, e.g. cauliflower, broccoli, spinach, green beans, onions.

Raw pineapple slices dusted with shredded coconut.

Light meal A jacket potato stuffed with sprouted seeds or grains and tofu dip made with: 1 cup tofu, juice of 1 lemon, 1 teaspoon wholegrain Meaux mustard, 1 tablespoon low-salt vegetable bouillon powder, a few leaves of fresh basil or some chopped parsley. Combine well in a food processor. This will keep for several days in the fridge.

Wednesday

Main meal Grilled fresh mackerel with garlic and lemon juice served with a selection of steamed vegetables. Or split-pea soup made with: 1 cup dried split peas, soaked overnight, 1 onion, 2 medium carrots, 2 sticks celery, 1 litre ($1^3/4$ pints) spring water, 1 tablespoon low-salt vegetable bouillon powder, 2 tablespoons chopped fresh herbs. Put the peas, vegetables and water into a pot, boil and simmer for $1^1/2$ hours until the peas are tender. Add the vegetable bouillon and fresh herbs 5 minutes before serving. If you want a smooth soup, put into a food processor and blend.

Salad of fresh young spinach leaves and sliced white mushrooms dressed with lemon and olive oil and sprinkled with toasted sunflower seeds.

Orange sorbet made from 8 oranges with skin and seeds removed and pulped in a processor. Add a tiny amount of honey to sweeten and some nutmeg, ginger or fresh mint. Pour the mixture into ice-cube trays or a plastic container and freeze. Remove from the freezer and leave to thaw slightly for about 10 minutes. Blend the mixture again immediately before serving.

Light meal 100 per cent buckwheat soba noodles in a bowl of miso broth (see p. 368). To cook soba noodles, bring a big pot of water to a firm boil and add the noodles slowly so the water continues to boil. When it begins to foam pour a cup of cold water into the pot. When it comes to the boil the second time add another cup of water, repeating this process three times. Once the noodles are *al dente*, drain them and rinse immediately under cold water to prevent their sticking together. Make the miso broth and place the cold noodles into it immediately and serve. You can cook more soba than you will eat at one meal and store them in the fridge for later. Doing this makes soba and miso broth an almost instant meal.

Thursday

Main meal Fresh vegetables either with tofu or chicken, wok-fried in a little olive oil or soy oil. Serve on a bed of steamed organic brown rice made from 1 cup brown rice, 2–3 cups spring water, 2 teaspoons vegetable bouillon powder, 3 tablespoons fresh parsley, 1 teaspoon marjoram and 2 cloves garlic. Wash the rice three times under running water and put into a saucepan. Boil the water in a kettle and pour over the rice. Add seasonings except for parsley. Bring to the boil and cook gently for 45 minutes or until all the liquid has been absorbed. Garnish with parsley and serve.

Apple ginger salad made from 6 green apples, 1/4 cup fresh orange juice, 1 teaspoon grated fresh ginger, 2 teaspoons clear honey and 3 tablespoons toasted sesame seeds. Baked apples made from 4 large apples, 1/2 cup date butter or raisins that have been soaked in water for 2 hours, 1/4 cup chopped almonds or pecans, 2 tablespoons vanilla essence, 2 tablespoons rum, 2 tablespoons fresh lime or lemon juice. Wash and core the apples. Mix other ingredients together in a small bowl and stuff the core of each apple. Place in a non-stick oven dish and pour remaining mixture over the apples, adding a tablespoon or two of water if necessary. Bake for 45 minutes at 180°C (350°F) Gas mark 4.

Light meal Corn soup made from 2 fresh corn on the cob, 1/2 pint warm spring water, 2 spring onions, 1 teaspoon low-salt vegetable bouillon powder, 1/4 red pepper, 1/4 green pepper, 1 tablespoon watercress, 1 tablespoon tahini. Wash the corn and cut off the kernels. Mix together with the water, spring onions and vegetable bouillon powder, season with tahini and blend until creamy in a blender or food processor. Add the chopped peppers and watercress. Toast made from rye bread and spread with soya cottage cheese made from 2 cups tofu, $3/4$ cup mayonnaise, 1 teaspoon low-salt vegetable bouillon powder, 1 teaspoon caraway seeds, 1 teaspoon mild curry powder, 1 clove garlic, handful fresh herbs and 2 tablespoons chopped chives. Mash the tofu well, add all the other ingredients and blend. This will keep for several days in the fridge.

Friday

Main meal Dahl stew made from $3/4$–1 cup red lentils or split peas, 1 large cauliflower broken into florets, 3 large carrots, pinch of turmeric, 3 cloves garlic, 2 tablespoons low-salt vegetable bouillon powder, 1 large onion, 1 red pepper, 1 yellow pepper, 2 teaspoons ground cummin, 2 teaspoons coriander, 2 teaspoons fresh ginger, 1–2 teaspoons mild curry powder, 1 large parsnip, 1 cup broccoli florets, 2 large tomatoes or 3 tablespoons tomato paste with $1/2$ cup water. Put the lentils or peas into a large pot and cover with 3 cups water and 1 tablespoon low-salt vegetable bouillon powder. Cook for 45 minutes until tender. Purée in a food processor and set them aside. While the peas are cooking, braise the onion in a little water with the garlic, turmeric, ginger and 1 tablespoon vegetable bouillon. When they have softened add the vegetables, except the broccoli, and other seasonings, and simmer until cooked. Pour the puréed legume mixture into the vegetables, add the broccoli and serve immediately.

Sunshine salad made from a few leaves of crisp lettuce, 1 medium-sized fresh pineapple, 2 coarsely grated carrots, 2 finely chopped sticks celery, 2 handfuls soaked sultanas, $1/2$ teaspoon celery seeds. Dress with an oil-free French dressing made from $3/4$ cup tomato juice, $1/4$ cup lemon juice or cider vinegar, 1 teaspoon wholegrain mustard, a little low-salt vegetable bouillon powder, 1 clove garlic and black pepper.

Carob and banana ice-cream made from 4 cups (about 1 litre or $13/4$ pints) soya milk, 4 ripe bananas, 3 tablespoons granular lecithin (optional), 1 cup unheated carob powder, $1/2$ cup pear concentrate and 1 teaspoon vanilla essence. Freeze the milk in a low, flat plastic container. When frozen, remove from the freezer and let it sit for about half an hour until it is just soft enough to slice into pieces. Put the bananas into the food processor, add about a cup of the frozen milk, the lecithin, carob powder, pear concentrate and vanilla, and blend until it is just mixed. Add the remainder of the soya milk. Should it become too liquid, return to the freezer for a few minutes then stir before serving.

Light meal Nut milk shake made from: $1/3$ cup almonds (blanched), $2/3$ cup soya milk, 5 pitted dates, a few drops vanilla essence and 1 teaspoon honey. Blend the almonds and the soya milk really well until the mixture is smooth. Add the other ingredients and process well. Serve immediately.
An orange or apple.

Saturday

Main meal Scrambled tofu made from $1/2$ cup diced onions, $1/2$ cup diced carrots, $1/2$ cup chopped celery, 2 cloves garlic, 1 teaspoon olive or soya oil, 2 cups mashed tofu, 1 tablespoon soy sauce, 2 teaspoons low-salt vegetable bouillon powder and 1 teaspoon mild curry powder.

Sprout salad made from 1 cup lentil sprouts, 1 cup fenugreek sprouts, 1 cup alfalfa sprouts, 1 cup shredded Chinese leaves, 3 sliced carrots and 4 diced tomatoes. Dress the salad with $1/2$ cup tofu or 3 medium-ripe tomatoes, $1/2$ cup fresh garden herbs, 1 tablespoon sesame seeds, 2 tablespoons lemon juice, 1 teaspoon onion powder and 1 teaspoon celery salt.

Fresh fruit salad with cashew cream made from $1/2$ cup cashews, $3/4$ cup soya milk and dash of cinnamon or nutmeg. Put all the ingredients in a food processor and blend well.

Light meal Sprouted lentil salad made from $11/2$ cups fresh lentil sprouts, 1 large red pepper, 100 g (4 oz) broccoli florets, 100 g (4 oz) cauliflower florets, 150 g (6 oz) button mushrooms garnished with $1/4$ cup of splintered raw almonds and dressed with $1/4$ cup tomato juice, 2 tablespoons cider vinegar, 1 teaspoon freshly grated root ginger, 2 tablespoons fresh orange juice, 2 teaspoons vegetable bouillon powder or soy sauce and 1 teaspoon mild curry powder.

Sunday

Main meal Spicy shish-kebab made from 1 large aubergine, chunks of tofu, 10 fresh tomatoes, 24 large mushrooms, 1 red pepper, 1 green pepper, 2 large onions, 1 large swede or 2 small turnips. Marinade: $1^1/4$ cups olive oil, juice of 3 lemons, 2 tablespoons red wine, 3 cloves garlic, 1 teaspoon coriander, 2 tablespoons parsley, $1/2$ teaspoon nutmeg, 1 tablespoon fresh basil and 1 teaspoon dried oregano. Place all the marinade ingredients together in a large bowl and mix thoroughly. Grill the aubergine until just soft and put with the rest of the vegetables into the marinade. Allow to sit for 2–4 hours. Skewer the vegetables and baste with the marinade as they are grilled. Serve with brown rice or kasha made from 2 cups buckwheat, spring water to cover, 2 teaspoons vegetable bouillon powder, and 2 tablespoons chopped fresh parsley or other herbs. Place buckwheat in a heavy-bottomed pan and roast it dry over a medium heat while stirring with a wooden spoon. As it begins to darken pour hot water over the buckwheat and add the vegetable bouillon powder and 1 tablespoon of the herbs. Cover and simmer very slowly for about 15 to 20 minutes until all the liquid has been absorbed. Serve with remaining herbs as a garnish.

Sliced tomato and fresh basil or parsley salad dressing with lemon, garlic and olive oil.

Raspberry ice-cream made from 4 tablespoons agar flakes, $2^1/2$ cups soya milk, $1/4$ cup apple juice concentrate and 450 g (1 lb) frozen raspberries. Place the agar flakes and soya milk in the top of a *bain-marie* and boil gently, stirring constantly until the agar is dissolved. Take off the heat and pour in the apple juice concentrate, while still stirring. Add the raspberries, stir and chill. Stir the mixture from time to time until it has thickened, then freeze until firm.

Light meal Dairy-free muesli made from 2 tablespoons oat flakes or a combination of oat, rye and wheat soaked overnight in a little spring water or fruit juice. A handful of raisins also soaked overnight, 1 grated apple or pear, juice of $1/2$ lemon, 3 tablespoons soya milk or yogurt, 1 tablespoon apple concentrate or pear or strawberry juice, and $1/2$ tea-

spoon powdered cinnamon or ginger. Mix together the
soaked oat flakes and raisins and combine with the grated
apple or pear, lemon juice and the soya milk or yogurt.
Drizzle with fruit juice and sprinkle with cinnamon or ginger.
You can also sprinkle with fresh ground pecans, hazelnuts or
three seeds (sesame, pumpkin and sunflower). Serve immediately.

Chapter Twenty-eight

The Professionals

There is no substitute for healthy eating. Throughout evolution your body has relied upon natural foods to supply it with the vitamins, minerals, trace elements, essential fatty acids and all the other elements of nutrition it needs to maintain health and life. All nutrients are synergistic – they work together in highly complex ways. The body is genetically set up to receive these elements bound together in plant complexes and a pill full of vitamins and minerals can never take the place of that. That being said, unless you have lived an exemplary life, eaten foods you have grown yourself organically and not been exposed to high levels of pollutants in the environment, you may well benefit by taking certain carefully chosen nutritional supplements. There are also some quite remarkable natural substances – L-pyroglutamic acid, DMAE, N-acetyl-carnitine and melatonin – which used as nutritional supplements can revolutionize the way the brain functions. Some of these cognitive enhancers can heighten intelligence and improve memory. Others enhance immune functions or neuroendocrine regulation. Still others improve the body's ability to relax or regulate body rhythms or help protect against premature ageing. All are life-enhancers capable in one way or another of improving the quality of life and the energy levels of healthy people who use them. They are the next generation of professional supplements and, as such, can be very useful to women in mid-life and beyond.

The Powerfoods

The first rank of nutritional supplements – the very best of all – are the powerfoods: dried green barley, wheat grass, alfalfa, spirulina or blue-green algae, chlorella, flaxseed, seaweeds and apple cider vinegar. Spirulina or blue-green algae is a fine source of easily assimilated protein, chlorophyll, beta-carotene and vitamin B12 plus many other important trace elements. Green barley is also full of vitamins, minerals, enzymes and chlorophyll as is wheat grass. Flaxseeds are the best single source of essential fatty acids (see p. 383) The green foods can be added to fresh vegetables or fruit juices, miso broth or salads. Seaweeds go well in soups, casseroles, stir-fries, salads and miso broth. They are just about the best source of minerals and trace elements you can find anywhere. A tablespoon a day of apple cider vinegar in a glass of spring water cures dietary indiscretions. Spirulina and green barley are the two most important green powerfoods.

Spirulina A rich source of an amazing variety of essential nutrients, spirulina contains significant quantities of the essential fatty acid, linoleic, plus GLA, B12, iron, RNA, DNA, chlorophyll, and a blue pigment called phycocyanin found only in blue-green algae, which has been shown to increase the survival rate of animals with liver cancer. It is also a rich source of essential amino acids being 60 to 70 per cent protein. Easy to digest, spirulina helps protect immunity and aids mineral absorption. It also helps to stabilize blood sugar and curb appetite. Spirulina is available in tablet form but is easiest to take either in powder stirred into broth or juice or (my favourite form) as flakes which I sprinkle over salads and soups. A teaspoon or two a day of this powerfood brings excellent nutritional support, but be careful about the kind that you buy. Some spirulina is not good quality and it must be pure – preferably organic (see Resources, p. 511).

Green Barley This is a dried form of the natural juice taken from young barley leaves. It needs to be organically grown and pesticide-free. Rich in proteins, flavonoids, minerals including iron, vitamins such as K and B15, as well as chlorophyll and other nutrients, green barley is also rich in thousands of enzymes, not all of which are destroyed in the digestive process and many of which can play important roles in supporting metabolic processes. It also contains a high concentration of superoxide dismutase (SOD) – an anti-oxidant enzyme. Sprinkle from $1/2$ to 1 teaspoon of green barley on to salads or mix into juices, miso broth or water.

Anti-oxidants

Free radicals are toxic species of atoms or molecules which are highly reactive simply because they are electrochemically unbalanced. They are common and necessary to all biological systems and are formed naturally during a wide variety of biological processes from respiration to the carrying out of enzyme activities which are a normal part of energy production and cell metabolism. The body has important anti-oxidant enzymes – superoxide dismutase, catalase and glutathione peroxidase – designed to de-activate free radicals before they can cause damage to the body. The problem is, when we are subjected to physical, chemical and electromagnetic stress, then our bodies create more free radicals than our anti-oxidant enzymes can handle. When free radicals get out of hand they can precipitate a relentless process of destruction and degeneration in the body as a whole. Recent findings in the field of free radical pathology – the study of free radicals 'gone wrong' – are nothing short of revolutionary. They make it possible for the first time in scientific terms to formulate a *unified* theory of disease.

Thanks to free radical biochemistry, doctors well versed in the subject are beginning to make sense of a lot of what until now appeared to be contradictory clinical and epidemiological observations and to create a scientific rationale both for the treatment and prevention of a number of the major causes of degeneration and death: arteriosclerosis, cancer, arthritis, dementia and other age-related diseases. We know now that free radical damage underlies the pathology of *all* of these conditions despite the difference in their manifestations in the body. Free radical damage is the very foundation of premature ageing. To counteract it, certain anti-oxidant nutrients can be enormously effective: vitamins C and E, beta-carotene or the mixed carotinoids, zinc, selenium, the flavonoids, co-enzyme Q10, and the sulphur-based amino acids such as methionine, cysteine, N-acetyl cysteine, glucose-cysteine and taurine.

Troublesome though it may seem, with the exception of the B complex vitamins, which are often best taken together, anti-oxidants and other specific nutrients are best taken singly

– each on its own. This is much better than using multivitamin and mineral supplements. It is also important to take only fresh supplements. Vitamins, minerals and other supplements which are not fresh are toxic to the body and can do harm. Always buy the best quality supplements you can find. Most will stay fresh for 12 weeks after you have opened the container. Never remove vitamins from bottles more than one day before you are going to take them and keep all supplements away from sunlight and warmth. It is a good idea to smell the bottle whenever you remove supplements. If it has a strong odour the vitamins may have gone off and should be thrown away.

Vitamin C A water-soluble anti-oxidant, vitamin C plays an important role in the formation of collagen and the building of connective tissue in skin, tendons and cartilage. It is also important in supporting the action of the adrenal glands in their manufacture of essential hormones such as cortisone, adrenalin and the oestrogens – particularly in the case of menopausal and postmenopausal women when the adrenals take over this task from the ovaries. Vitamin C is also important for the health of other glands in the body as well as for the strength of teeth and gums, bones and organs, and it looks after immunity, helping to protect from the common cold, physical and mental stress, and the toxic effects of drugs, pollutants, and chemicals in food and water. Vitamin C is found in fresh fruits and vegetables, especially rose hips, blackcurrants, acerola cherries, green peppers, turnip greens and watercress. Tables of recommended daily doses of vitamin C will tell you that you need no more than 30 to 70 mg of the vitamin a day. However most nutritionists recommend 1,000 to 2,000 mg (1 to 2 g a day), and most women find that at such levels they look and feel better and have more energy. A good form of vitamin C as a supplement is so-called 'buffered' vitamin C – calcium ascorbate or magnesium ascorbate – together with the bioflavonoids (see Resources, p. 510).

Vitamin E This vitamin might be said to be the fat-soluble counterpart of vitamin C. It protects the unsaturated fatty acids, sex hormones and fat-soluble vitamins from free radical destruction. This is why it is often added to oils. It is also used as a base for the sub-lingual drops of progesterone – to protect against rancidity and degradation. Vitamin E supports good circulation, guards the lungs from free radical damage as a result of pollution, counters blood clots and helps retard ageing. It is also used to prevent and counter menstrual and menopausal problems, blood sugar problems, heart conditions, arthritis, varicose veins and benign breast lumps. Vitamin E is found in whole grains, dark green leafy vegetables, nuts, seeds, brown rice and wheatgerm. The recommended daily allowance of vitamin E is a mere 15 to 30 iu. Most nutritionists, however, use 100–200 iu for a healthy person and between 200–2,000 iu a day for therapeutic purposes. People with high blood pressure need to be careful when taking vitamin E since the dosage has to be increased gradually under the watchful eye of a practitioner trained in nutrition or it can exacerbate the condition.

Beta-carotene and the mixed carotinoids The carotinoids, of which beta-carotene is the best known and most widely studied, are precursors to vitamin A. They occur naturally in vegetables and can be turned into this vitamin in the body. This makes them a safe source of vitamin A since the body will metabolize only as much as it needs. Vitamin A is another important anti-oxidant which helps make the body resistant to infection by enhancing immunity. It is also needed to enhance the repair of epithelial tissue and to make strong bones. It helps prevent premature ageing (most so-called ageing is premature), fights free radical damage, improves the permeability of capillaries and protects against infection and cancer. Either vitamin A or the carotinoids are found in fish liver oils, animal livers, green and yellow fruits and vegetables, especially alfalfa, apricots, dandelion greens, garlic, parsley, watercress, yams and carrots. The recommended daily allowance for vitamin A (or vitamin A activity present in beta-carotene or the mixed carotinoids) is 5,000 iu per day. It is important not to take too much vitamin A itself – doses over 25,000 iu a day taken over a long time can cause toxicity. The same is not true of the carotinoids. Many nutritionists recommend a supplement of beta-carotene or mixed carotinoids giving an activity of 15,000 iu of vitamin A a day or even more.

Zinc Necessary for protein synthesis and the health of skin and bones, zinc is a co-factor in many of the body's enzymic processes involved in hormonal activities. It is also essential for the formation of DNA and RNA, and is needed for the production and health of the sex organs. Like all the anti-oxidant nutrients this mineral helps rid the body of toxic levels of pollutants including carbon dioxide, accelerates the healing of wounds, and supports the metabolism of vitamin A. Zinc is found in legumes, oysters, poultry, seafood, egg yolks, liver, food yeast, pecans, mushrooms, soy beans, sunflower seeds, pumpkin seeds, onions and herring. The recommended daily allowance of zinc is 15 mg. Most western diets are low in zinc and supplements of 30 to 45 mg a day are commonly used. The best form of zinc to take as a supplement is either zinc citrate or zinc picolinate since they are most readily absorbed.

Selenium Another important anti-oxidant, selenium is at the centre of the enzyme glutathione peroxidase which inactivates the excessive free radicals that destroy tissue. Selenium also helps protect the immune system and acts synergistically with vitamin E in the production of antibodies and to support a healthy heart. This trace element is also important for tissue elasticity and pancreatic deficiency while a deficiency in selenium has been consistently linked with the development of cancer and heart disease. Selenium is found in meats and grains – depending upon its presence in the soils on which they have been raised – in Brazil nuts, food yeast, brown rice, chicken, garlic, liver, molasses, onions, deep sea fish, wheatgerm and whole grains, mushrooms and sea plants. The recommended daily allowance of selenium is estimated to be 50 to 200 mcg. Very high doses of the mineral – above 3,000 mcg a day – are known to be toxic and can result in hair loss, nail loss and impairment of the nervous system.

D-glucose-L-cysteine This compound which is taken as a nutritional supplement for its anti-oxidant properties is one of two substances known to man that acts as a precursor to intracellular glutathione peroxidase – the most important anti-oxidant enzyme in the body. When you take glyco-cysteine it increases intracellular glutathionine peroxidase and has powerful anti-oxidant properties. Like most amino acids this should be taken on an empty stomach. Nutritionists recommend 500–1,000 mg a day.

Gamma Linolenic Acid (GLA) This fatty acid which is found in blackcurrant seed oil, borage oil, starflower oil and evening primrose oil is another regulator of T-lymphocyte functions in the immune system. Borage and starflower oil can be extracted without chemicals or refining. In a healthy body GLA can be made from the essential fatty acid linoleic acid. However, if a woman is deficient in magnesium, vitamins A, C, B3, B6 or zinc, her body may be unable to make the conversion. Junk fats in the diet can also block this conversion. GLA has been shown to have a positive effect on the production of steroid hormones including progesterone and the stress hormones, oestrogen and testosterone. GLA is also important in helping to prevent heart disease, arteriosclerosis, PMS and high blood pressure. In addition to being found in the natural plant oils, GLA is produced by biotechnology in a pure form. Nutritionists generally recommend between 500 and 1,500 mg of GLA a day when it is used as a supplement.

Co-enzyme Q10 A vitamin-like substance related to Vitamin E, CoQ10 is a powerful anti-oxidant found in human tissue. Its concentration diminishes with age. In Japan it is used in the treatment of heart disease. It has also shown itself to be useful in the treatment of allergies, asthma and respiratory complaints as well as anomalies of brain function. CoQ10 is believed by many to be a major step forward in the prevention of cancer and premature ageing. It is also used by athletes. CoQ10 is found in mackerel, salmon and sardines. In supplement form it must be protected from light and heat as it readily deteriorates.

Women-Power Nutrients

In addition to the anti-oxidants and powerfood supplements there are three more nutrients which are particularly important to menstruating and menopausal women and which you might consider taking as supplements: the B complex, B6 and magnesium.

B complex This group of water-soluble vitamins work together in the body and can profitably be taken together in the form of a B complex to help keep the nervous system and circulation functioning well, help build red blood cells, and look after the health of the skin. B complex vitamins are co-enzymes involved in energy production and can be useful to counter depression and anxiety. Buy only a top quality well-balanced B complex with 50 mg of B1, B2, B6, B3, pantothenic acid, choline, PABA and inositol, with 400 mcg of folic acid, 50 mcg of B12 and 50 mcg of biotin (see Resources, p. 510).

Vitamin B6 B6 works together with magnesium as a co-factor in a great many enzyme reactions in the body. It is involved in the production of antibodies, is essential for the synthesis and actions of DNA and RNA in the cells, and aids in assimilation, fat metabolism (including essential fatty acids) and protein metabolism. It also facilitates the body's manufacture of progesterone and reduces inflammatory reactions as well as preventing nervous disorders. B6 is needed for the production of hydrochloric acid in the stomach and for the absorption of vitamin B12 from foods. Anti-depressant drugs, oestrogen and oral contraceptives all increase the need for B6, and carpal tunnel syndrome, where the hands and fingers grow numb, is linked to a B6 deficiency. B6 is found in food yeast, wheatgerm, soy beans, blackstrap molasses, leafy vegetables, egg yolks, walnuts and carrots. Raw food contains much higher quantities of this vitamin since cooking and food processing destroys it. The recommended daily allowance for B6 is a mere 2 mg. However, virtually every doctor who is nutritionally aware, and all nutritionists, insist that for optimal health we need a great deal more than this. As John Lee says, 'Since this vitamin is inexpensive and remarkably safe at effective levels (50 mg once or twice a day) it is wise to supplement it along with magnesium.' An intake above 200 mg of B6 a day taken over long periods of time – i.e. two years – may cause neurological problems.

Magnesium This mineral is also an important catalyst in a huge number of enzyme reactions particularly those involved in energy production and the metabolism of sugars. It helps the body make use of B vitamins and vitamin E as well as essential fatty acids, calcium and other minerals. Magnesium is needed for a healthy heart, to regulate acid-alkaline balance and as a natural tranquillizer. It also helps prevent the build-up of cholesterol in the arteries. Adequate magnesium in the body increases calcium absorption and helps its role in mineralizing bones. Deficiencies of this mineral are common since non-organic farming, where fields are spread with lots of potassium which is an antagonist to magnesium, food processing and long-term storage of food all deplete our diet of this mineral.

Sugar and alcohol rob the body of magnesium too. A deficiency of magnesium causes loss of calcium and potassium from the body and can lead to premature ageing of the skin, depression, irritability, epileptic seizures, arteriosclerosis, muscle cramps, impaired metabolism and confusion. Good food sources of magnesium include alfalfa, apples, kale, seafood, seaweeds, tofu, green leafy vegetables, whole grains, sunflower seeds, brown rice, unsulphured black molasses and sesame seeds. The recommended daily allowance of magnesium is generally considered to be 350 mg. Up to 750 mg of magnesium is used daily for therapeutic purposes, split into three 250 mg doses. As part of his osteoporosis treatment and prevention programme John Lee uses 300 mg supplements of magnesium a day. The best form of magnesium is chelated magnesium since it is well absorbed and many other forms are not.

Hydrochloric acid (HCL) In normal conditions the stomach secretes adequate amounts of HCL and pepsin for the digestion of food and to prepare it for further enzymic actions. For all of this to happen the pH needs to be around 2 which is optimum for pepsin activity. In many women, as they get older, levels of hydrochloric acid in the stomach decrease so that they do not digest foods as efficiently and neither are they able to assimilate important minerals into their bloodstream. A supplement of HCL and pepsin taken with each meal can provide optimal conditions for pepsin activity as well as acidifying important minerals such as calcium, iron and zinc for bonding to other compounds for use by the body.

Next Generation Helpers

This is where the whole business of nutritional supplements gets exciting since most of these supplements are capable of taking healthy people to even greater levels of energy, wellbeing and clarity of mind. These are substances which in one way or another affect brain functioning. The brain's biochemistry is more complex than that of any other organ in the body. It functions in highly elaborate ways to regulate an enormous range of control mechanisms mostly by transmitting (together with the nervous system as a whole) electrical impulses. Only recently have the biochemical mechanisms which underlie the transmission of these electrical impulses begun to be explained by science. The many billions of functional units in the brain – the neurones – are rarely close enough to each other to be able to communicate directly. Instead they communicate by chemical means through specialized structures called *synapses* which lie at the end of an axon or nerve branch. The chemicals which carry the electrical impulses from synapse to synapse are known as *neurotransmitters*. Each neurotransmitter has its own characteristic. Some are excitatory in character. They rapidly trigger electrical discharge. Others are inhibitory. Science has so far isolated scores of neurotransmitters but there could turn out to be hundreds as yet undiscovered. They are made in the body out of nutrients from the foods you eat and there is very good evidence that many of the most important neurotransmitters are diet-dependent – the levels of them in your brain are directly related to how many of the specific nutrients such as amino acids, vitamins and minerals needed for their manufacture are supplied through the diet. There is also much evidence that there is no reason for brainpower to decline with age. Neither should anyone expect that feelings of depression or apathy or even long-standing fatigue are 'normal'. But when the nuts and bolts of neurotransmitter manufacture are not present in adequate quantities in the body or when they are unable to pass through the blood-brain barrier any of this can occur. Most of the next generation supplements are able with remarkable speed and efficiency to restore high-level energy, clarity of mind and brain function by supplying these nuts and bolts. That is why you will sometimes find them referred to as 'smart drugs' although they have nothing to do with drugs. With all of the next generation supplements experts insist it is important to start small and go slow, gradually increasing the amounts you are taking for maximum effects. Everyone is different. If you take more than your body considers optimal then the benefits from them begin to decrease. The trick is to find just the right amount for you. When it comes to the brain stimulants, if you take more than one they can be taken together first thing in the morning on an empty stomach. I use them often. For when the brain functions well you feel so much more alive and positive, not to mention all the body's other organs and systems which can be affected for the good. Melatonin needs to be taken in the evening.

L-Pyroglutamic Acid One of the major mood-enhancing and stimulating neurotransmitters for the brain is glutamic acid. Unfortunately glutamic acid taken as a nutritional supplement does not easily cross the blood-brain barrier so it is not useful as a cognitive enhancer. L-pyroglutamic acid, however, is. It is one of the best supplements for elevating mood and energizing mental functions. Alcoholics have less than normal amounts of glutamic acid in the brain. L-pyroglutamic acid is frequently given to alcoholics to help them break the addiction. Doses vary between 1,000 mg and 3,000 mg a day.

DMAE (dimethylaminoethanol) This is a precursor to choline which in turn becomes acetylcholine – an important brain neurotransmitter. DMAE when taken on an empty stomach is able to cross the blood-brain barrier and deliver choline to brain neurons, stimulating concentration and enhancing memory and alertness. It can improve the ability to learn, raise physical energy and improve intelligence. It also has a wonderful effect on mood, helping people without confidence to feel more confident and outgoing. Doses vary between 130 mg and 500 mg a day.

Acetyl-L-carnitine This helps the transfer of lipids and fats and also acts as a precursor to acetylcholine, improving concentration, memory and alertness. It is often taken with DMAE. Doses vary between 120 mg and 240 mg a day.

N-acetyl-L-tyrosine This is a precursor to the important brain chemical noradrenaline – the stimulating neurotransmitter which is a mood elevator. Athletes have a naturally high level of noradrenaline while chronically depressed people are known to have low levels. N-acetyl-L-tyrosine is useful in breaking addictions and is widely used for withdrawal from drugs. Doses vary between 300 and 900 mg a day.

Melatonin Melatonin is the most interesting and the most broadly useful of all the new generation supplements. It is a key element in the maintenance of the body's hormonal balance, in the regulation of immune integrity, and in the control of the body's daily metabolic functions or circadian rhythms. Melatonin is secreted by the tiny pinecone-shaped pineal – what the mystics call the 'third eye' – which sits deep within the brain. The pineal is a kind of neuro-endocrine transducer. It converts incoming nerve impulses received as bioelectrical messages about the outside environment into outgoing hormones. Even the way in which electromagnetic fields affect the body is mediated through the pineal gland and melatonin. During the daylight hours the pineal, which is highly responsive to the amount of light to which you are exposed, releases very little melatonin. However, with the coming of darkness, levels rise two-to-three-fold to help regulate the circadian rhythms or bodily processes that depend upon our internal 'clocks'. As melatonin rises you begin to experience a hypnotic-like state which helps bring sleep on. Then in the morning when the daylight returns melatonin production decreases again.

When you are subjected to much bright sunlight during the day, melatonin secretion is stimulated in the hours of darkness that follow. When, however, enough full spectrum sunlight is not available during the day melatonin production declines in the evenings. In some people this can produce Seasonal Affective Disorder (SAD) or chronic depression. This can be counteracted either by the use of artificial full-spectrum light boxes during the day or by taking melatonin supplements in the evening, or both. In recent years melatonin supplements have been used to counter jet lag, clear away SAD and even to treat cancer.

One of the most effective treatments for insomnia in women over the age of 40 is to take between 3 and 20 mg of melatonin as a nutritional supplement in the evening. When you suffer from jet lag after crossing several time zones this is largely because melatonin secretions become temporarily out of sync with the rhythms of day and night in the new time zone. Much jet lag can be eliminated by taking from 3 to 15 mg of melatonin at around 9 p.m. each evening, local time. Start this three days before you leave home and continue for up to 10 days at your new destination – depending on how many time zones you have crossed.

Researchers such as Dr Steve Levine and his colleague John Fontenot, who have looked closely at melatonin, have discovered both that its production tends to decline with age and also that a melatonin deficiency may be a critical starting point for degeneration. Studies have shown that the pineal gland inhibits the growth of tumours through the release of melatonin. As a result, melatonin is one of the compounds used in the natural treatment of cancer by some practitioners. There is also a strong indication that supplements of this important hormone can exert anti-ageing effects on the body, enhance the immune system, help to normalize menstrual cycles, lift depression, and (most important of all for women who awaken regularly in the night) counteract insomnia. In numerous studies it has been shown that when people with insomnia take melatonin in the evening, both their total sleep time as well as daytime alertness is improved within a couple of weeks.

Like all next-generation supplements melatonin demands that you experiment for a while to find the right dose and the right time to take it. Some people find within an hour of taking it they are ready to go to sleep. Others need to take it early on in the evening, just after dusk, and a few respond best to it being taken just before going to bed. There is also a wide range of optimal doses depending upon individual biology. Most of the studies of melatonin used 20 mg of the substance a day. However, as a nutritional supplement, it is usually sold in 3 mg doses. Most people find that 5 of these 3 mg capsules (i.e. 15 mg) at night work well although some do better on very low doses of 3 to 9 mg. Nutritionists advise that you monitor its effects and also how you feel the next day. You should feel bright and good. If you feel sluggish try reducing the dose and see what happens.

Chapter Twenty-nine
Second Coming

What a woman can accomplish through exercise is impressive not only in terms of protecting her body from the ravages of female troubles and even from time itself but also in protecting her from illness and in rejuvenating her body in medically measurable ways. But exactly what kind of exercise *is* the right kind? It is an important question to answer because so much of what has become fashionable – fancy clothing and tossing weights around in a gym – is mostly the *wrong* kind. Walking or running along roads filled with air pollution and subjecting your body to the stress this brings can also do more harm than good.

Aware of the benefits of exercise, most people who exercise regularly do aerobic movement – swimming, cycling, running or walking. There is much to be said for this kind of exercise. It improves the functioning of the heart, lowers cholesterol and shifts brain chemistry so that you produce natural opiates which make you feel good. It also increases noradrenaline – a brain chemical which improves your self-image and confidence. Aerobic exercise can also enhance your body's ability to burn fat not only while you are working out but for many hours afterwards as well. This makes aerobic exercise an important part of any good exercise programme. So get out and walk briskly as often as you can. But aerobic exercise doesn't go far enough. It does not offer the body enough weight resistance to maintain muscle mass.

One interesting study compared the Lean Body Mass (LBM) to fat ratio in three groups of women – non-exercisers, aerobic exercisers and weight trainers. Researchers found significant differences. In sedentary women 21.8 per cent of their body weight was fat. Among the aerobic exercisers 16.2 per cent was fat while among resistance trainers only 14.7 per cent of their body weight was fat. This, and the kind of research looked at in Body Heat (p. 179), is revolutionizing fitness advice. Exercise physiologists have come to realize that although aerobic exercise has a place as *part* of an exercise programme it does not maintain bones and muscle the way resistance exercise does. The bottom line is that we need both, although resistance exercise is the more important of the two. As a member of the advisory board of the American College for Sports Medicine (which has in the past promoted aerobic exercise as the best form for overall health and fitness) said: 'Done correctly, weight training is the most efficient, effective and safest form of exercise there is, and it won't be long before people realize it.'

Let's Get Started

What does a confirmed lounge lizard do once she decides she wants to explore how exercise can change her life? First she gets approval from her doctor to make sure that there is no reason she should not start on a simple graded programme. Then go easy. If you start small and work up you will win. If you start big you can not only wear out your body but also lose your taste for movement. The whole effort will then have become counter-productive since you will end up hating exercise and getting nowhere. For exercise to work it has to become an ordinary part of your daily life. It needs to be done regularly at least three times a week. Begin with only 15 minutes in the morning when you get up or at any other time of the day that is convenient. The great news is that right from that very first session your body will begin to rejuvenate itself. Exercise routines progress well when you work out at the same time each day. Try to do this if you can. Your body will get used to the routine and love it. When it comes to resistance training you don't need to own a lot of fancy equipment either. Nor do you need to join a gym. A couple of dumb bells will do. Later on, if you catch the exercise bug, you might like to have a bar bell as well. Dumb bells and bar bells are what are known as *free weights* as opposed to the kind of gym equipment you find in a multitude of sizes and shapes and glitzy finishes these days. They are also far simpler since you can tuck them under the bed out of sight when they are not in use and you can make use of them any time you want without having to dress in special clothes and go to the gym.

Choose the kind of dumb bells – each of which fits into one hand – that have six removable weights on each so that you can add and then take off weights as needed for each exercise. Your body and their weight against gravity offer all the resistance you need to work muscles deeply. The machines you find in gyms are designed to mimic the effects of free-weight exercises but, with a couple of minor exceptions, no matter how flash they look, they are not as good as simple free weights because the range of movement which you go through in each exercise is restricted by the machine. Free weights should form the basis of any good weight-training routine, whether you are a complete beginner or a professional weightlifter.

There are three things you want to accomplish in your exercise programme. First, you want to maintain and to improve your heart and lung fitness. For this you will use weights plus some form of aerobic activity for warming up and cooling down. Secondly, you want to maintain and increase your muscle mass. Finally, you want to maintain and improve your flexibility and for this you need some kind of slow stretching afterwards.

Warm Up

It is important at the beginning of any exercise session that you spend a few minutes doing an aerobic activity. (You must never pick up a weight when your muscles are cold.) This can be running on the spot, slow steady jumping jacks, using a rowing machine (my favourite) or bouncing on a rebounder (mini trampoline). In the beginning your total exercise session may last only 15 to 20 minutes in which case you will want to devote five minutes at the beginning to the aerobic warm up. Later on it can be longer. I generally row on a Concept II rowing machine for about 10 minutes at a slow steady pace to get my heart and lungs moving and to warm up before beginning my weights. As the length of your exercise session grows week by week, until it is ideally 45 minutes to an hour at a time, so will the time you spend on your aerobic activities at the beginning and end of the session and perhaps in the middle too.

Stretch Out

After this initial period which should last long enough so that you feel fully warmed up, you should then spend 5 to 10 minutes stretching. Stretch slowly and smoothly towards the ceiling, towards your toes, to the side. Never jerk when stretching and breathe deeply. Stretching before a workout but after a warm up is done to allow major muscle groups along with associated tendons and ligaments to be gently stretched, ensuring possible injuries are greatly reduced. Now you are ready for your muscle work.

Weights Workout

To work with weights properly you need to split your sessions into different body parts and work one or two body parts per session, leaving at least 48 hours between that session and the next time you work that body part. The muscle and bone strengthening that comes with resistance training does not take place *while* you are using the weights. In fact working out stresses the muscles and bones causing tiny breakdowns in the cells to occur. It is during the *rest* that comes after a workout that new muscle and bone is built in direct response to the piezoelectric stimulation at a molecular level. If you come to the point of using quite heavy weights and training five times a week then it is important to work out each body part only once a week for it can take about 48 hours for the breakdown process to take place and between 48 and 72 hours to build new strong tissue to replace it. Ignorant of these facts, many gung-ho body builders and weight trainers overtrain their muscles and end up undermining their immune system, while getting nowhere near the benefits in terms of strengthening LBM that they should. Exercising a particular muscle group every 5 to 8 days is ideal for optimum progress.

Stand in any gym and watch weight trainers do their stuff. It can be highly instructive in showing you how *not* to work with weights. Ninety per cent of the men and women who use weights let their bodies swing all over the place and, when they are doing an exercise such as a dumb bell curl, they let the weight just fall back after each movement instead of being in control. When you do your movements be sure to keep your body absolutely centred with each movement, only using the particular muscle group that is supposed to be working, and emphasize the *eccentric* contraction or return movement, where you are returning the weight to its original position. Resist the movement all the way back. It is the stress placed on your muscles of lengthening again when they are under resistance load that brings about most of the gains in strength and LBM you are after. Be sure while you are working out that you drink lots of water between each set and eat plenty of alkaline-forming foods (see p. 302) since any kind of exercise tends to make your system more acid.

The Cool Down

It is important to spend a few minutes at the end of a weights session again doing some kind of aerobic activity to cool down. How long depends on the length of your weights session. You can go through the same kind of activity you have used in the beginning of your session or even take a brisk walk, but make sure you stay warm by adding an extra sweater for your body will cool down fast and you don't want to become chilled.

The Stretch Out

Then do some more stretching for a couple of minutes. You will find that your body stretches more easily now since your muscles are full of blood and energized. Go slow and enjoy the feeling. It can be wonderful.

Beginner's Programme

All of the exercises here are classic weight-training movements. They are simple and straightforward. They require nothing more than a couple of dumb-bells (the kind that have six weights on each). Start with the lightest weights. You will be able to tell for yourself if something feels right. Never strain. As your body becomes accustomed to the lighter weight you can add a bit more. The object of the exercise is not to use heavy weights but simply to provide your body with enough weight to create resistance against which your muscles do their work. You will find pictures of the movements given below in any standard book on weight training or you can ask a fitness instructor to show them to you. Each exercise is done smoothly and with complete control both on the contraction of the muscle group and on the relaxation. While one muscle group is working, the rest of the body remains still and centred. Start off by doing only three training sessions a week with one set per exercise. A set is the same exercise repeated a certain number of times: so 2x10 would mean ten repetitions of the movement, rest for two to three minutes, then ten more repetitions of the movement; 3x10 means the ten repetitions are done three times with two minutes rest between each set. Work up to longer by adding more exercises for each muscle group you are working with and doing one warm-up set of easy repetitions (10–15) followed by a heavier set using a little more weight (5–10 repetitions). Begin with very light weights – just enough for you to feel that your muscles are being worked as you near the end of your repetitions. Then by the time you are ready to add your second set, put on a little more weight until at the end of your repetitions your muscles feel tired.

Session One: Shoulders and Arms

Dumb bell press 2x10
Side lateral raise 2x10
Single arm tricep extension 2x10
Tricep kickback 2x10
Dumb bell curl 2x10
Concentration curl 2x10

Session Two: Chest and Back

Dumb bell bench press 2x10
Dumb bell flies 2x10
Single arm rowing 2x10
Dumb bell shrug 2x10
Floor hyperextensions 2x10

Session Three: Legs and Abdominal Muscles

Dumb bell squat 2x10
Dumb bell lunge 2x10
Calf raise 2x10
Abdominal crunch 2x10–15
Reverse crunch 2x10–15

The Result

Each woman is in reality two women, an outer woman and an inner counterpart, that is an individual self that is utterly unique. Each woman has a stable centre of strength and growth. Each inner woman sees the world in her own way, has her own brand of creativity, her own needs and desires, and is a law unto herself. The inner self holds the power to create, change, build, nurture and transform. The outer woman is the vehicle for what the self creates. When her self is allowed free expression, then a woman is truly beautiful for she is fully alive. Her body is strong, her skin is clear and healthy, and her movements, speech and actions radiate a kind of vitality that is unmistakably charismatic because it is *real*, an outward expression of who she truly is. Many of the secrets to calling forth this kind of aliveness are to be found within the body itself – secrets which are best learned by working with muscle. Once you get the hang of it, working with weights is like meditation – one of the most mind-stilling activities in the world. Meanwhile as your LBM begins to develop you will find your muscles and whole body have come alive. Then, as you work out, your muscles will begin to glow until after a few months your body often begins to feel the way it did when you were a child – radiant with life and spirit.

Chapter Thirty
Magnum Force

As far back as the 1940s natural progesterone – chemically the exact same molecule produced by the corpus luteum in a woman's body – was known to offer protection against the dangers of excess oestrogen including miscarriage. It was also considered to be a natural contraceptive believed to offer protection against pregnancy without harmful side-effects via a completely different mechanism than that which would be later developed as drug-based contraceptives. So important is progesterone to a woman's health that the body produces it not in micrograms or picograms, as in the case of the oestrogens and other hormones, but in milligrams. Since 1948 in Britain and 1981 in the United States natural progesterone has been used in the treatment of PMS. In 1953 Dr Katherina Dalton and Dr Raymond Green in Britain published the first paper on PMS in medical literature, 'The Premenstrual Syndrome'. Dalton, who describes premenstrual syndrome as the commonest of endocrine disorders, was the first to test the use of progesterone on women as a treatment for the condition. She was soon to become the leading investigator on PMS and the use of progesterone for its treatment in the world. Dalton's work is always quoted by later investigators who have further explored the use of natural progesterone not only in the treatment of PMS but menopausal problems and other conditions.

Progesterone is a natural hormone, that is, chemically identical to the hormone naturally found in a woman's body, not a chemically altered patentable drug as are the progestogens or progestins. Progesterone is available under prescription in oral form, by injection, and as a suppository or implant. It is also available without prescription in most countries (Britain is presently excluded, although it can be ordered for personal use from abroad by any woman wanting to buy it) in the form of a cream to rub on the surface of the body or in a vitamin E oil. In both cases the progesterone has been derived from diosgenin found in the wild yam – usually either *Dioscorea villosa* or *Dioscorea Mexicana*. Some doctors who frequently use progesterone prefer tablets or the injectable form (this is what Dalton still does). Increasingly, however, for ease and economy, the cream and oil are preferred. There are a number of creams and oils available. The best (see Resources, pp. 505–507) have been on the market for a long time and have been well tested by doctors and the women who have used them. A 50 g (2 oz jar) of the cream – technically marketed as a cosmetic in many countries – contains between 900–1,000 milligrams of progesterone. Natural progesterone oil in d-alpha tocopherol (vitamin E) is more potent than the cream; a 25 g (1 oz) bottle of the oil, technically a food supplement, contains between 2,500 and 3,000 milligrams of progesterone.

There follow some of the most frequently asked questions about natural progesterone as well as a few general protocols following the practices of doctors who frequently use it: Dr John Lee in California, Barry Durrant-Peatfield and Shamim Daya in Britain; Joel T. Hargrove, Director of the PMS and Menopause Clinics at Vanderbilt University in Nashville; Neils Lauersen, Professor of Obstetrics and Gynaecology at New York Medical College and author of *PMS: Premenstrual Syndrome and You*; and others including investigative biochemist Dr Ray Peat. Many have long experience in the use of the natural hormone: orally, by injection or by topical application, in the treatment of PMS, osteoporosis, menopausal disturbances, infertility and for skin care.

In many ways progesterone cream and oil have advantages over other forms of the hormone. A typical patient on injected progesterone therapy may need 10 or more injections a month which can mean trips to the doctor's surgery, expense and inconvenience. Some of the solvents in which progesterone by injection is dissolved can have toxic side-effects. The oil – which is placed under the tongue and allowed to absorb through the mucosa of the mouth for five minutes rather than swallowed – is able to by-pass breakdown by the liver. Like the cream it can enter the bloodstream directly so that far less is needed than when given orally.

Apart from its reported actions in countering so many

female ailments (unlike the synthetic progestogens which are end-product molecules incapable of being converted to other hormones by the body) natural progesterone is directly in the path of the biosynthesis of all of the adrenal corticosteroids and all the other sex hormones such as testosterone and the oestrogens. It is a precursor for them. This means the body can transform progesterone into all these other hormones when needed (see diagram p. 75). When you lack progesterone, by following the arrows in the diagram you will see which biosynthetic pathways are eliminated and which hormones will have to be produced via an alternative pathway (such as DHEA) for your body to have them at all. When progesterone is adequately supplied, the body is able to make all of whatever else it needs. On the other hand, when there is not enough progesterone present this can be a major reason why people wake up with morning stiffness or suffer arthritis, injury to a joint, carpal tunnel syndrome, or tendonitis – conditions which never seem to get better since the body is simply not making all the cortisone that is needed to suppress inflammation and arrest the deleterious action in the joints. Doctors working with the progesterone cream report that such conditions frequently clear up when the cream is used for other purposes.

How Does Natural Progesterone Differ from the Synthetic Progestogens?

Natural progesterone, which was first crystallized in 1934, is now derived from plant sources and is an exact molecular match of the progesterone produced in a woman's body. It is not known to have any side-effects except for altering the menstrual cycle temporarily in some women and bringing about a state of relaxation. By contrast, pharmaceutical manufacturers' product information on the various synthetic progestogens or progestins commonly used as oral contraceptives and in HRT carry a long list of small print cautions, contra-indications and adverse reactions, which include life-threatening pulmonary embolism, cerebral haemorrhage, cerebral thrombosis and cancers as well as dozens of minor complaints such as depression, migraine, fibroid enlargement, loss of hair, nausea and vomiting. To quote Dr Neils Lauersen, 'Progestogens are chemically formulated from progesterone, but rather than duplicating the properties of progesterone, these synthetic hormones react differently. When a woman is treated with synthetic progestogens, her body becomes confused and produces less natural progesterone, causing salt build up, fluid retention and hypoglycaemia . . . synthetic progestogens generally make PMS symptoms worse, so if a woman is about to be treated with progesterone, she should be sure that it is *natural* progesterone.' The synthetic progestogens can also cause breast cancer and hirsutism, while natural progesterone counters both.

What are the Side-Effects of Synthetics

Here are a few side-effects of one of the most commonly prescribed synthetic progestogens – Provera – medroxyprogesterone acetate as reported in the 1995 edition of Physicians' Desk Reference.

Warnings Increased risk of birth defects. Beagle dogs given the drug have been reported to develop malignant nodules in the mammary glands; must be discontinued if sudden or partial loss of vision occurs, may contribute to thrombophlebitis. Usage in pregnancy is not recommended.

Contra-indications Thrombophlebitis, thromboembolic disorders, cerebral apoplexy, liver dysfunction or disease, known or suspected malignancy of breast or genital organs, undiagnosed vaginal bleeding, missed abortion, or known sensitivity.

Precautions May cause fluid retention, epilepsy, migraine, asthma, cardiac or renal dysfunction, breakthrough bleeding or menstrual irregularities and may cause or contribute to depression. The effect of prolonged use of this drug on pituitary, ovarian, adrenal, hepatic or uterine function is unknown. May decrease glucose tolerance – diabetic patients must be carefully monitored – may increase thrombotic disorders associated with oestrogens.

Adverse reactions May cause breast tenderness, sensitivity reactions such as urticaria, pruritus, oedema, or rash; may cause acne, alopecia and hirsutism, oedema, weight changes, cervical erosions and changes in cervical secretions, cholestatic jaundice, mental depression, nausea, insomnia or somnolence, anaphylactiod reactions and anaphylaxis (severe allergic reactions), thrombophlebitis and pulmonary embolism, breakthrough bleeding, spotting, menorrhea or changes in menses.

When taken with oestrogens, the following have been observed Rise in blood pressure, headaches, dizziness, nervousness, fatigue, changes in libido, hirsutism and loss of scalp hair, decrease in T-3 uptake values, premenstrual-like syndrome, changes in appetite, cystitis-like syndrome, erythema multiform, erythema, haemorrhagic eruption, itching.

Besides Its Use in the Treatment of Female Complaints, Is Natural Progesterone Good for Other Things Too?

Apart from its well-known reproductive functions, progesterone – unlike the progestogens which are end-molecules – is a precursor to a whole family of other molecules (of steroid hormones) which are not easily made without it: the cortisone that your adrenal gland makes for instance. In men, who make progesterone in their testes, it is also a precursor to testosterone. So progesterone is needed for the production of other hormones such as the oestrogens as well as cortisol which is often called the 'fight or flight' hormone since it comes into play when you are under stress. At such times your body diverts progesterone away from being converted into the oestrogens needed for female functions, changing it instead into cortisol. This can result in a deficiency in female hormones including progesterone itself if the stress is prolonged enough and produces symptoms such as hot flushes at or near menopause and PMS earlier on. That is the down side. The up side is that when enough natural progesterone is available to the body it can be turned into other steroids (including the oestrogens) which help balance emotions, increase your ability to handle stress, counter hot flushes and vaginal dryness and do so many other things for some women that when you attempt to list them it makes progesterone look like a panacea, while in reality it is only part of a total approach to natural health care for women. As a result of its remarkable ability to provide the raw materials for the production of other steroid hormones, to counter the dangers implicit in oestrogen dominance in the body, and its interaction on other glands, organs and systems of the body, here are a few of the symptoms which doctors and women using it claim respond to progesterone therapy.

- anxiety
- black circles under the eyes
- blurred vision
- breast pain and problems
- cold hands and feet
- constipation
- cyclic acne
- depression
- disturbances in appetite
- dry skin
- exhaustion
- fibroids
- infertility
- insomnia
- irritability
- lack of sex drive
- lethargy
- low blood sugar
- migraines
- mood swings
- muscle and joint pains
- panic attacks
- poor concentration
- poor digestion
- sciatica
- spontaneous abortion
- spontaneous bruising
- stiffness
- thinning hair
- water retention

How Do You Use a Cream?

That partly depends on what it is being used for (see below for specific protocols). All gonadal hormones, being small, fat-soluble molecules, are easily absorbed through the skin – in fact better than when given orally. Natural progesterone dissolved in a moisturizing emulsion is readily absorbed through the skin and taken into the bloodstream. It can be applied to the face, belly, breasts, back, thighs – almost anywhere on the body. Go for the largest possible areas of relatively thin skin. It is rapidly taken up and after a few minutes leaves no trace on the skin surface. At the beginning in progesterone-deficient women a lot of the progesterone is absorbed into body fat. After a while, as the receptors in the fatty tissues become saturated, successive doses of progesterone bring about an increase in blood levels and physiological effects. This is why it can take three months of use for some women to begin to experience the benefits of progesterone cream. Others, however, seem to experience results much more quickly. Transdermal progesterone by-passes the liver (where breakdown of oral progesterone occurs) and travels to specific receptor sites where it is needed. Only small quantities of progesterone are needed to make big changes in the body and mind. Where doctors who prescribe oral progesterone or injectable progesterone are working with doses of from 200 mg to as much as 500 mg or even 800 mg a day, the dose you need to have the same effect absorbed from a cream is likely to be at least 10 times less than that – more in the order of 20 mg to 25 mg a day.

When applying the cream – which you can do once or twice a day – it is a good idea to rotate its application around different areas of the body. When the cream is taken through the skin it is absorbed into the fat cells and if the receptors there become saturated they can't absorb any more. So it is advisable to apply it to the abdomen one day, on the thighs the next, on the breasts the next and so forth, returning to the original site every four or five days. Many women discover that the progesterone cream is just about the best thing you can use as a skin moisturizer. It has such a good effect on the face that they want to use it every day. It is probably not necessary to use it every day but only a couple of times a week. There is also always the danger that you could develop an allergic reaction to some ingredient any cream contains if you use it every day in the same place.

How Much of a Cream Should I Use?

Most doctors suggest you start with $1/4$ to $1/2$ teaspoon a day then monitor how rapidly it is absorbed. Every woman's requirement for natural progesterone is unique to her. In a menstruating woman natural progesterone is usually used for 14 days a month starting on about day 13 or 14 of her menstrual cycle (counting the first day of a period as day one), then stopping on day 27 or 28 and increasing the amounts used in the last week or so before a period begins. A woman who is anovulatory would use the cream in a cyclical way each month from day 12 to day 26 for three months. Anovulation can result from lack of synchronous timing between the hypothalamus, the pituitary and the ovaries so the chemical messages are not arriving at the right time. If a woman cycles this way, using progesterone cream for three months and then withdrawing it sometimes allows the normal ovulation to return. (This is the way it is used in treating infertility.)

After using the cream for a few months many women no longer need to use as much and the amount can be decreased, all the while monitoring the effect on symptoms. If symptoms increase you use more. When they decrease you need less. As biochemist Ray Peat says, 'Since progesterone is not known to have any side-effects except for alteration of the menstrual cycle and production of euphoria . . . the basic procedure should be to use it in sufficient quantity to make the symptoms disappear, and to time its use so that menstrual cycles are not disrupted. This normally means using it only between ovulation and menstruation unless symptoms are sufficiently serious that a missed period is not important.' In menopausal women doctors usually recommend using the cream 21 days a month and leaving it off for 7 before beginning again. Although there is no reason why a woman cannot use it continuously, if you do, the progesterone receptor sites may become accustomed to a continual supply of progesterone so they lose some of their receptivity to it. This is no more than a variation on the principle of natural medicine that says that the body thrives on change and that it is best – even with herbal supplements or brain stimulants or vitamins and minerals – to have periodic short breaks away from using them. John Lee recommends that, instead of trying to measure $^1/_4$ to $^1/_2$ teaspoon each time you open the jar, simply begin by using a 50 g (2 oz) jar each month – whether or not you are using the cream for 14 days a month or 21 days – for the first three or four months of use. Once it has been established – either by a doctor taking blood levels of progesterone or by an improvement in symptoms – that the problems being treated are responding, you can gradually decrease amounts down to half a jar a month. Some women absorb progesterone more easily through the skin than others. And because oestrogen and progesterone have so very many mutually antagonistic effects, how much oestrogen there is in a woman's body will also to some extent determine the quantity of progesterone needed to balance it. In PMS the dose usually needs initially to be high in order to counter the effects of previously unopposed oestrogen. After menopause, when oestrogen levels are low and a woman is using the progesterone for protection against osteoporosis, the effective doses are usually far lower. Blood progesterone levels can be taken by a doctor, but Lee insists – and the many women I have spoken to confirm this – that women themselves are the best judge of how much they need. Thanks to the great safety of natural progesterone, considerable latitude is allowed.

What is the Difference Between the Natural Progesterone Creams and the Sub-lingual Granules and Oil?

The sub-lingual granules and oil have at least three times the concentration of progesterone found in the creams. They are taken sub-lingually by putting a few drops of the oil or several of the pellets in the mouth and holding them there under the tongue – usually for five to eight minutes – until they have been absorbed by the mucosa in the mouth. I personally believe that the sub-lingual pellets or granules are preferable to the oil; they are easier and more pleasant to use and you have a greater control over how you are taking them, particularly since the oil can be hard to squeeze from the bottle. The oil can also be applied intra-vaginally by putting a few drops of it on the finger and introducing the finger into the vagina. The creams are effective for long-term use and maintenance, the granules and the oil are more immediate in their actions. Sometimes – in the case of severe PMS or hot flushes – it can be helpful to use both cream and sub-lingual applications together. Some suppliers make two varieties of the oil, one of which has the addition of essential oil of peppermint in an attempt to improve the flavour (in my opinion it doesn't!). Use only the oil *without* the peppermint for vaginal application. Some companies produce a cream without alcohol which can also be applied directly to the vagina and vulva.

Should Application of a Cream Be Cycled?

Yes. When the body is continually exposed to signals from a hormone such as progesterone or any other compound there is always the chance that this can lead to reduced receptor sensitivity as receptors in effect tune down the volume. During regular monthly menstruation there occurs a week or so each month during which hormone levels are low. Doctors recommend that progesterone be cycled monthly. In postmenopausal women it can be used for 2 to 3 weeks a month and then discontinued for a week before beginning again so that at least 5 to 7 days a month remain hormone free. In menstruating or perimenopausal women the timing of progesterone use is made to coincide with the normal luteal phase of menstruation – from about day 12 or 13 of the cycle to day 26 or 27. Sometimes this can be difficult to do if a woman's periods are irregular. Occasionally, too, some spotting occurs mid-month when progesterone is started. Should this happen, John Lee recommends that the progesterone be halted for 12 days and then started anew.

How Long Do I Have to Use Natural Progesterone to See Results?

This varies enormously. In the case of hot flushes or PMS some women notice relief immediately. In general, meno-pausal and menstrual difficulties will be relieved within 3 months. The action of the progesterone oil taken sub-lingual-ly is much faster than the cream in its actions since it gets into the bloodstream right away. This is why it can be so helpful to use the oil every 15 minutes or so when a woman is experienc-ing hot flushes. The oil can also be useful in this way for migraine. In the case of osteoporosis, bone scans taken 6 months after beginning progesterone treatment and follow-ing a good nutritional regime generally show an increase of at least 5 per cent in bone density – often much greater depending upon the state of the bones at the beginning of treatment.

How Do I know When to Use Progesterone Cream More or Less Frequently?

By keeping an eye on the symptoms for which you have been using the cream and by keeping an eye on how quickly the cream is absorbed into the skin from day to day. If you find it is absorbed in less than a minute – which often happens 5 to 7 days before a period – then increase the number of applica-tions a day to 2, 3 or 4 times. Similarly, if symptoms are pre-sent use more until they abate, increasing the quantity slightly until menstruation. As for how long to use the cream this depends on your own body and on what you are using it for. Some women find that after 3 or 4 months they can cut down on the cream and gradually stop it altogether. Others – partic-ularly menopausal and postmenopausal women – choose to use it permanently in whatever dose they themselves find appropriate to protect against osteoporosis, care for skin and improving the body's ability to handle stress. Each woman's biochemistry is unique. It is a question of listening to your own body and feelings.

Can Progesterone Be Used to Enhance Fertility?

Infertility now affects 1 in 6 women in the West. Many women who have difficulty conceiving or who have had several unexplained miscarriages in the first trimester of pregnancy are low progesterone producers – a condition known as *luteal phase deficiency* – where the corpus luteum in the second half of the menstrual cycle produces so little progesterone that the endometrium (the womb lining) is not properly prepared for secured implantation of a fertilized egg. Others, because of oestrogen dominance, are not ovulating normally. It is worth trying progesterone for three months as a means of conceiving. John Lee recommends that such a woman use a progesterone cream starting with day 10 or 12 of her menstrual cycle – just before ovulation should take place – through to day 28 of the cycle. Then she should stop using the cream and begin counting again from day 1 when her period begins. This is done for three months. Cycling in this way suppresses ovulation and ensures that hormonal cycles become regular. On the fourth month he tells the woman to stop using the cream, anticipating that the follicles and ovulation will proceed at the right timing and that the woman will now have a better chance of becoming pregnant. Lee has had this happen so successfully with so many women that he knows it works. They ring him to say, 'Hey, I'm pregnant. We're going to name it after you!' Lee believes that oestrogen dominance and the inability to get pregnant probably have a common cause – that a woman may not be completing ovulating and this may be putting her ovaries at risk. The progesterone that such a woman is given helps bring about full follicle development and ovulation, making becoming pregnant less difficult.

Is it Okay to Use a Progesterone Cream When I am Pregnant?

There is generally no reason to take progesterone when a woman is pregnant since the production of progesterone rises dramatically during pregnancy anyway. However, unlike the synthetic progestogens, natural progesterone is completely safe in pregnancy. It is even used by doctors to help protect against threatened miscarriage. During pregnancy the body's own production of progesterone rises from 15, 20 or 25 mg a day during luteal peak periods to 350–400 mg a day. Progesterone plays an important role in the development of the baby. Studies carried out in the 1950s show that the subsequent IQ of a child as it grows can be related to whether the mother was making sufficient progesterone. Human milk from healthy mothers contains significant quantities of progesterone. This appears to be important for the development of the child's nervous system. John Lee often recommends progesterone to women just after birth – especially to those with postnatal depression. Progesterone is at its highest level in a woman's body just before birth, then it falls close to zero. It appears that the rapid fall of progesterone that occurs with birth and the elimination of the placenta which produces progesterone during pregnancy tends to precipitate depression in some women.

Does Natural Progesterone Cream Help Vaginal Dryness?

Vaginitis and a tendency to recurrent urinary tract infections can occur in women of all ages but especially after menopause when the production of oestrogen and progesterone decreases. Natural progesterone cream used on the perineum and intra-vaginally is generally successful in treating both vaginal dryness and vulvar dystrophy, both of which tend to return to normal after 3 or 4 months of using the cream. In a very few women for whom progesterone itself does not completely solve the problem, a small quantity of oestrogen cream applied topically (on the skin) is useful.

Is There a Relationship Between Progesterone and Good Thyroid Function?

Yes. Optimal levels of progesterone help thyroid hormones work. Many women who are told by their doctors that they have symptoms of hypothyroidism get to a point where their body is still making oestrogen but not progesterone. Then they can have trouble with weight gain. They tend to be tired and to be easily affected by the cold. Often the doctor believes this to be hypothyroidism and will prescribe thyroid hormones. Doctors who regularly use progesterone with their patients have found that many of these women are simply not making enough progesterone. Adding progesterone improves thyroid function so that many women who would otherwise need thyroid hormones do not require them while others on thyroid hormones generally need to reduce the dose once progesterone levels are improved. It is important to monitor the TSH (thyroid-stimulating hormone) levels of any woman on thyroid hormones who uses a progesterone cream since the continued use of thyroid medication once the progesterone level in the body has improved cellular utilization of thyroid hormone could lead to a woman becoming *hyper*-thyroid.

Are There Any Side-effects to Using Natural Progesterone?

To quote biochemist Ray Peat, 'Progesterone is not known to have any side-effects except for alteration of the menstrual cycle and production of euphoria . . . the basic procedure should be to use it in sufficient quantity to make symptoms disappear, and to time its use so that menstrual cycles are not disrupted.' Joel Hargrove MD, Director of the PMS and Menopause Clinics at Vanderbilt University in Nashville in the United States, has been using 300-400-500 – even 1,000 mg – of oral progesterone a day and has found no undesirable side-effects. 'I've been prescribing progesterone for 12 years and I haven't seen any long-term effects . . . it doesn't affect cholesterol levels, it doesn't affect Mother Nature – basically it is a wonderful thing.' The levels of progesterone that enter the body through the cream are far lower (usually in the realm of 10 to 15 mg a day) than are produced by a woman's body. When progesterone is being used for PMS by menstruating women too much over a few months it can occasionally delay a period a day or so. Stopping its use for a week and then resuming it at a lower dose clears this up. Sometimes women with irregular periods get some spotting at ovulation when they start progesterone use. Doctors say that the period is attempting to regulate to a 28-day cycle. In time periods become regular and spotting is alleviated. Women who are starting menopause sometimes see some spotting when they start using progesterone which also clears. Very occasionally a postmenopausal woman using progesterone will get a small period for the first month or two then this stops permanently. Should this happen it is a sign that the progesterone is causing the body to eliminate excess stored oestrogen which can trigger a shedding of the endometrium or breakthrough bleeding. It can be a big help to work with a doctor who is familiar with natural progesterone use if you feel you need reassurance about anything (the vast majority are not at all, unfortunately). If any kind of breakthrough bleeding continues past three months or so it is important to consult a doctor. Unlike the synthetic hormones, no human cancer has ever been reported as a result of natural progesterone treatment. There are, however, reports in the scientific literature that natural progesterone has been used to protect from and even to treat uterine cancer. In using the cream you are getting very small amounts of progesterone. As John Lee says, 'During pregnancy the placenta makes as much as 300 to 400 mg of progesterone a day. You will be lucky using the cream or the oil to even get to the level of the corpus luteum production in a menstruating woman which is about 20 to 25 milligrams a day. This is why I maintain without exception that there is no way that progesterone supplementation can cause anyone any harm. If that were to happen it would mean that a woman's own menstrual monthly production of progesterone would also be harmful. I don't believe that there is a supplement that has the safety record that progesterone does.'

Is There a Test to Determine If a Woman is Anovulatory?

The only way to know for sure is to have a laboratory test done for low serum progesterone – that is low levels of progesterone in the blood – between day 18 and 26 of your menstrual cycle. A normal serum progesterone level after ovulation is in the range of 7–28 picograms. If a woman does not ovulate that month then the level tends to be around 0.3 picograms. However, many experts in the use of natural progesterone, such as John Lee, claim that the only real test comes not from laboratory results but from how a woman feels.

Is There a Test to Determine Optimal Progesterone Levels in a Postmenopausal Woman?

Again serum levels of progesterone can be taken. Generally a progesterone level of about 9 is optimal for most women. It is far more important, however, that a woman judge for herself how much she needs by being aware of her symptoms or lack of them.

Can Natural Progesterone Supplementation Help Protect Me from Heart Disease and Cancer?

The latest study on hormone therapy for older women – the results of which have been called 'dramatic' by the President of the American Heart Association – shows that natural progesterone used with oestrogen is better than oestrogen and Provera in relation to protection from the risks of heart disease. The nationwide study of 875 women including 147 at Stanford University in California has produced a gold mine of information about what combinations work best. However, experts on the use of natural progesterone have commented that it is a shame the study did not look at the use of *progesterone alone.* In the mid-1940s an interesting study was begun by Johns Hopkins University in the United States in a clinic established for women with possible hormone problems. Among the many things measured were progesterone levels. Almost 30 years later, in 1978, researchers looked up the cancer incidence of women who had normal progesterone levels and compared it with women who had low levels. They discovered that the cancer rate was 10 times higher in the women who were low in progesterone. Their findings were reported in the prestigious *American Journal of Epidemiology* in 1981 but, like so many important findings, they disappeared without a trace. The cancer-protective capacities of progesterone were not restricted to breast cancer or uterine cancers either – they applied to all cancer. Mounting levels of xenoestrogens in the environment and oestrogen dominance which is much more widespread now than it was 30 years ago make it important for women in the industrialized world to be aware of the protective actions they can take. At least we now have a chance.

How Does a Woman in Perimenopause Begin Using the Cream?

In the years just preceding menopause when women are experiencing changing patterns of menstruation such as irregular flows or missed periods, using a progesterone cream can bring menstruation back to normal and keep it that way until the moment at which menopause arrives and periods cease altogether. When you first add progesterone in this case sometimes *oestrogen rebound* can take place. This is a temporary phenomenon where the sensitivity of the oestrogen receptors is heightened by the presence of progesterone. A woman can get a temporary worsening of her symptoms such as tender breasts or PMS symptoms. She may also get an irregular or unexpected period where the endometrial proliferation which has built up because of the oestrogen in her body is now able to be shed thanks to sufficient progesterone being present. This is normal and will soon clear away once the extra sensitivity of oestrogen receptors settles down. The progesterone cream is used between day 12 or 13 and day 26 or 27 of the menstrual cycle beginning with half a jar a month during this period but be careful to adjust the dose according to the relief from symptoms which you get. Some women need to use a whole jar of the cream each month during this period. Stopping the use of the cream at day 26 or 27 usually brings on a normal period within the next 48 hours.

If Someone Is on HRT Already and Wants to Stop, How Does She Go About It?

HRT means that some sort of oestrogen is being given to a woman, generally with a progestogen of some kind. Since oestrogens contribute to oestrogen dominance with all that implies and the progestogens are known to have many negative side-effects and natural progesterone none, if a woman is taking both synthetic oestrogen and a progestogen the first step is generally to substitute natural progesterone for the progestogen, then gradually to decrease the synthetic oestrogen allowing the progesterone to take whilst monitoring symptoms. When a woman on HRT wishes to get off it, there are a few things that need to be kept in mind. The first is that the progestogens and progesterone compete for receptor sites in the body so that the full benefits of progesterone will be reduced until the progestogens have been cleared from the body. Second, blood levels of progesterone will not rise to optimal levels until 2 or 3 months after you begin to use the cream. Third, the use of a progesterone cream may temporarily sensitize oestrogen receptors leading to an experience of high-oestrogen effects – fluid retention, tenderness and swelling in the breasts or even the appearance of scant vaginal bleeding. These are only temporary and will soon clear. John Lee tells his patients that when they start progesterone he wants them to use a 50 g (2 oz) jar a month for 2 or 3 months, leaving off 7 days a month then beginning again the next month. He reduces the oestrogen they are taking by 50 per cent the moment they start on the progesterone and also the progestogen they have been taking by 50 per cent. Then the next month they can reduce each of those again by 50 per cent, and the same the next month, then they stop. It is important to allow time for the progesterone to reach physiological equilibrium as the synthetic hormones are reduced, because if they are stopped abruptly women will tend to be flooded with hot flushes and think, 'Oh, I can't stop.' By the end of the third month the HRT can safely be completely discontinued. If natural progesterone does not clear up any symptoms completely within 3 or 4 months then Lee considers adding a small amount of oestrogen. However, with most women, natural progesterone is enough to handle everything.

How Does a Woman Who Has Had a Hysterectomy Use the Cream?

She can go by the calendar month, using the cream for 21 days and leaving off for the last week. In three months the hypothalamus will have linked into the monthly cycles since the business of the ovaries following the cycle, intricate though it is, is remarkably *plastic*. This should enable her body to handle any hot flushes and bring protection against osteoporosis.

Why Not Use a Progesterone Cream Continuously After Menopause?

Progesterone is best used in a cyclic fashion over the course of a month and postmenopausal women should leave a minimum of 4 or 5 days when they are not using the cream. The reason for this is that hormones work by combining with a receptor which is already in the cell which then migrates to the nucleus and to a DNA gene to create the response. It is like a key in a lock activating some response. If you occupy or stimulate a receptor continually it will eventually tune down the response. It is as if you were working in a noisy street – at first the noise bothers you until you get used to it and you shut it out. Then if you go on holiday and come back again the noise will be noticed again. Similarly, if you go out in bright sunlight then come into a darkened room it takes a few minutes for your eyes to see since the bright sun has tuned down your receptor response for light. Then if you go back out into the bright sun it will be so bright you cannot stand it. Using progesterone cream and then stopping it for a few days helps keep the receptor sites sensitive to it. If you used it continually you would end up with reduced benefit from it.

Do You Get A Build-up of Progesterone or Do You Have to Use a Progesterone Cream Forever?

How long you use a progesterone cream depends upon your response to it. Using it for 3 or 4 months you can monitor the improvement in the condition for which you have taken it. Often menstruating women can then greatly reduce the amount they are using, always monitoring symptoms to see that they do not return. Similar advice applies to postmenopausal women. However, because of the protection natural progesterone offers a woman from osteoporosis, hirsutism and so many other things, you may like to use a progesterone cream on an ongoing basis. It is likely that once any symptoms have been cleared up you will need very little of the cream to maintain the benefits. When John Lee's patients ask him, 'How long should I go on using this?' he says, 'Do it until you are 96 and then we will reconsider.' For, sadly, in the world we live in, the causes for women's oestrogen dominance and progesterone deficiency are not likely to go away.

Further Reading

Highly Recommended Books on the Science of Menopause

Brown, Ellen and Lynne Walker, *Breezing Through the Change*, Frog Ltd, Berkeley, CA, USA, 1994.

Coney, Sandra, *The Menopause Industry*, Penguin Books, London, 1991.

Dalton, Dr K., 'The Premenstrual Syndrome', *British Medical Journal*, 1953, 1, 1007.

Dumble, Lynette, and Renate Klein, 'Hormone Replacement Therapy: Hazards, Risks and Tricks', Proceedings of *Menopause: The Alternative Way: Facts and Fallacies of the Menopause Industry*, 1993, Australian Women's Research Centre, Deakin University, Australia.

Lee, John R., MD, *Natural Progesterone*, BLL Publishing, California, USA, 1993.

Lee, John R., MD, *Optimal Health Guidelines*, BLL Publishing, California, USA, 1994.

Northrup, Christiane, *Women's Bodies, Women's Wisdom*, Bantam Books, New York, 1994.

Pearl, W., *Keys to the Inner Universe. The Encyclopedia on Weight Training*, Bill Pearl Enterprises, Phoenix, Oregon, 1982.

Reitz, Rosetta, *Menopause, a Positive Approach*, Unwin Paperbacks, London, 1985.

Vines, Gail, *Raging Hormones*, Virago, London, 1993.

Weed, Susun S., *Menopausal Years, The Wise Woman Way*, Ash Tree Publishing, New York, 1992.

Highly Recommended Books on the Mythology of Menopause

Achterberg, Jeanne, *Woman as Healer*, Shambhala, Massachusetts, USA, 1990.

Baring, Anne, and Jules Cashford, *The Myth of the Goddess*, Viking Arkana, London, 1991.

Becker, Ernest, *The Denial of Death*, The Free Press, New York, 1973.

Campbell, Joseph, *The Hero With a Thousand Faces*, Bollingen Foundation, New York, USA, 1972.

Campbell, Joseph, *Transformations of Myth Through Time*, Harper and Row, New York, USA, 1990.

Campbell, Joseph, *Primitive Mythology, The Masks of God*, Arkana, Penguin, New York, USA, 1991.

Downing, Christine, *Psyche's Sister*, Continuum Publishing Company, New York, 1988.

Downing, Christine, *Women's Mysteries*, The Crossroad Publishing Company, New York, USA, 1992.

Downing, Christine, *The Goddess*, The Crossroad Publishing Company, New York, USA, 1992.

Ereira, Alan, *The Heart of the World*, Jonathan Cape, London, 1990.

Foley, Helene P., *The Homeric Hymn to Demeter*, Princeton University Press, New Jersey, USA, 1994.

Franz, Marie-Louise, von, *Patterns of Creativity Mirrored in Creation Myths*, Spring Publications, Zürich, Switzerland, 1972.

Franz, M. L., von, *Shadow and Evil in Fairytales*, Spring Publications, New York, 1974.

George, Demetra, *Asteroid Goddesses*, ACS Publications Inc., CA, USA, 1986.

George, Demetra, *Mysteries of the Dark Moon*, HarperSanFrancisco, USA, 1992.

Gimbutas, Marija, *The Civilization of the Goddess*, HarperSanFrancisco, USA, 1991.

Gleason, Judith, *Oya, In Praise of the Goddess*, Shambhala Publications Inc., Massachusetts, USA, 1987.

Graves, Robert, *The White Goddess*, Faber and Faber, London, 1961.

Grof, Stanislav, and Christina Grof (eds), *Spiritual Emergency*, Jeremy Tarcher Inc., Los Angeles, USA, 1989.

Grof, Stanislav, and Christina Grof, *The Stormy Search for the Self*, Jeremy Tarcher Inc., Los Angeles, USA, 1990.

Hall, Nor, *The Moon and the Virgin*, The Women's Press, London, 1980.

Harding, Esther M., *A Woman's Mysteries Ancient and Modern*, Rider and Company, London, 1971.

Ingerman, Sandra, *Soul Retrieval*, HarperSanFrancisco, USA, 1991.

Ingerman, Sandra, *Welcome Home*, HarperSanFrancisco, USA, 1993.

Lovelock, J. E., *Gaia*, Oxford University Press, Oxford, 1979.

Manheim, Ralph, *Grimm's Tales for Young and Old*, Victor Gollancz Ltd, London, 1977.

Mookerjee, Ajit, *Kali, The Feminine Force*, Thames and Hudson, London, 1988.

Morgan, Elaine, *The Descent of Woman*, Souvenir Press, London, 1972.

Murdock, Maureen, *The Heroine's Journey*, Shambhala Publications Inc, Massachusetts, USA, 1990.

Owen, Lara, *Her Blood is Gold*, HarperSanFrancisco, USA, 1993.

Pinkola Estés, Clarissa, *Women Who Run With the Wolves*, Rider, London, 1992.

Redgrave, Peter, *The Black Goddess and the Sixth Sense*, Bloomsbury, London, 1987.

Shuttle, Penelope, and Peter Redgrave, *The Wise Wound*, Victor Gollancz Ltd, London, 1978.

Walker, Barbara G., *The Crone, Woman of Age, Wisdom and Power*, HarperSanFrancisco, USA, 1988.

Wolkstein, Diane, and Samuel Noah Kramer, *Inanna, Queen of Heaven and Earth*, Rider and Company, London, 1983.

References

Chapter One: Bloodless Revolution

Campbell, Joseph, *The Hero With a Thousand Faces*, Bollingen Foundation, New York, USA, 1972.

Campbell, Joseph, *Transformations of Myth Through Time*, Harper and Row, New York, USA, 1990.

Campbell, Joseph, *Primitive Mythology, The Masks of God*, Arkana, Penguin, New York, USA, 1991.

Coney, Sandra, *The Menopause Industry*, Penguin Books, London, 1991.

Dumble, Lynette, and Renate Klein, 'Hormone Replacement Therapy: Hazards, Risks and Tricks', Proceedings of *Menopause: The Alternative Way: Facts and Fallacies of the Menopause Industry*, 1993, Australian Women's Research Centre, Deakin University, Australia.

Durrant-Peatfield, Barry, 'The Premenstrual Syndrome', Monograph. Received December 1994.

George, Demetra, *Asteroid Goddesses*, ACS Publications Inc., CA, USA, 1986.

George, Demetra, *Mysteries of the Dark Moon*, HarperSanFrancisco, USA, 1992.

Ingerman, Sandra, *Soul Retrieval*, HarperSanFrancisco, USA, 1991.

Ingerman, Sandra, *Welcome Home*, HarperSanFrancisco, USA, 1993.

Khaw, K.T., 'The Menopause and Hormone Replacement Therapy', *Postgraduate Medical Journal*, 1992, 68, 615–623.

Khaw, K.T., (ed.), *Hormone Replacement Therapy*, Churchill Livingstein, London, 1992.

Lee, J.R., MD, 'Understanding Osteoporosis'. Summary.

Lee, J.R., MD, 'Osteoporosis reversal; the role of progesterone', *International Clinical Nutritional Review*, 1990, June, Sydney, Australia.

Lee, J.R., MD, 'Osteoporosis reversal with transdermal progesterone', *The Lancet*, 1990, November, Letter. 336.

Lee, J.R., MD, 'Is natural progesterone the missing link in osteoporosis prevention and treatment?' *Medical Hypotheses*, 1991, 35, 314, 318.

Lee, J.R., MD, 'Hormonal and nutritional aspects of osteoporosis', *Health and Nutrition*, 1991, Winter, Vol. 6, Issue 4.

Lee, J.R., MD, *Natural Progesterone*, BLL Publishing, California, USA, 1993.

Lee, J.R., MD, 'The Theory of Estrogen Dominance', Seminar given at St Thomas's Hospital, London, 4 June 1994.

Lee, J.R., MD, 'Clinical Uses of Natural Progesterone', Seminar given at St Thomas's Hospital, London, 4 June 1994.

Lee, J.R., MD, 'Dr John Lee speaking at the Chelsea Hotel, London, 5 June 1994', Video.

Lee, J.R., MD, 'Effects of Progesterone on Osteoporosis and Menopausal Symptoms', Seminar given at St Thomas's Hospital, London, 4 June 1994.

Lee, J.R., MD, 'Successful Menopausal Osteoporosis Treatment Restoring Osteoclast/Osteoblast Equilibrium', *The Townsend Letter for Doctors*, 1994, August/September, 900.

Peat, R., 'Progesterone: Safe Antidote for P.M.S.', *McCall's*, 1990, October, 152–156.

Peat, R., 'The Progesterone Deception', *Ray Peat's Newsletter*, 1986, 4 May, 44.

Peat, R., 'Blocking Tissue Destruction', Unpublished Paper.

Peat, R., PhD., 'Progesterone in Orthomolecular Medicine', Blake College Booklet, Eugene, Oregon. Available from Foundation for Hormonal and Nutrition Research, 8150 SW, Barnes Road, Portland, OR 97225, USA.

Peat, R., 'Progesterone Can Be Taken Orally', Letter to the Editor, *The Townsend Letter for Doctors*, 1994, November.

Peat, R., *Nutrition for Women*, Kenogen, Eugene, Oregon, USA, 1981.

Pinkola Estés, Clarissa, *Women Who Run With the Wolves*, Rider, London, 1992.

Prior, J.C., 'Progesterone as a bone-trophic hormone', *Endocrine Review:* 11:386–398, 1990.

Prior, J.C., 'Spinal bone loss and ovulatory disturbances', *New England Journal of Medicine*, 323, 18, 1990.

Prior, J.C., Y. Vigna, and R.N. Alojado, 'Progesterone and the prevention of osteoporosis', *Canadian Journal of Obstetric/Gynecology & Women's Health Care*, 3, 4, 1991.

Prior, J.C., 'Progesterone and its relevance for osteoporosis', *Bulletin for Physicians,* 1993, March, vol. 2, no. 2.

Prior, J.C., Y. Vigna, and R. Burgess, 'Medroxyprogesterone increases trabecular bone density in women with menstrual disorders', University of British Columbia, Vancouver. Paper presented at annual meeting of the Endocrine Society, 11 June, 1987, Indianapolis, IN, USA.

Prior, J.C., Y.M. Vigna, and D. W. McKay, 'Reproduction for the athletic woman: new understandings of physiology and management', *Sports Medicine,* 1992, 14, 190–199.

Shaffer, Willa, *Wild Yam, Birth Control Without Fear,* Woodland Health Books, Utah, USA, 1986.

Shaffer, Willa, *Midwifery and Herbs,* Woodland Books, Utah, USA, 1986.

Weed, Susun S., *Menopausal Years, The Wise Woman Way,* Ash Tree Publishing, New York, 1992.

Chapter Two: Cry Freedom

Aitken, M., D.M. Hart, and R. Lindsay, 'Oestrogen replacement therapy for prevention of osteoporosis after oophorectomy', *British Medical Journal,* 1973, 3, 515–518.

Barrett-Connor, E., 'Postmenopausal estrogen replacement and breast cancer', *New England Journal of Medicine,* 1989, 5, 321.

Barzel, U.S., 'Estrogens in the prevention and treatment of postmenopausal osteoporosis: a review', *American Journal of Medicine,* 1988, 85: 847–850.

Begley, S., and D. Glick, 'The Estrogen Complex', *Newsweek,* 21 March 1994.

Berkgvist, L., H.O. Adami, I. Persson, R. Hoover, and C. Schairer, 'The risk of breast cancer after estrogen and estrogen-progestin replacement', *New England Journal of Medicine,* 1989, 5, 321.

Biller, B.M., J.F. Coughlin, V. Saxe, et al., 'Osteopenia in women with hypothalmic amenorrhea: a prospective study', *Obstetrics and Gynecology,* 1991, 78, 996–1001.

Bonnar, J., et al., 'Coagulation system changes in postmenopausal women receiving oestrogen preparations', *Post Graduate Medical Journal,* 1976, 52, 30.

Boston Collaborative Drug Surveillance Program, 'Surgically confirmed gallbladder disease, venous thromboembolism, and breast tumours in relation to menopausal oestrogen therapy', *New England Journal of Medicine*, 1974, 15, 290.

Bullen, B.A., G.S. Skriniar, I.Z. Beitins, et al., 'Introduction of menstrual disorders by strenuous exercise in untrained women', *New England Journal of Medicine*, 1985, 312, 1349–1353.

Coney, Sandra, *The Menopause Industry*, Penguin Books, London, 1991.

Durrant-Peatfield, Barry, 'The Premenstrual Syndrome', Monograph. Received December 1994.

Felson, D.T., Y. Zhang, M.T. Hannan, D.P. Kiel, P.W.F. Wilson, and J.J. Anderson, 'The effect of postmenopausal estrogen therapy on bone density in elderly women', *New England Journal of Medicine*, 1993, 329:1141–1146.

Gambrel, R.D., 'The menopause: benefits and risks of estrogen-progestogen replacement therapy', *Fertility Sterility*, 1982, 37, 457–474.

Grant, Dr Ellen, *Sexual Chemistry, Understanding Our Hormones, The Pill and HRT*, Cedar Original, Mandarin Paperbacks, London, 1994.

Guyton, Arthur C., *Textbook of Medical Physiology*, Sixth Edition, W.B. Saunders Company, Philadelphia, USA, 1981.

Hargrove, Joel T., et al., 'Menopausal hormone replacement therapy with continuous daily oral micronized estradiol and progesterone', *Obstetrics and Gynaecology*, 1989, 73, 606–612.

Hargrove, Joel T., et al., 'Progesterone: Safe Antidote for PMS', *McCall's*, October 1990.

Henderson, B.E., R.K. Ross, M.C. Pike, and J.T. Casagrande, 'Endogenous hormones as a major factor in human cancer', *Cancer Research*, 1982, 42, 3232–3239.

Hileman, Bette, 'Environmental estrogens linked to reproductive abnormalities, cancer', *C&EN Washington*.

Hoover, R., L.A. Gray Sr., P. Cole, B. MacMahon, 'Menopausal estrogens and breast cancer', *New England Journal of Medicine*, 1976, 295, 401–405.

Inman, W.H.W., et al., 'Thromboembolic disease and the steroidal content of oral contraceptives. A report to the committee on Safety of Drugs', *British Medical Journal*, 1970, 203

Kamen, Betty, *Startling New Facts About Osteoporosis*, Nutrition Encounter Inc., California, USA, 1989.

Kamen, Betty, *Hormone Replacement Therapy, Yes or No?* Nutrition Encounter Inc., California, USA, 1993.

Lee, J.R., MD, 'Understanding Osteoporosis'. Summary.

Lee, J.R., MD, 'The Theory of Estrogen Dominance', Seminar given at St Thomas's Hospital, London, 4 June 1994.

Lee, J.R., MD, 'Osteoporosis reversal with transdermal progesterone', *The Lancet*, Letter. 336. November 1990.

Lee, J.R., MD, 'Is natural progesterone the missing link in osteoporosis prevention and treatment?, *Medical Hypotheses*, 1991, 35, 314, 318.

Lee, J.R., MD, 'Hormonal and nutritional aspects of osteoporosis', *Health and Nutrition*, 1991, Winter, Vol. 6, Issue 4.

Lee, J.R., MD, *Natural Progesterone*, BLL Publishing, California, USA, 1993.

Lee, J.R., MD, *Optimal Health Guidelines*, Second Edition, BLL Publishing, California, USA, 1993.

Lee, J.R., MD, Endocrinology Notes: Progesterone and Estrogen. 6 February 1993.

Lee, J.R., MD, 'The Theory of Estrogen Dominance', Seminar given at St Thomas's Hospital, London, 4 June 1994.

Lee, J.R., MD, 'Clinical Uses of Natural Progesterone', Seminar given at St Thomas's Hospital, London, 4 June 1994.

Lee, J.R., MD, 'Dr John Lee speaking at the Chelsea Hotel, London, 5 June 1994', Video.

Lee, J.R., MD, 'Effects of Progesterone on Osteoporosis and Menopausal Symptoms', Seminar given at St Thomas's Hospital, London, 4 June 1994.

Lee, J.R., MD, 'The Multiple Effects of Progesterone', Seminar given at St Thomas's Hospital, London, 4 June 1994.

Lee, J.R., MD, 'The Theory of Estrogen Dominance', Seminar given at St Thomas's Hospital, London, 4 June 1994.

Lees, B., et al., 'Differences in proximal femur bone density over two centuries', *Lancet*, 1993, 341:673-675.

McKinlay, John, Sonja McKinlay and Donald Brambilla, 'Health Status and utilisation behaviour associated with menopause', *American Journal of Epidemiology*, 1987, 125, 1, 110–121.

McKinlay, John, Sonja McKinlay and Donald Brambilla, 'The relative contributions of endocrine changes and social circumstances to depression in mid-aged women', *Journal of Health and Social Behaviour*, 28, 4, 345–363.

McKinlay, Sonja, and John McKinlay, 'Selected studies of the menopause: a methodological critique', *Journal of Biosocial Science*, 1973, 5, 533–555.

Metcalf, M.G., 'Incidence of ovulatory cycles in women approaching the menopause', *Biosocial Science*, 1979, 11, 39–48.

Nabulsi, A.A., A.R. Folsom, A. White, et al., 'Association of hormone replacement therapy with various cardiovascular risk factors in postmenopausal women', *New England Journal of Medicine*, 1993, 328, 1069–1075.

Peat, R., PhD., 'Estrogen in 1990', *Blake College Newsletter*, 1990, Eugene, Oregon, USA.

Peat, R., PhD., 'Progesterone in Orthomecular Medicine', Booklet.

Prior, J.C., Y. Vigna, and R. Burgess, 'Medroxyprogesterone increases trabecular bone density in women with menstrual disorders', University of British Columbia, Vancouver. Paper presented at annual meeting of the Endrocine Society, 11 June, 1987, Indianapolis, IN, USA.

Prior, J.C., 'Progesterone as a bone-trophic hormone', *Endocrine Review:* 11:386–398, 1990.

Prior, J.C., 'Spinal bone loss and ovulatory disturbances', *New England Journal of Medicine*, 323, 18, 1990.

Prior, J.C., Y. Vigna, and R.N. Alojado, 'Progestone and the prevention of osteoporosis', *Canadian Journal of Obstetric/Gynecology & Women's Health Care*, 3, 4, 1991.

Prior, J.C., Y.M. Vigna, D.W. McKay, 'Reproduction for the athletic woman: new understandings of physiology and management', *Sports Medicine*, 1992, 14, 190–199.

Prior, J.C., 'Progesterone and its relevance for osteoporosis', *Bulletin for Physicians*, 1993, March, vol. 2, no. 2.

Shapiro, S., 'Oral contraceptives – a time to take stock', *New England Journal of Medicine*, 1986, 315, 450.

Stadel, B.V., 'Oral contraceptives and cardiovascular disease', *New England Journal of Medicine*, 1981, 305, 612.

Stevenson, J.C., P.C. Michael, F.G. Gangar, T.C. Hillard, B. Lees, and M.J. Whitehead, 'Effects of transdermal versus oral hormone replacement therapy on bone density in spine and proximal femur in postmenopausal women', *The Lancet*, vol. 336, 2265–2269.

Stryer, Lubert, *Biochemistry*, W.H. Freeman and Company, San Francisco, 1975.

Studd, John, and Rod Barber, 'Mastering the Menopause', Leaflet presented with the compliments of Organon Laboratories Ltd, Cambridge, 1994.

Swenerton, K.D., P. Fugere, A.B. Miller, et al., 'Menopausal progestins and breast cancer', *JSOCG*, 1991, 13, 7–9.

Tietz, Norbert W., PhD., *Textbook of Clinical Chemistry*, W.B.
Saunders Company, Philadelphia, USA, 1986.

Vollman, R.F., 'The Menstrual Cycle', in *Major Problems in Obstetrics
and Gynecology*, vol. 7, (ed.) E. A. Friedman, W.B. Saunders
Company, Toronto, Canada, 1977.

Wise, P.W., 'Influence of estrogen on ageing of the central nervous
system: its role in declining female reproductive function',
Menopause: Evaluation, Treatment and Health Concerns, 1989,
53–70.

Chapter Three: Sleeping with the Enemy

The work of the following researchers is referred to in J. Raloff's
'The Gender Benders': Michael Fry, Devra Lee-Davis, Louis J.
Guillette, Neils Skakkebaek, Ana Soto, John P. Sumpter and
Mary S. Wolff. Raloff's 'Eco-Cancers' refers to the work of David
E. Blask and Steven M. Hill, and Robert Liburdy. R. Weiss's
'Estrogen in the environment' refers to the work of David Crews
and Herman Aldercreutz.

Begley, S., and D. Glick, 'The Estrogen Complex', *Newsweek*, 21
March 1994.

Berkgvist, L., H.O. Adami, I. Persson, R. Hoover, and C. Schairer,
'The risk of breast cancer after estrogen and estrogen-progestin
replacement', *New England Journal of Medicine*, 1989, 5, 321.

Colborn, T., vom Saal F.S. Soto A.M., 'Developmental Effects of
Endocrine-disrupting chemicals in wildlife and humans', in
Environmental Health Perspectives, 1993, 101: 378–384.

'Environmental Estrogens: Pathway to Extinction', xenoestrogen
conference held 13 May, 1995 in Santa Rosa, California, USA.
Speakers: Howard A. Bern PhD, tumor and comparative
endocrinologist at UC, Berkeley in the Department of
Integrative Biology and Cancer Research Laboratory; Theo
Colborn PhD, Senior Scientist and Manager of Wildlife &
Contaminants Project at World Wildlife Fund and editor of
*Chemically Induced Alterations in Sexual & Functional Development:
Wildlife/Human Connection*; Donald Michael Fry PhD, Professor
at UC, Davis in Department of Avian Sciences – researches toxic
effects of airborne and waterborne organochlorine pesticides

on development and reproduction in birds; Louis Guillette Jr PhD, Professor of Zoology, University of Florida, and expert adviser for Environmental Protection Agency in US and US Fish and Wildlife Department – focuses on endocrine disrupting contamination in endangered species, reptiles and other wildlife; John McLachlan, PhD, Chief of National Institute of Environmental Health Sciences (NIEHS), 1972–1994, in laboratory of reproductive and developmental toxicology – now director of Tulane/Xavier Centre for Bioenvironmental Research; Marion Moses MD, President of San Francisco's Pesticide Education Centre who is both board certified in occupational medicine and an expert on the impact of chemical exposures, especially pesticides, on human health.

Gambrell, R.D., 'The menopause: benefits and risks of estrogen-progestogen replacement therapy', *Fertility Sterility*, 1982, 37, 457–474.

Guillette, L.J. Jr., 'Endocrine-disrupting environmental contaminants and reproduction: lessons from the study of wildlife, published in Woman's Health Today: Perspectives on Current Research and Clinical Practice, 1994, 201–207.

Guyton, Arthur C., *Textbook of Medical Physiology*, Sixth Edition, W.B. Saunders Company, Philadelphia, USA, 1981.

Hiatt, R.A., R. Bawol, G.D. Friedman, and R. Hoover, 'Exogenous estrogen and breast cancer after bilateral oopherectomy', *Cancer*, 1984, 54, 139–144.

Hileman, Bette, 'Environmental estrogens linked to reproductive abnormalities, Cancer', *C&EN*, *Washington*, 31 January 1994, 19–23.

La Vecchia, C., A. Decarli, F. Parazzini, A. Gentile, C. Liberati, and S. Franceschi, 'Non-contraceptive oestrogens and the risk of breast cancer in women', *International Journal of Cancer*, 1986, 38, 853–858.

Lee, J.R., MD, 'Osteoporosis reversal; the role of progesterone', *International Clinical Nutritional Review*, Sydney, Australia, June 1990.

Lee, J.R., MD, 'Is natural progesterone the missing link in osteoporosis prevention and treatment?' *Medical Hypotheses* 1991, 35, 316–318.

Lee, J.R., MD, *Natural Progesterone*, BLL Publishing, California, USA, 1993.

Lee, J.R., MD, Endocrinology Notes: Progesterone and Estrogen. 6 February 1993.

Lee, J.R., MD, 'The Theory of Estrogen Dominance', Seminar given at St Thomas's Hospital, London, 4 June 1994.

Lee, J.R., MD, 'Dr John Lee speaking at the Chelsea Hotel, London, 5 June 1994', Video.

Medical Tribune, 'Sperm-count drop tied to pollution rise', 26 March 1992.

McLachlan, I.A., 'Functional Toxicology: a new approach to detect biologically active xenobiotics', in *Environmental Health Perspectives*, 1993, 10: 386–387.

Moses, Marion, MD, 'Pesticides and Human Health – An Interview with Dr Marion Moses by Cincy Deuhring', in *Informed Consent*, May/June 1994, 21-24; also Moses, M., 'Pesticides and Breast Cancer' in *Pesticide News*, December 1994, 23: 3–5.

Peat, R., PhD., 'Estrogen in 1990', *Blake College Newsletter*, 1990, Eugene, Oregon, USA.

Peat, R., PhD., 'Progesterone in Orthomolecular Medicine', Booklet.

Raloff, J., 'Eco-Cancers, do environmental factors underlie a breast cancer epidemic?', *Science News*, 3 July 1993.

Raloff, J., 'The Gender Benders' Part Two 'That Feminine Touch', *Science News*, 8 January 1994 and 22 February 1994.

Skakkebaek, Neils E., et al., *British Medical Journal*, 1992, January.

Soto, Ana, et al., *Science News*, 3 July 1993, 12.

Soto, Ana, et al., *Science News*, 8 January 1994, 24.

Stadel, B.V., 'Oral contraceptives and cardiovascular disease', *New England Journal of Medicine*, 1981, 305, 612.

Stevens, Richard G., *American Journal of Epidemiology*, 1987, April.

Stone, Richard, 'Environmental Toxicants Under Scrutiny at Baltimore Meeting – meeting brief review' in *Science*, 24 March 1995, 267: 1770–1771. And 'Dioxins Dominate Denver Gathering of Toxicologists – meeting brief review' in *Science*, 18 November 1994, 266: 1162–1163.

Stryer, Lubert, *Biochemistry*, W.H. Freeman and Company, San Francisco, 1975.

Tietz, Norbert, W., PhD., *Textbook of Clinical Chemistry*, W.B. Saunders Company, Philadelphia, USA, 1986.

von Kaulla, F., et al., 'Conjugated oestrogens and hypercoagulability', *American Journal of Obstetrics and Gynecology*, 1975, 122, 688.

Weiss, R., 'Estrogen in the environment', *Washington Post*, 1994, 25th January, p. 10–13.

Wolff, Mary S., Devra Lee-Davis, et al., *Science News*, 24 April 1993, 262.

Chapter Four: Search for the Grail

Austin, Phylis, Agatha Thrash, and Calvin Thrash, *Natural Remedies, A Manual*, Yuchi Pines Institute, Seale, Al, USA, 1983.

Barrett-Connor, E., 'Postmenopausal estrogen replacement and breast cancer', *New England Journal of Medicine*, 1989, 5, 321.

Begley, S., and D. Glick, 'The Estrogen Complex', *Newsweek*, 21 March 1994.

Berkgvist, L., H.O. Adami, I. Persson, R. Hoover, C. Schairer, 'The risk of breast cancer after estrogen and estrogen-progestin replacement', *New England Journal of Medicine*, 1989, 5, 321.

Brown, Ellen and Lynne Walker, *Breezing Through The Change*, Frog Ltd, Berkeley, CA, USA, 1994.

Christiansen, C., B.J. Riis, L. Nilas, P. Rodbro, and L. Deftos, 'Uncoupling of bone formation and resorption by combined oestrogen and progestogen therapy in postmenopausal osteoporosis', *Lancet*, 1985, October.

Coney, Sandra, *The Menopause Industry*, Penguin Books, London, 1991.

Felson, D.T., Y. Zhang, M.T. Hannan, D.P. Kiel, P.W.F. Wilson, and J.J. Anderson, 'The effect of postmenopausal estrogen therapy on bone density in elderly women', *New England Journal of Medicine*, 1993, 329:1141–1146.

Guyton, Arthur C., *Textbook of Medical Physiology*, Sixth Edition, W.B. Saunders Company, Philadelphia, USA, 1981.

Hudson, Tori, *Gynecology and Naturopathic Medicine*, TK Publications, Oregon, USA, 1992.

Kamen, Betty, *Hormone Replacement Therapy, Yes or No?*, Nutrition Encounter Inc., California, USA, 1993.

Lee, J.R., MD, 'Understanding Osteoporosis'. Summary.

Lee, J.R., MD, 'Osteoporosis reversal; the role of progesterone', *International Clinical Nutritional Review*, 1990, June, Sydney, Australia.

Lee, J.R., MD, 'Osteoporosis reversal with transdermal progesterone', *The Lancet*, 1990, November, Letter. 336.

Lee, J.R., MD, 'Is natural progesterone the missing link in osteo-porosis prevention and treatment?' *Medical Hypotheses* 1991, 35, 314, 318.

Lee, J.R., MD, 'Hormonal and nutritional aspects of osteoporosis', *Health and Nutrition*, 1991, Winter, Vol. 6, Issue 4.

Lee, J.R., MD, *Natural Progesterone*, BLL Publishing, California, USA, 1993.

Lee, J.R., MD, 'The Theory of Estrogen Dominance', Seminar given at St Thomas's Hospital, London, 4 June 1994.

Lee, J.R., MD, 'Clinical Uses of Natural Progesterone', Seminar given at St Thomas's Hospital, London, 4 June 1994.

Lee, J.R., MD, 'Dr John Lee speaking at the Chelsea Hotel, London, 5 June 1994', Video.

Lee, J. R., MD, 'Effects of Progesterone on Osteoporosis and Menopausal Symptoms', Seminar given at St Thomas's Hospital London, 4 June 1994.

Lee, J.R., MD, 'Successful Menopausal Osteoporosis Treatment Restoring Osteoclast/Osteoblast Equilibrium', *The Townsend Letter for Doctors*, 1994, August/September, 900.

Medical Research Publishers, *Amazing Medicines The Drug Companies Don't Want You To Discover!* Tempe, Arizona 85281, USA, 1993.

Peat, R., PhD., 'Progesterone in Orthomolecular Medicine', Blake College Booklet, Eugene, Oregon. Available from Foundation for Hormonal and Nutrition Research, 8150 SW, Barnes Road, Portland, Oregon, 97225, USA.

Peat, R., 'Origins of Progesterone Therapy', *The Townsend Letter for Doctors*, 1992, November, 112, 1016.

Shaffer, Willa, *Wild Yam, Birth Control Without Fear*, Woodland Health Books, Utah, USA, 1986.

Stevenson, J.C., P.C. Michael, F.G. Gangar, T.C. Hillard, B. Lees, M.J. Whitehead, 'Effects of transdermal versus oral hormone replacement therapy on bone density in spine and proximal femur in postmenopausal women', *Lancet* Vol. 336, 2265–2269.

Studd, John and Rod Barber, 'Mastering the Menopause', Leaflet presented with the compliments of Organon Laboratories Ltd, Cambridge, 1994.

Williams, David G., 'The forgotten hormones', *Alternatives for the Health Conscious Individual*, 1991, Vol. 4, No 6, 41–46.

Whitehead, M.I., D. Fraser, L. Schenkel, D. Crook, J.C. Stevenson, 'Transdermal administration of oestrogen/progestogen hormone replacement therapy', *Lancet*, 1990, Vol. 335, 310–311.

Chapter Five: Cycles of the Moon

Coney, Sandra, *The Menopause Industry*, Penguin Books, London, 1991.

Guyton, Arthur C., *Textbook of Medical Physiology*, Sixth Edition, W.B. Saunders Company, Philadelphia, USA, 1981.

Lee, J.R., MD, 'The Theory of Estrogen Dominance', Seminar given at St Thomas's Hospital, London, 4 June 1994.

Lee, J.R., MD, 'Is natural progesterone the missing link in osteoporosis prevention and treatment?' *Medical Hypotheses* 1991, 35, 314, 318.

Lee, J.R., MD, *Natural Progesterone*, BLL Publishing, California, USA, 1993.

Lee, J.R., Endocrinology Notes: Progesterone and Estrogen. 6 February 1993.

Lee, J.R., MD, 'Clinical Uses of Natural Progesterone', Seminar given at St Thomas's Hospital, London, 4 June 1994.

Peat, R., PhD., 'Estrogen in 1990', *Blake College Newsletter*, 1990, Eugene, Oregon, USA.

Peat, R., PhD., 'Progesterone in Orthomolecular Medicine', Blake College Booklet, Eugene, Oregon.

Stryer, Lubert, *Biochemistry*, W.H. Freeman and Company, San Francisco, 1975.

Thomas, J. Hywel, and Brian Gillham, *Wills' Biochemical Basis of Medicine*, Butterworth Heinemann Ltd, Oxford, 1989.

Tietz, Norbert W., PhD., *Textbook of Clinical Chemistry*, W.B. Saunders Company, Philadelphia, USA, 1986.

Vollman, R.F., 'The Menstrual Cycle,' in *Major Problems in Obstetrics and Gynecology*, vol. 7, (ed.) E.A. Friedman, W.B. Saunders Company, Toronto, Canada, 1977.

Williams, David G., 'The Forgotten Hormone', *Alternatives for the Health Conscious Individual*, 1991, Vol. 4, No. 6, 41–46.

Chapter Six: Crazed Woman

The Amarant Trust Newsletter, 'Feeling Good', The Amarant Centre, London, 1993, Spring Issue.

Bewley, S., and T.H. Bewley, 'Drug Dependence with Oestrogen Replacement Therapy', *The Lancet*, 1992. 339, 290–291.

Boston Collaborative Drug Surveillance Program (A Report), 'Surgically confirmed gallbladder disease, venous thromboembolism and breast tumours in relation to postmenopausal estrogen therapy', *New England Journal of Medicine,* 290(1), 15–19.

Brown, Ellen and Lynne Walker, *Breezing Through The Change,* Frog Ltd, Berkeley, CA, USA, 1994.

Cabot, Sandra, *Don't Let Your Hormones Ruin Your Life,* Women's Health Advisory Service, NSW, Australia, 1991.

Colditz, Graham A., Kathleen Egan, and Meir J. Stampfer, 'Hormone replacement therapy and risk of breast cancer: Results from epidemiologic studies', *American Journal of Obstetrics and Gynecology,* 186(5), 1473–1479.

Collings, Jill, 'Suffering in Silence', *The Guardian,* 24 November 1988.

Coney, Sandra, *The Menopause Industry,* Penguin Books, New Zealand, 1991.

Cunningham, Gary, and Marshall D. Lindheimer, 'Hypertension in pregnancy', *New England Journal of Medicine,* 1992, 326, 927–932.

Davis, Peter, *For Health or Profit? Medicine, the Pharmaceutical Industry, and the State in New Zealand,* Oxford University Press, Auckland, New Zealand, 1992.

Dumble, Lynette J., 'Hormone Replacement Therapy: The Big Myth of Modern Medicine', *Healthsharing Women Research Issues Forum II: Hormone Replacement Therapy,* 1992, April, Melbourne, Australia.

Dumble, Lynette, and Renate Klein, 'Hormone Replacement Therapy: Hazards, Risks and Tricks', Proceedings of *Menopause: The Alternative Way: Facts and Fallacies of the Menopause Industry,* 1993, Australian Women's Research Centre, Deakin University, Australia.

Dyerassi, C., 'The Making of the Pill', *Science,* 1984, 84, 127–129.

Ehrenreich, Barbara, and Deirdre English, *For Her Own Good: 150 Years of the Expert's Advice to Women,* Anchor Books, New York, USA, 1979.

Gaby, Alan R., 'Premarin and Animal Cruelty', *Townsend Letter for Doctors,* 1994, November.

Gaby, Alan R., *Preventing and Reversing Osteoporosis,* Prima, USA, 1994.

Gangar, Kevin, and Elizabeth Key, 'Individualising HRT', *The Practitioner,* 1993, April, 237, 358–360.

Garnett, Timothy J., John Studd, A.F. Henderson, N.R. Watson, M.

Savvas, and A. Leather, 'Hormone Implants and Tachyphylaxis', *British Journal of Obstetrics and Gynaecology*, 1990, 97, 917–921.

Gorman, Theresa and Malcolm Whitehead, *The Amarant Book of Hormone Replacement Therapy*, Pan Books, London, 1989.

Greer, Germaine, *The Change*, Penguin Books, London, 1991.

Hall, C., 'Caution Urged on Hormone Therapy', *The Independent*, 3 June 1993.

Hoover, Robert, et al., 'Menopausal estrogens and breast cancer', *New England Journal of Medicine*, 1976, 295(8), 401–405.

Kaufert, R., 'Myth and Menopause', *Sociology of Health and Illness*, 1982, 4, 141–166.

Khaw, K.T., 'The Menopause and Hormone Replacement Therapy', *Postgraduate Medical Journal*, 1992, 68, 615–623.

Khaw, K.T. (ed.), *Hormone Replacement Therapy*, Churchill Livingstein, London, 1992.

Klein, Renate, and Lynette J. Dumble, 'Disempowering Mid-Life Women: The Science and Politics of Hormone Replacement Therapy', Women's Studies International Forum, Australia, 1994.

The Lancet, Editorial: 'Dangers in Eternal Youth', 1975, 2, 1135.

Lee, J.R., MD, 'Understanding Osteoporosis'. Summary.

Lee, J.R., MD, 'Osteoporosis reversal; the role of progesterone', *International Clinical Nutritional Review*, Sydney, Australia, June, 1990.

Lee, J.R., MD, 'Osteoporosis reversal with transdermal progesterone', *Lancet*. Letter. 336. November, 1990.

Lee, J.R., MD, 'Is natural progesterone the missing link in osteoporosis prevention and treatment?, *Medical Hypotheses*, 1991 35, 314, 318.

Lee, J.R., MD, 'Hormonal and nutritional aspects of osteoporosis', *Health and Nutrition*, Vol. 6, Issue 4, Winter 1991.

Lee, J.R., MD, *Natural Progesterone*, BLL Publishing, California, USA, 1993.

Lee, J.R., MD, *Optimal Health Guidelines*, Second Edition, BLL Publishing, California, USA, 1993.

Lee, J.R., MD, Endocrinology Notes: Progesterone and Estrogen. 6 February 1993.

Lee, J.R., MD, 'The Theory of Estrogen Dominance', Seminar given at St Thomas's Hospital, London, 4 June 1994.

Lee, J.R., MD, 'Clinical Uses of Natural Progesterone', Seminar given at St Thomas's Hospital, London, 4 June 1994.

Lee, J.R., MD, 'Dr John Lee speaking at the Chelsea Hotel, London, 5 June 1994', Video.

Lee, J.R., MD, 'Effects of Progesterone on Osteoporosis and Menopausal Symptoms', Seminar given at St Thomas's Hospital London, 4 June 1994.

Lee, J.R., MD, 'The Multiple Effects of Progesterone', Seminar given at St Thomas's Hospital, London, 4 June 1994.

Lee, J.R., MD, 'Successful Menopausal Osteoporosis Treatment Restoring Osteoclast/Osteoblast Equilibrium', *The Townsend Letter for Doctors*, 1994, August/September, 900.

Lewis, Jane, 'Feminism, the Menopause and Hormone Replacement', *Feminist Review*, 1993, 43, 38–56.

Lindgren, R., G. Berg, M. Hammer, and E. Zuccon, 'Hormone Replacement Therapy and Sexuality in a Population of Swedish Postmenopausal Women', *Acta Obstet. Gynecol. Scand.*, 1993, 72, 292–297.

McCrea, F., 'The Politics of Menopause: The Discovery of a Deficiency Disease', *Social Problems*, 1983, 31, 111–123.

McCrea, F., and G. Markle, 'The Estrogen Replacement Controversy in the USA and the UK: Different Answers to the Same Question?', *Social Studies of Science*, 1984, 14, 1–26.

Mack, Thomas, et al., 'Estrogens and endometrial cancer in a retirement community', *New England Journal of Medicine*, 1976, 294(23), 1262–1267.

Mannen, E.F., 'Oral contraceptives and blood coagulation: a critical review', *American Journal of Obstetrics and Gynecology*, 1982, 142, 781–790.

National Advisory Committee on Core Health and Disability Support Services, 'Hormone Replacement Therapy', Consensus Development Conference Report, Wellington, New Zealand, December, 1993.

Northrup, Christiane, *Women's Bodies, Women's Wisdom*, Bantam Books, New York, 1994.

Peat, Ray, 'The Progesterone Deception', *Ray Peat's Newsletter*, 1986, May.

Psaty, Bruce M., et al., 'A review of the association of estrogens and progestins with cardiovascular disease in postmenopausal women', *Archives of Internal Medicine*, 153, 1421–1427.

Reitz, Rosetta, *Menopause, A Positive Approach*, Unwin Paperbacks, London, 1985.

Rinzler, Carol Ann, *Estrogen and Breast Cancer: A Warning to Women . . .*, Macmillan Publishing Company, New York, USA, 1993.

Rochon Ford, Anne, 'Hormones: Getting Out of Hand', in *Adverse Effects: Women and the Pharmaceutical Industry*, (ed.) Kathleen McDonnell, IOCU, Penang, Malaysia, 1986.

Rowland, Robyn, *Living Laboratories. Women and Reproductive Technology*, Pan Macmillan, Sydney, Australia, 1992.

Sadgrove, Judy, 'HRT: older women's friend or foe?' *The Guardian*, 20 February 1990.

Saul, Helen, 'The bad news about ``good' cholesterol'', *New Scientist*, 14 August 1993.

Seaman, Barbara, and Gideon Seaman, *Women and the Crisis in Sex Hormones*, Bantam Books, New York, 1977.

Silberstein, Stephen D., and George R. Merriam, 'Estrogens, progestins and headaches', *Neurology*, 1991, 41, 786–793.

Smith, Donald C., et al., 'Association of exogenous estrogen and endometrial carcinoma', *New England Journal of Medicine*, 1975, 293(23), 1164–1167.

Sporrong, T., L.A. Mattsson, E. Stradbert, and M. Uvebrant, 'Continuous combined HRT: long-term effects on the endometrium', Abstract 337. 7th International Congress on the Menopause, Stockholm, Sweden, June 20–24, 1993.

Stampfer, Meir, et al., 'Postmenopausal estrogen therapy and cardiovascular disease', *New England Journal of Medicine*, 1991, 325, 756–762.

Studd, J., and M. Thom, 'Letter to the Editor', *New England Journal of Medicine*, 1979, 300, 922–923.

Vines, Gail, 'The Challenge to HRT', *New Scientist*, 23 October 1993.

Vines, Gail, *Raging Hormones*, Virago Press, London, 1993.

Whitecroft, S.I.J., M.C. Ellerington and M.I. Whitehead, 'Routes of estrogen administration', *Annual Progress in Reproductive Medicine*, (eds) R.H. Asch and J. Studd, The Parthenon Publishing Group, Carnforth, UK, 1993.

Whitehead, M.I., T.C. Hillard, and D. Crook, 'The role and use of progestogens', *Obstetrics and Gynecology*, 1990, 75(4), 59S–76S.

Wilson, R., *Feminine Forever*, M. Evans, New York, 1966.

Wilson, R.A., and T.A. Wilson, 'The Fate of the Non-Treated Postmenopausal Woman: A Plea for Maintenance of Adequate Estrogen from Puberty to the Grave', *Journal of the American Geriatrics Society*, 1963, 11, 346–362.

Ziel, H.K., and Finkle, W.D., 'Increased risk of endometrial carcinoma among users of conjugated estrogens', *New England Journal of Medicine*, 1975, 293(23), 1167–1170.

Chapter Seven: Dark Gods

Abraham, G.E., and J.T. Hargrove, 'Effect of Vitamin B on Premenstrual Tension Syndrome: A double blind crossover study', *Infertility*, 1980, vol. 3, 155.

Abraham, G.E., 'Nutritional factors in the etiology of the Premenstrual Tension Syndromes', *Journal of Reproductive Medicine*, 1983, vol. 28, 446.

Aldercreutz, H., 'Diet and Plasma Androgens in Postmenopausal Vegetarian and Omnivorous Women and Postmenopausal Women with Breast Cancer', *American Journal of Clinical Nutrition*, 1989, vol. 49, 433.

Aldercreutz, H., et al., 'Determination of urinary lignans and phytoestrogen metabolites, potential antiestrogens and anticarcinogens in urine of women on various habitual diets', *J. Steroid, Biochem*, 1986, 25, 791–797.

Aldercreutz, H., et al., 'Dietary phytoestrogens and the menopause in Japan', *The Lancet*, 1992, vol 339, 1233.

Balch, James F., and Phyllis A. Balch, *Prescription for Nutritional Healing*, Avery Publishing Group Ltd, New York, USA, 1990.

Barrett-Connor, E., 'Postmenopausal estrogen replacement and breast cancer', *New England Journal of Medicine*, 1989, 5, 321.

Barzel, U., 'Estrogens in the prevention and treatment of postmenopausal osteoporosis: A review', *American Journal of Medicine*, 1988, 85, 847–850.

Begley, S., and D. Glick, 'The Estrogen Complex', *Newsweek*, 21 March 1994.

Berkgvist, L., H.O. Adami, I. Persson, R. Hoover, C. Schairer, 'The risk of breast cancer after estrogen and estrogen-progestin replacement', *New England Journal of Medicine*, 1989, 5, 321, 293–297.

Biskind, M.S., 'The Effect of Vitamin B Complex Deficiency on the Inactivation of Estrone in the Liver', *Endocrinology*, 1942, vol. 31, 109–114.

Bloom, H., 'The influence of delay on the natural history and prognosis of breast cancer', *British Journal of Cancer*, 1965, 19, 228–262.

Borysenko, Joan, *Guilt is the Teacher: Love is the Lesson*, Warner Books, New York, 1991.

Botez, M.I., 'Neurologic Disorders Response to Folic Acid Therapy', *Canadian Medical Association Journal*, 1976, vol. 15, 217.

Boyd, N., 'Effect of a Low-Fat, High-Carbohydrate Diet on Symptoms of Clinical Mastopathy', *Lancet*, 1988, vol. 2, 128.

Brown, Ellen, and Lynne Walker, *Breezing Through The Change*, Frog Ltd, Berkeley, CA, USA, 1994.

Brown, R.R., et al., 'Correlation of serum retinol levels with response to chemotherapy in breast cancer', *American Journal of Obstetrics and Gynecology*, vol. 148, no. 3, 309–312.

Buell, P., 'Changing incidence of breast cancer in Japanese-American women', *Journal of the National Cancer Institute*, 1973, vol. 51, 1479–1483.

Bulbrook, P.D., M.C. Swain, and D.Y. Wang, et al., 'Breast Cancer in Britain and Japan: Plasma Oestradiol-17B Oestrone, and Progesterone, and their Urinary Metabolites in Normal British and Japanese Women', *European Journal of Cancer*, 1976, vol. 12, 725–735.

Carol, K.K., 'Dietary factors in immune-dependent cancers', in M. Winick, ed., *Current Concepts in Nutrition*, vol. 6, *Nutrition and Cancer*, John Wiley and Sons, New York, USA, 1977.

Colditz, G.A., et al., 'Prospective Study of Estrogen Replacement Therapy and Risk of Breast Cancer in Postmenopausal Women', *Journal of the American Medical Association*, 1990, vol. 264, 2648–252.

Colditz, G.A., et al., 'Type of postmenopausal hormone use and risk of breast cancer: 12 year follow-up from the Nurse's Health Study', *Cancer Causes and Control*, 1992, 3, 433–439.

Cowan, L.D., L. Gordis, et al., 'Breast cancer incidence in women with a history of progesterone deficiency', *American Journal of Epidemiology*, 1981, 114:209–217.

Cowley, G., et al., 'In pursuit of a terrible killer', *Newsweek*, 10 December 1990, 66–68.

Cramer, D.W., et al., 'Dietary Animal Fat and Relationship to Ovarian Cancer Risk', *Obstetrics and Gynecology*, 1984, vol. 63, no. 6, 833–838.

DHHS publication no. (PHS) 90-1101, 'Mortality', Part A, Washington D.C., U.S. Government Printing Office, 1990.

Dickinson, L.E., et al., 'Estrogen Profiles of Oriental and Caucasian Women in Hawaii', *New England Journal of Medicine*, 1974, vol. 291, 1211–1213.

Documenta Geigy, Scientific Tables, sixth edition, 493.

Facchinetti, F., et al., 'Oral magnesium successfully relieves premenstrual mood changes', *Obstetrics and Gynecology*, 1991, vol. 78, no. 2, 177–181.

Follingstad, Alvin, 'Estriol, The Forgotten Estrogen?', *Journal of the American Medical Association*, 1978, January 2, vol. 239, no. 1, 29–30.

Gambrell, R.D., 'The menopause: benefits and risks of estrogen-progestogen replacement therapy', *Fertility Sterility*, 1982, 37, 457–474.

Gambrell, R.D., 'Complications of Estrogen Replacement Therapy' in D.P. Swartz, ed., *Hormone Replacement Therapy*, Williams and Watkins, Baltimore, MD, U.S.A., 1992.

Goci, G.S., and G.E. Abraham, 'Effect of Nutritional Supplement . . . on Symptoms of Premenstrual Tension', *Journal of Reproductive Medicine*, 1982, vol. 83, 527–531.

Goldin, B., and J. Gorsback, 'The effect of milk and lactobacillus feeding on human intestinal bacterial enzyme activity', *American Journal of Clinical Nutrition*, 1984, vol. 39, 756–761.

Goodman, L., et al., *Pharmacological Basis of Therapeutics*, Macmillan Publishing Co., New York, USA, 1975.

Guyton, Arthur C., *Textbook of Medical Physiology*, Sixth Edition, W.B. Saunders Company, Philadelphia, USA, 1981.

Heimer, G.M., D.E. Englund, 'Effects of Vaginally-Administered Oestriol on Postmenopausal Urogenital Disorders: a Cytohormonal Study', *Maturitas*, 14 March 1992, vol. 3, 171–179.

Henderson, B.E., R.K. Ross, M.C. Pike, and J.T. Casagrande, 'Endogenous hormones as a major factor in human cancer', *Cancer Research*, 1982, 42, 3232–3239.

Hiatt, R.A., R. Bawol, G.D. Friedman, and R. Hoover, 'Exogenous estrogen and breast cancer after bilateral oopherectomy', *Cancer*, 1984, 54, 139–144.

Hileman, Bette, 'Environmental estrogens linked to reproductive abnormalities, cancer', *C&EN Washington*.

Hill, P., 'Diet, Lifestyle and Menstrual Activity', *American Journal of Clinical Nutrition*, 1980, vol. 33, 1192.

Hoeh, S.K., and K.K. Carroll, 'Effects of dietary carbohydrate in the incidence of mammary tumors induced in rats by 7, 12-dimethylbenzanthracene', *Nutrition and Cancer*, 1979, vol. 1, no. 3, 27–30.

Holl, M.H., et al., 'Gut bacteria and aetology of cancer of the breast', *Lancet*, 1971, vol. 2, 172–173.

Hoover, R., L.A. Gray Sr, P. Cole, and B. MacMahon, 'Menopausal estrogens and breast cancer' *New England Journal of Medicine*, 1976, 295, 401–405.

Hughes, R.E., 'Hypothesis: a new look at dietary fiber in human nutrition', *Clinical Nutrition*, 1986, vol. 406, 81–86.

Hunter, D.J., et al., 'A prospective study of the intake of vitamins C, E and A, and the risk of breast cancer', *New England Journal of Medicine*, 1993, July 22, vol. 324, no. 4, 234–240.

Huppert, L., 'Hormonal replacement therapy: Benefits, risks, doses', *Medical Clinics of North America*, 1987, 71, 23–39.

Ingram, D., 'Effect of Low-Fat Diet on Female Sex Hormone Levels', *Journal of National Cancer Institute*, 1987, vol. 79, 1225.

Iosif, C.S., 'Effects of Protracted Administration of Estriol on the Lower Urinary Tract in Postmenopausal Women', *Archives of Gynecology and Obstetrics*, 1992, vol. 3, no. 251, 115–120.

IpC, 'Dietary Vitamin E Intake and Mammary Carcinogenesis in Rats', *Carcinogenesis*, 1982, vol. 3, 1453–1456.

Journal of the National Cancer Institute, 'Author of Canadian breast cancer study retracts warnings', 3 June 1992, 84, 832–834.

Kato, I., et al., 'Alcohol consumption in cancers of hormone related organs in females', *Japan Journal of Clinical Oncology*, 1989, vol. 19, no. 3, 202–207.

Kellis, T.T., and L.E. Vickery, 'Inhibition of Human Estrogen Synthetase (Aromatase) by Flavonoids', *Science*, 1984, vol. 255, 1032–1034.

Kelly, M., 'Hypercholesterolemia: The cost of treatment in perspective', *Southern Medical Journal*, 1990, 83, 1421–1425.

Kinlen, L., 'Meat and fat consumption and cancer mortality: a study of strict religious orders in Britain', *The Lancet*, 1982, 946–949.

Kirkengen, A.L., P. Anderson, E. Gjersoe, G.R. Johannessen, N. Johnsen, and E. Bodd, 'Oestriol in the Prophylactic Treatment of Recurrent Urinary Tract Infection in Postmenopausal Women', *Scandinavian Journal Primary Health Care*, 10 June 1992, 139–142.

Kolata, G., 'Studies say Mammograms fail to help many women', *New York Times*, 26 February 1993.

Kolata, Gina, 'Breast cancer screening under 50: experts disagree if benefit exists', *New York Times*, 14 December 1993.

Kushi, M., *The Cancer Prevention Diet*, St Martin's Press, New York, 1983.

Landau, R.S., et al., 'The effect of alpha tocopherol in premenstrual symptomatology: a double-blind trial', *Journal of the American College of Nutrition*, 1983, vol. 2, 115–123.

La Vecchia, C., A. Decarli, F. Parazzini, A. Gentile, C. Liberati, S. Franceschi, 'Non-contraceptive oestrogens and the risk of breast cancer in women' *Int J Cancer*, 1986, 38, 853–858.

Lee, H.P., et al., 'Dietary effects on breast cancer risk in Singapore', *The Lancet*, 18 May 1991, vol 337, 1197–1200.

Lee, J.R., MD, 'Osteoporosis reversal; the role of progesterone', *International Clinical Nutritional Review*, Sydney, Australia, June, 1990.

Lee, J.R., MD, 'Is natural progesterone the missing link in osteoporosis prevention and treatment?, *Medical Hypotheses* 1991, 35, 316–318.

Lee, John R., MD, *Natural Progesterone*, BLL Publishing, California, USA, 1993.

Lee, J.R., MD, Endocrinology Notes: Progesterone and Estrogen. 6 February 1993.

Lee, J.R., MD, 'The Theory of Estrogen Dominance', Seminar given at St Thomas's Hospital, London, 4 June 1994.

Lee, J.R., MD, 'Dr John Lee speaking at the Chelsea Hotel, London, 5 June 1994', Video.

Lee, J.R. MD, *Optimal Health Guidelines*, Second Edition, BLL Publishing, California, USA, 1993.

Lemon, H.M., 'Oestiol and Prevention of Breast Cancer', *The Lancet*, 10 March 1973, vol. 1, no. 802, 546–547.

Lemon, H.M., 'Estriol Prevention of Mammary Carcinoma Induced by 7, 12-Dimethylbenzanthracene and Procarbazine', *Cancer Research*, 1975, vol. 35, 1341–1353.

Lemon, H.M., 'Clinical and Experimental Aspects of Anti-Mammary Carcinogenic Activity of Estriol', *Frontiers of Hormonal Research*, 1977, vol. 5, no. 1, 155–173.

Lemon, H.M., 'Pathophysiologic Considerations in the Treatment of Menopausal Patients with Oestrogens; The Role of Oestriol in the Prevention of Mammary Carcinoma', *Acta Endocrinologica*, 1980, vol. 233, 17–27

Lemon, H.M., H.H. Wotiz, L. Parsons, and P.J. Mozden, 'Reduced estriol excretion in patients with breast cancer prior to endocrine therapy', *Journal of the American Medical Association*, 1966, 196, 112–120.

Levy, J.A., et al., *Basic and Clinical Immunology*, 4th edn, Lange Medical Books, Los Angeles, CA, USA, 1982.

London, R.S., et al., 'Endocrine Parameters and Alpha-Tocopherol Therapy of Patients with Mammary Dysplasia', *Cancer Research*, 1981, vol. 41, 3811–3813.

Lubran, M., and G. Abraham, 'Serum and red cell magnesium levels in patients with Premenstrual Tension', *American Journal of Clinical Nutrition*, 1982, vol. 34, 2364.

McConnell, K.P., et al., 'The relationship between dietary selenium and breast cancer', *Journal of Surgical Oncology*, 1980, vol. 5, no. 1, 67–70.

McCormick, J., 'Cervical smears: A questionable practice?' *The Lancet*, 22 July 1989, 207–209.

McDougall, J., *McDougall's Medicine, A Challenging Second Opinion*, New Century Publishers, Piscastaway, NJ, USA, 1985.

McKenna, T., 'Pathogenesis and Treatment of Polycystic Ovary Syndrome', *New England Journal of Medicine*, 1988, vol. 318, 558.

MacMahon, B., et al., 'Urine Estrogen Profiles in Asian and North American Women', *International Journal of Cancer*, 1974, vol. 14, 161–167.

Medical Tribune, 'Sperm-count drop tied to pollution rise', 26 March 1992.

Medical Tribune, 'Late-cycle mastectomies may reduce recurrences', May 1992.

Michnovicz, J.,and H. Bradlow, 'Altered estrogen metabolism and excretion in humans following consumption of Indole-3-Carbinol', *Nutrition and Cancer*, 1991, vol. 16, 59–66.

Miller, A., et al., 'Canadian National Breast Screening Study: 1. Breast cancer detection and death rates among women aged 40–49 years', *Canadian Medical Association Journal*, 1992, 147, 1459–1476.

Moss, R., *The Cancer Industry: Unravelling the Politics*, Paragon House, New York, USA, 1989.

National Centre for Health Statistics, 'Vital statistics of the United States', 1987, vol. 2.

Nielson, M., et al., 'Breast cancer and atypia among young middle-aged women: a study of 110 medical-legal autopsies', *British Journal of Cancer*, 1987, vol. 56, 814–819.

Norris, Ronald, 'Progesterone for Premenstrual Tension', *Journal of Reproductive Medicine*, 1983, August, vol. 28, no. 8, 509–515.

Peat, R., PhD., 'Estrogen in 1990', *Blake College Newsletter*, 1990, Eugene, Oregon, USA.

Peat, R., PhD., 'Progesterone in Orthomolecular Medicine', Booklet.

Physicians' Desk Reference, Medical Economics Co., Oradell, New Jersey, USA, 1989.

Polson, D., 'Polycystic Ovaries – A Common Finding in Normal Women', *Lancet*, 1988, vol. 1, 870.

Poyduck, M.E., 'Inhibiting Effect of Vitamin C and B12 on the Mitotic Activity of Acites Tumors', *Experimental Cell Biology*, 1979, vol. 47, no. 3, 210–217.

Price, F., 'Theoretical Involvement of Vitamin B6 in Tumor Initiation', *Medical Hypothesis*, 1985, vol. 15, 421–428.

Punnonen, R., S. Vilsak, and L. Rauramo, 'Skinfold Thickness and Long-Term Postmenopausal Hormone Therapy', *Maturitas*, 5 April 1984, vol. 4, 259–262.

Raloff, J., 'Eco-Cancers, do environmental factors underlie a breast cancer epidemic?', *Science News*, 3 July 1993, 144, 10–13.

Raloff, J., 'The Gender-Benders' Part Two 'That Feminine Touch', *Science News*, 8 January 1994, and 22 February 1994.

Robin, E., MD, *Matters of Life and Death: Risks vs. Benefits of Medical Care*, W.H. Freeman & Co., New York, 1984.

Rose, D., 'Effect of a Low-Fat Diet on Hormone Levels in Women with Cystic Breast Disease, I: Serum Steroids and Gonadotropins', *Journal of the National Cancer Institute*, 1987, vol. 78, 623.

Rose, D., 'Effect of a Low-Fat Diet on Hormone Levels in Women with Cystic Breast Disease, II: Serum Radioimmunoassayable Prolactin and Growth Hormone and Bioactive Lactogenic Hormones,' *Journal of the National Cancer Institute*, 1987, vol. 78, 627.

Rosenberg, L., et al., 'Breast cancer and alcoholic beverage consumption', *The Lancet*, 1982, vol. 1, 267.

Rosenthal, Elisabeth, 'Cancer Surgeons Debate Timing of Breast Operations', *Health*, Wednesday 5 February 1992.

Rossignol, A.M., 'Caffeine-Containing Beverages and Premenstrual Syndrome in Young Women', *American Journal of Public Health*, 1985, vol. 75, no. 11, 1335–1337.

Sanchez, A., 'A Hypothesis on the Etiologic Role of Diet on the Age of Menarche', *Medical Hypotheses*, 1981, vol. 7, 1339.

Sattilaro, Anthony, and Tom Monte, *Living Well Naturally*, Houghton Mifflin, Boston, USA, 1984.

Schwartz, S., 'Dietary Influences on the Growth and Sexual Maturation in Premenarchal Rhesus Monkeys', *Hormones and Behavior*, 1988, vol. 22, 231.

Scott, J., 'Hormones may increase cancer risk, study says', *Los Angeles Times*, 2 August 1989, 1–15.

Seely, S., and D.F. Horrobin, 'Diet and breast cancer: the possible connection with sugar consumption', *Medical Hypotheses*, 1983, vol. 3, 319–327.

Sillero-Arenas, M., et al., 'Menopausal Hormone Replacement Therapy and Breast Cancer: A meta-Analysis', *Obstetrics and Gynecology*, 1992, February, vol. 79, no. 2, 286–293.

Skrabanek, P., 'False premises and false promises of breast cancer screening', *The Lancet*, 10 August 1985, 316–320.

Snowden, D.A., Letter to the Editor, *Journal of the American Medical Association*, 1985, vol. 3, no. 254.

Speroff, L., 'The Breast as an Endocrine Target Organ', *Contemporary Obstetrics and Gynecology*, 1977, vol. 9, 69–72.

Stadel, B.V., 'Oral contraceptives and cardiovascular disease', *New England Journal of Medicine*, 1981, 305, 612.

Stampfer, M., et al., 'A prospective study of postmenopausal estrogen therapy and coronary heart disease', *New England Journal of Medicine*, 313, 1044–1049.

Stryer, Lubert, *Biochemistry*, W.H. Freeman and Company, San Francisco, 1975.

Thomas, J. Hywel, and Brian Gillham, *Will's Biochemical Basis of Medicine*, Second Edition, Butterworth Heinemann Ltd, Oxford, 1992.

Tietz, Norbert, W. PhD., *Textbook of Clinical Chemistry*, W.B. Saunders Company, Philadelphia, USA, 1986.

Tzingounis, V.A., M.F. Aksu and R.B. Greenblatt, 'Estriol in the Management of the Menopause', *Journal of the American Medical Association*, 1978, vol. 239, 1638–1641.

van Haaften, M., G.H. Donker, A.A. Haspeis, and J.H. Thijssen, 'Oestrogen Concentrations in Plasma, Endometrium, Myometrium, and Vagina of Postmenopausal Women, and Effects of Vaginal Oestriol (E3) and Oestradiol (E2)

Applications', *Journal of Steroid Biochemistry*, 1989, vol. 4A, 647–653.

von Kaulla, F., et al., 'Conjugated oestrogens and hypercoagulability', *American Journal of Obstetrics and Gynecology*, 1975, 122, 688.

Wattenberg, L.W., 'Inhibition of neoplasia by minor dietary constituents', *Cancer Research* (supp), 1983, May, 43, 2448–2453.

Weiss, R., 'Estrogen in the environment', *Washington Post*, 25 January 1994, p. 10–13.

Welch, H. Gilbert, and William Black, 'Advances in Diagnostic Imaging', *New England Journal of Medicine*, 1993, April, vol. 328, 1237–1243.

Werbach, Melvyn R., *Nutritional Influences on Illness*, Second Edition, Third Line Press, California, 1987.

Willet, W., et al., 'Dietary fat and risk of breast cancer', *New England Journal of Medicine*, 1987, vol. 316, no. 22.

Williams, D.G., 'The Forgotten Hormone', *Alternatives*, 1991, vol. 4, no. 6, 11.

Woods, M., 'Low-Fat, High-Fiber Diet and Serum Estrone Sulfate in Premenopausal Women', *American Journal of Clinical Nutrition*, 1989, vol. 49, p. 1179.

Wotiz, H.H., D.R. Beebe, and E. Muller, 'Effect of Estrogens on DMBA-Induced Breast Tumors', *Journal of Steroid Biochemistry*, 1984, vol. 20, 1067–1075.

Wynder, E.L., et al., 'Diet and Breast Cancer. Causation and Therapy', *Gynecology and Obstetrics*, 1986, Springer-Verlag, 558–561.

Yang, C., et al., 'Noncontraceptive hormone use and risk of breast cancer', *Cancer Causes and Control*, 1992, 3, 475–479.

Yuesheng, Z., et al., 'A major inducer of anticarcinogenic protective enzymes from broccoli: isolation and elucidation of structure', *Proc. Natl. Acad. Sci.*, 1992, 89, 2399–2403.

Zussman, L., et al., 'Sexual response after hysterectomy-oopherectomy: Recent studies and reconsideration of psychogenesis', *American Journal of Obstetrics and Gynecology*, 1981, 140, 725–729.

Chapter Eight: Gremlins in the Architecture (and Chapter Twenty-two: Angels in the Architecture)

Abraham, G.E., 'The Importance of Magnesium in the Management of Primary Postmenopausal Osteoporosis', *The Journal of Nutritional Medicine*, 1991, 2, 165–178

Abraham, G.E., and Harinder Grewal, 'A Total Dietary Program Emphasizing Magnesium Instead of Calcium', *Journal of Reproductive Medicine*, 1990, May, vol. 35, no. 5, 503–507.

Aihara, Herman, *Acid and Alkaline*, George Ohsawa Macrobiotic Foundation, Oroville, CA, USA, 1980.

Aitken, M., D.M. Hart, and R. Lindsay, 'Oestrogen replacement therapy for prevention of osteoporosis after oopherectomy', *British Medical Journal*, 1973, 3, 515–518.

Albanes, A.A., et al., *Nutr Rep Internat*, 1985, 1093–1115.

Albright, F., et al., 'Postmenopausal osteoporosis: its clinical features', *JAMA*, 1941, 116, 2465–2474.

Allen, L.H., 'Protein-induced hypercalcuria: A longer term study', *American Journal of Clinical Nutrition*, 1974, 32, 741.

American Journal of Medicine, 1969, 46, 197.

Anand, C., and H.M. Linkswiler, 'Effect of protein intake on calcium balance of young men given 500mg calcium daily', *J. Nutr*, 1974, 104, 695.

Avioli, L.V., 'Rationale for the use of cacitonin in postmenopausal osteoporosis', *Annale Chirugiae et Gynaecologiae*, 1988, 77, 224.

Bain, C., W. Willet, C.H. Hennekens, et al., 'Use of Postmenopausal Hormones and Risk of Myocardial Infarction', *Circulation*, 1981, 64, 42–46.

Barzel, U.S., 'Estrogens in the prevention and treatment of postmenopausal osteoporosis: a review', *American Journal of Medicine*, 1988, 85, 847–850.

Berkgvist, L., H.O. Adami, I. Persson, R. Hoover, and C. Schairer, 'The risk of breast cancer after estrogen and estrogen-progestin replacement', *New England Journal of Medicine*, 1989, 5, 321.

Block, G.D., et al., *American Journal of Clinical Nutrition*, 1980, 33, 2128–2136.

Briscoe, A.M., and C. Ragan, *American Journal of Clinical Nutrition*, 1966, 19, 296.

British Medical Journal, 1984, 289, 1103.

Brockis, J.G., A.S. Levitt, and S.M. Cruthers, 'The effects of vegetable and animal protein diets on calcium, urate and oxalate excretion', *British Journal of Urology*, 1982, 54, 590.

Bryce-Smith, Professor D., 'Boron: A Candidate for Essentiality', *Green Library Offprint*, Green Library Ltd, Surrey, No. 46.

Carlisle, E.M., 'Silicon as an Essential Trace Element in Animal Nutrition', *Ciba Foundation Symposium*, 1986, 121, 123.

Cecil's Textbook of Medicine, 18th Edition, 1988, p. 1514.

Cohen, L., A. Laor, and R. Kitzes, 'Bone Magnesium Crystallinity Index and State of Body Magnesium in Subjects with Senile Osteoporosis, Maturity-onset Diabetes and Women Treated with Contraceptive Preparations', *Magnesium,* 1983, 2, 70–75.

Christiansen, C., M.S. Christiansen, and I. Transbol, 'Bone mass in postmenopausal women after withdrawal of oestrogen/progestogen replacement therapy', *The Lancet,* 28 February 1981, 459–461.

Christiansen, C., B.J. Riis, L. Nilas, P. Rodbro, and L. Deftos, 'Uncoupling of bone formation and resorption by combined oestrogen and progestogen therapy in postmenopausal osteoporosis', *The Lancet,* October 1985, 800–801.

Coats, C., 'Negative effects of a high-protein diet', Family Practice Recertification, 1990, 12, 80–88.

Coney, Sandra, *The Menopause Industry',* Penguin Books, London, 1991.

Cooper, C., C.A.C. Wickham, D.J.R. Barker, and S.J. Jacobsen, 'Water fluoridation and hip fracture', *JAMA* 1991, 266, 513–514.

Cowan, L.D., L. Gordis, et al., 'Breast cancer incidence in women with a history of progesterone deficiency', *American Journal of Epidemiology,* 1981, 114:209–217.

Cramer, D.W., et al., *American Journal of Epidemiology,* 1994, 139, 282–289.

Crane, Milton G., 'The Use of Progpesterone and/or an Estrogen in Osteoporosis', Unpublished, available from Weimar Institute, Weimar, CA 95736.

Cummings, S.R., 'Are Patients with Hip Fractures More Osteoporotic?', *American Journal of Medicine,* 1985, 78, 487.

Cummings, S.R., et al., 'Epidemiology of Osteoporosis and Osteoporotic Fractures', *Epidemiology Reviews,* 1985, 7, 178.

Cundy, T., M. Evans, H. Roberts, et al., 'Bone density in women receiving depo-medrosyprogesterone acetate for contraception', *British Medical Journal,* 1991, 303, 13–16.

Danielson, C., J.L. Lyon, M. Eger, and G.K. Goodenough, 'Hip fractures and fluoridation in Utah's elderly population', *JAMA,* 1992, 268, 746–747.

DeLuca, H.F., *Vitamin D: Metabolism and Function,* Springer-Verlag, New York, USA, 1979.

DeLuca, H.F., 'The Latest Information on Vitamin D and Bone Status', *Complementary Medicine*, May/June 1986, 14.

Donaldson, C.L., et al., *Metabolism*, 1970, 19, 1071–1084.

Doppelt, S., *Harvard Medical School Newsletter*, 3–4 November, 1981.

Dudl, R.J., et al., 'Evaluation of Intravenous Calcium as Therapy for Osteoporosis', *American Journal of Medicine*, 1973, 55, 631.

Dyckner, T., and P.O. Wester, 'Effect of Magnesium on Blood Pressure', *British Medical Journal*, 1983, 286, 1847.

Edgren, R.A., 'Progestogens', reprinted from *Clinical Use of Sex Steroids*, Year Book Medical Publishers, Inc. USA, 1980.

Ellis, F.R., S. Holesh, and J.W. Ellis, 'Incidence of osteoporosis in vegetarians and omnivores', *Am Clin Nutr*, 1972, 25, 555.

Ettinger, B., H.K. Genant, and C.E. Cann, 'Long-term estrogen replacement therapy prevents bone loss and fractures', *Ann Intern Med*, 1985, 102, 319–324.

Francis, R.M., and D.M. Beaumont, letters to the editor, 'Involutional Osteoporosis', *New England Journal of Medicine*, 1987, 316, 216.

Fisken, R.A., 'Osteoporosis: A Clinical Guide. Review of Books', *The Lancet*, 1988, 2, 996.

Friedman, G.L., 'Diet in the Treatment of Diabetes', in *Modern Nutrition in Health and Disease*, (eds) R.S. Goodhart and M.E. Shils, 6th edition, Lea and Febiger, Philadelphia, USA, 1980.

Gaby, A.R., *Preventing and Reversing Osteoporosis*, Prima Publications, Rocklin, CA, USA, 1994.

Gaby, A.R., and J.V. Wright, 'Nutrients and bone health', *JAMA*, 1988, 4, 2–6.

Gambrell, R.D., 'The Menopause: Benefits and Risks of Estrogen-progestogen Replacement Therapy', *Fertility Sterility*, 1982, 37, 457–474.

Gambrell, R.D., C.A. Bagnell, and R.B. Greenblatt, 'Role of estrogens and progesterone in the etiology and prevention of endometrial cancer. Review', *American Journal of Obstetrics and Gynecology*, 1983, 146, 696–707.

Gambrell, R.D., R.C., and Maier, S.L., 'Decreased Incidence of Breast Cancer in Postmenopausal Estrogen-progestogen Users', *Obstetrics and Gynecology*, 1983, 62, 435–443.

Genant, H.K., G.S. Gordon, and P.G. Hoffman Jr, 'Osteoporosis: Part II, Prevention of bone loss and fracture in women and risks of menopausal estrogen therapy', Medical Staff Conference, U. of Cal. SF. *West J Med*, 1983, 139, 204–211.

Gonzalez, E.R., *Journal of the American Medical Association*, 1980, 243, 309–316.

Goulding, A., *New Zealand Medical Journal*, 1990, 103, 120.

Gordon, G.S., J. Picchi, and B.S. Roots, 'Antifracture efficacy of long-term estrongens for osteoporosis', *Trans Assoc Am Physicians*, 1973, 86, 326–332.

Guyton, Arthur C., *Textbook of Medical Physiology*, Sixth Edition, W.B. Saunders Company, Philadelphia, USA, 1981.

Halioua, L., and J.J.B. Anderson, 'Lifetime Calcium Intake and Physical Activity Habits: Independent and Combined Effects on the Radial Bone of Healthy Premenopausal Caucasian Women', *American Journal of Clinical Nutrition*, 1989, 49, 534.

Hall, F.M., M.A. Davis, and D.T. Baran, 'Sounding Board: Bone Mineral Screening for Osteoporosis', *New England Journal of Medicine*, 1987, 316, 212.

Hammond, C.B., F.R. Jelvsek, K.L. Lee, W.T. Creasman, and R.T. Parker, 'Effects of long-term estrogen replacement therapy. I Metabolic effects', *American Journal of Obstetrics and Gynecology*, 1979, 133, 525–536.

Hargrove, Joel T., et al., 'Menopausal hormone replacement therapy with continuous daily oral micronized estradiol and progesterone', *Obstetrics and Gynaecology*, 1989, 73, 606–612.

Hargrove, Joel T., et al., 'Progesterone: Safe Antidote for PMS', *McCalls*, October 1990.

Harrison's Principles of Internal Medicine, 12th Edition, 1991, p. 1925.

Harvard Medical School Health Letter, 1976, March.

Heaney, R., et al., *American Journal of Clinical Nutrition*, 1986, 43, 299.

Hedlund, L.R., and J.C. Gallagher, 'Increased incidence of hip fracture in osteoporitic women treated with sodium fluoride', *J Bone Miner Res*, 1989, 4, 223–225.

Hegsted, M., S.A. Schuette, M.B. Zemel, et al., 'Urinary calcium and calcium balance in young men as affected by level of protein and phosphoros intake', *J Nutr*, 1981, 111, 553.

Holl, M.G., and L.H. Allen, 'Comparative Effects of Meals High in Protein, Sucrose, or Starch on Human Mineral Metabolism and Insulin Secretion', *American Journal of Clinical Nutrition*, 1988, 48, 1219.

Holst, J., S. Cajander, and B. von Shoultz, 'Endometrial effects of a continuous percutaneous estrogen/low dose progestogen regimen for climacteric complaints', *Maturitas*, 1987, 9, 63–67.

Hudleston, A.L., et al., *Journal of the American Medical Association*, 1980, 244, 1107–1109.

Human Nutrition Information Service, C.S.F. II, 'Nationwide Food Consumption Survey Continuing Survey of Food Intakes by Individuals', 85–81, Washington, D.C., US Department of Agriculture, 1985.

Hutchinson, T.A., S.M. Polansky, and A.R. Feinstein, 'Postmenopausal oestrogens protect against fractures of hip and distal radius: a case control study', *The Lancet*, 1979, II, 705–709.

Jacobsen, S.L., et al., *JAMA*, 1990, 264, 500–502.

Johansen, J.S., S.B. Jensen, B.J. Riis, et al., 'Bone formation is stimulated by combined estrogen, progestogen', *Metabolism*, 1990, 39, 1122–1126.

Johnston, F.A., et al., *Journal of American Dietary Association*, 1952, 28, 933–938.

Journal of the American Medical Association 'National Institutes of Health, Consensus Conference: Osteoporosis', 1984, 252, 799.

Kabayashi, A., et al., *American Journal of Clinical Nutrition*, 1975, 28, 681–683.

Kamen, Betty, *Startling New Facts About Osteoporosis*, Nutrition Encounter Inc., California, USA, 1989.

Kleerekoper, M.E., E. Petersen,E. Phillips, D. Nelson, et al., 'Continuous sodium fluoride therapy does not reduce vertebral fracture rate in postmenopausal osteoporosis', *J Bone Miner Res*, 1989, Res. 4 (Suppl. 1), S376.

Kilner, B., and Pors Nielsen, S. *Clinical Science*, 1982, 62, 329–336.

Lane, N., et al., *Med Sci Sport Exer*, 1988, 20, suppl. 51.

Lee, J.R., MD, 'Understanding Osteoporosis'. Summary.

Lee, J.R., MD, 'Osteoporosis reversal; the role of progesterone', *International Clinical Nutritional Review*, Sydney, Australia, June 1990.

Lee, J.R., MD, 'Osteoporosis reversal with transdermal progesterone', *The Lancet*, November 1990, Letter 336.

Lee, J.R., MD, 'Is natural progesterone the missing link in osteoporosis prevention and treatment?' *Medical Hypotheses*, 1991, 35, 314, 318.

Lee, J.R., MD, 'Hormonal and nutritional aspects of osteoporosis', *Health and Nutrition*, 1991, Winter, Vol 6, Issue 4.

Lee, J.R., MD, *Natural Progesterone*, BLL Publishing, California, USA, 1993.

Lee, J.R., MD, *Optimal Health Guidelines*, Second Edition, BLL Publishing, California, USA, 1993.

Lee, J.R., MD, 'Dr John Lee speaking at the Chelsea Hotel, London, 5 June 1994', Video.

Lee, J.R., MD, 'Effects of Progesterone on Osteoporosis and Menopausal Symptoms', Seminar given at St Thomas's Hospital, London, 4 June 1994.

Lee, J.R., MD, 'The Multiple Effects of Progesterone', Seminar given at St Thomas's Hospital, London, 4 June 1994.

Lee, J.R., MD, 'Successful Menopausal Osteoporosis Treatment Restoring Osteoclast/Osteoblast Equilibrium', *The Townsend Letter for Doctors*, 1994, August/September, 900.

Lees, B., and J.C. Stevenson, 'An evaluation of dual-energy X-ray absorptiometry,' *Osteoporosis Int*, 1992, 2, 146–52.

Lees, B., T. Molleson, T.R. Arnett, and J.C. Stevenson, 'Differences in proximal femur bone density over two centuries', *The Lancet*, 1993, 341:673–675.

Leichsenring, J.M., et al., *Journal of Nutrition*, 1957, 63, 425–435.

Lindsay, R., D.M. Hart, C. Forrest, and C. Baird, 'Prevention of spinal osteoporosis in oopherectomized women', *The Lancet*, 1980, II, 1151–1154.

Lindsay, R., D.M. Hart, D. Purdie, M.M. Ferguson, A.S. Clark, and A. Karaszewski, 'Comparative effects of oestrogen and a progestogen on bone loss in postmenopausal women', *Clin Sc & Mol Med*, 1978, 54, 193–195.

Linksilver, H.M., et al., *Trans NY Acad Sci*, 1974, 36, 333.

Lufkin, E.G., et al., 'Treatment of postmenopausal osteoporosis with transdermal oestrogen', *Annals of Int Med*, 1992, July, 117, 1–9.

McDougall, *McDougall's Medicine, A Challenging Second Opinion*, New Century Publishers, Piscataway, NJ, USA, 1985.

MacIntyre, I., M.I. Whitehead, L.M. Banks, et al., 'Calcitonin for prevention of postmenopausal bone loss,' *The Lancet*, 1988, 1, 900.

Margen, S., et al., *American Journal of Clinical Nutrition*, 1974, 27, 584.

Marsh, A.G., et al., 'Vegetarian Lifestyle and Bone Mineral Density', *American Journal of Medicine*, 1987, 82, 73.

Mazess, R.B., 'On aging bone loss', *Clin Orthop*, 1982, 165, 239–252.

Mazess, R.B., H.S. Barden, M. Ettinger, and E. Schultz, 'Bone Density of the radius, spine and proximal femur in osteoporosis', *J Bone Min Res*, 1988, 3, 13–18.

Monte, T., *New Age Journal*, 1991, September/October, 25.

Munk-Jensen, N., S.P. Nielsen, E.B. Obel, and P.B. Eriksen, 'Reversal of postmenopausal vertebral bone loss by oestrogen and progestogen: a double-blind placebo-controlled study', *British Medical Journal*, 1988, 296, 1150–1152.

National Osteoporosis Foundation, *Medications and Bone Loss*, Washington DC, USA, 1994.

National Osteoporosis Society, *Osteoporosis, A Decision-Making Document for Diagnosis and Prevention*, PO Box 10, Radstock, Bath, BA3 3YB.

National Osteoporosis Society, *Osteoporosis, A Guide to its Causes, Treatment and Prevention*, Number 1 in a series of Information Booklets, PO Box 10, Radstock, Bath, BA3 3YB, January 1993.

National Research Council, *Recommended Dietary Allowances*, 10th edition, National Academy Press, Washington DC, 1989.

Nielsen, F.H., et al., *Trace Element Research*, 1990, 9, 61.

Nilas, L., et al., *British Medical Journal*, 1984, 289, 1103–1106.

O'Mally, B.W., 'Progesterone: Mechanism of Action', in *Metabolic effects of gonadal hormones and contraceptive steroids*, H.A. Salhanick, D.M. Kipnis, R.L. Vande Wiele, Plenum Press, New York, 1969.

Oski, Frank A., *Don't Drink Your Milk!* 9th edition, Teach Services, Brushton, New York, USA, 1989.

Osteoporosis, *Yoga Journal*, 1988, March/April, 44.

Ott, P., 'Should Women Get Screening Bone Mass Measurements?', *Annals of Internal Medicine*, 1986, 104, 874.

Pak, C.Y.C., 'Nutrition and Metabolic Bone Disease' in *Nutritional Diseases: Research Directions in Comparative Pathobiology*, Alan R. Liss, New York, 1986.

Peat, R., PhD., 'Progesterone in Orthomolecular Medicine', Blake College Booklet, Eugene, Oregon. Available from Foundation for Hormonal and Nutrition Research, 8150, SW Barnes Road, Portland, OR 97225, USA.

Peat, R.F., *Nutrition for Women*, Blake College Publishers, Eugene, Oregon, USA, 1978.

Pfeiffer, C.C., *Mental and Elemental Nutrients: A Physician's Guide to Nutrition and Health Care*, Keats Publishing, New Canaan, 1975.

Pizzorno, Joseph E., and Michael T. Murray, *A Textbook of Natural Medicine,* John Bastyr College Publications, Seattle, Washington, 1985.

Prior, J.C., 'Progesterone as a bone-trophic hormone', *Endocrine Review:* 1990, 11:386-398.

Prior, J.C., 'Spinal bone loss and ovulatory disturbances', *New England Journal of Medicine,* 1990, 323, 18.

Prior, J.C., 'Progesterone and its relevance for osteoporosis', *Bulletin for Physicians,* 1993, March, vol. 2, no. 2.

Prior, J.C., Y. Vigna, and R.N. Alojado, 'Progesterone and the prevention of osteoporosis', *Canadian Journal of Obstetrics/Gynecology & Women's Health Care,* 1991, 3, 4.

Prior, J.C., Y. Vigna, and R. Burgess, 'Medroxyprogesterone increases trabecular bone density in women with menstrual disorders', University of British Columbia, Vancouver. Paper presented at annual meeting of the Endocrine Society, 11 June, 1987, Indianapolis, IN, USA.

Rambaut, P.C., A.W. Goode, *The Lancet,* 1985, 2, 1050–1052.

Recker, R.R., *New England Journal of Medicine,* 1985, 313, 70.

Riggs, B.L., H.W. Wahner, L.J. Melton, L.S. Richelson, H.L. Judd, and W.M. O'Fallon, 'Dietary calcium intake and rate of bone loss in women', *Journal of Clinical Investigation,* 1987, 80, 979–982.

Riggs, B.L., et al., 'Effect of Fluoride Treatment on the Fracture Rate in Postmenopausal Women with Osteoporosis', *New England Journal of Medicine,* 1990, 322, 802–809.

Riis, B.R., et al., 'Does calcium supplementation prevent postmenopausal bone loss?' *New England Journal of Medicine,* 1987, 316, 173–177.

Rowe, J.W., and R.D. Kahn, *Science,* 1987, 237, 143.

Rudy, D.R., 'Hormone replacement therapy', *Postgraduate Medicine,* 1990, Dec, 157–164.

Scientific American Medicine, updated, chapter 15, section X, p. 9.

Saltman, P., et al., *Journal of Nutrition,* 1986, 116, 134.

Shapiro, J.R., et al., *Aren Intern Med,* 1975, 135, 563–567.

Sheikh, M.S., et al., 'Gastrointestinal Absorption of Calcium from Milk and Calcium Salts', *New England Journal of Medicine,* 1987, 317, 532.

Smith, D.C., R. Prentice, D.J. Thompson, and W.L. Hermann, 'Association of exogenous estrogen and endometrial carcinoma', *New England Journal of Medicine,* 1975, 293, 1164–1167.

Smith, E.L., et al., *Calcified Tissue International*, 1984, 36, Suppl. 129.

Smith, E.L., and C. Gilligan, *Physician Sportsmed*, 1987, 15, 91–100.

Sowers, M.F.R., M.K. Clark, M.L. Jannausch, and R.B. Wallace, 'A prospective study of bone mineral content and fracture in communities with differential fluoride exposure', *Am J Epidemiol*, 1991, 134, 649–660.

Spencer, H., et al., *American Journal of Clinical Nutrition*, 1978, 31, 2167.

Spencer, H., et al., *American Journal of Clinical Nutrition*, 1982, 36, 32.

Spencer, H., et al., *Arch Intern Med*, 1983, 143, 657.

Spencer, H., et al., *Clinical Orthopaedics*, 1984, 184, 270.

Stepan, J.J., et al., 'Castrated men exhibit bone loss: effect of calcitonin treatment on biochemical indices of bone remodeling,' *J Clin Endocrinal Metab*, 1989, 69, 523–527.

Stevenson, J.C., B. Lees, M. Davenport, M.P. Cust, and K.F. Gangar, 'Determinants of bone density in normal women: risk factors for future osteoporosis', *British Medical Journal*, 1989, 298, 924–928.

Stevenson, J.C., 'Dietary Calcium and Hip Fracture', *The Lancet*, 1988, 1318.

Stevenson, J.C., P.C. Michael, F.G. Gangar, T.C. Hillard, B. Lees, and M.I. Whitehead, 'Effects of transdermal versus oral hormone replacement therapy on bone density in spine and proximal femur in postmenopausal women', *The Lancet*, Vol. 336, 2265–2269.

Stevenson, J.C., M.I. Whitehead, M. Padwick, et al., 'Dietary intake of calcium and post-menopausal bone loss,' *British Medical Journal*, 1988, 297, 15–17.

Stryer, Lubert, *Biochemistry*, W.H. Freeman and Company, San Francisco, USA, 1975.

Thorne Research Inc, 'Osteoporosis: Calcium and Beyond', *Capsulations*, 1990.

Tietz, Norbert W., PhD., *Textbook of Clinical Chemistry*, W.B. Saunders Company, Philadelphia, USA, 1986.

Underwood, E., *Trace Elements in Human and Animal Nutrition*, 4th edition, Academic Press, New York, 1977.

Vikkanski, L., 'Magnesium May Slow Bone Loss', *Medical Tribune*, 1993, July 22, 9.

Virvidakis, K., et al., *International Journal of Sports Medicine*, 1990, 11, 244–246.

Watts, N.B., T.H. Steven, H.K. Genant, et al., 'Intermittent cyclical etidronate treatment of postmenopausal osteoporosis,' *New England Journal of Medicine*, 1990, 323, 73–79.

Weiss, N.S., C.L. Ure, J.H. Ballard, A.R. Williams, and J.R. Darling, 'Decreased risk of fracture of hip and lower forearm and post-menopausal use of estrogen', *New England Journal of Medicine*, 1980, 303, 1195–1198.

Whitaker, Dr Julian, 'Your Program for Healthy Bones', *Health and Healing*, 1994, January, Vol. 4, No 1, 4–8.

Will's Biochemical Basis of Medicine, 1989, ch. 22, p. 258.

Yoshioka, T., B. Sato, K. Matsumoto, and K. Oso, 'Steroid receptors in osteoblasts,' *Clin Orthop*, 1980, 148, 297–303.

Zetterberg, C., and G.B.J. Andersson, 'Fractures of the proximal end of the femur in Goteberg, Sweden, 1940–1979', *Acta Orthopaed Scand*, 1980, 54, 681–686.

Ziel, H.K., and W.D. Finkle, 'Increased risk of endometrial carcinoma among users of conjugated estrogens', *New England Journal of Medicine*, 1975, 293, 1167–1170.

Chapter Nine: Phoenix in the Fire

Beyene, Y., 'Cultural significance and physiological manifestations of menopause: a biocultural analysis', *Cult. Med. Psychiatry*, 1986, 10:47–71.

Burrows, Harold, *Biological Actions of Sex Hormones*, 2nd edition, 1949, Cambridge University Press.

Coney, Sandra, *The Menopause Industry*, Penguin Books, London, 1991.

Cooper, J.C., *An Illustrated Encyclopaedia of Traditional Symbols*, Thames and Hudson Ltd, London, 1982.

DeFazio, J., D.R. Meldrum, J.H. Winer, and H.L. Judd, 'Direct action of androgen on hot flushes in the human male', *Maturitas*, 1984, 6:3–8.

Erlik, Y., D.R. Meldrum, and H.L. Judd, 'Estrogen levels in postmenopausal women with hot flushes', *Obstet Gynecol*, 1982, 59:403–407.

Feldman, G.M., A. Voda, and E. Gronseth, 'The prevalence of hot flushes and associated variables among perimenopausal women', *Res. Nurs. Hlth*, 1985, 8:261–268.

Feldman, J.M., R.W. Postlethwaite, and J.F. Glenn, 'Hot flashes and sweats in men with testicular insufficiency', *Arch. Intern. Med.*, 136:606–608.

Ginsburg, J., J. Swinhoe and B. O'Reilly, 'Cardiovascular responses during the menopausal hot flush', *Br. J. Obstet. Gynaecol,* 1981, 88:925–930.

Grant, Dr Ellen, *Sexual Chemistry, Understanding Our Hormones, The Pill and HRT,* Cedar Original, Mandarin Paperbacks, London, 1994.

Greenwood, Dr Sadja, *Menopause The Natural Way,* Macdonald & Co., London, 1987.

Hudson, Tori, *Gynecology and Naturopathic Medicine,* TK Publications, Oregon, 1992.

Kaufert, Pat, 'Anthropology and the menopause: the development of a theoretical framework', *Maturitas,* 1982, 4, 181–193.

Kronenberg, F., 'Hot flashes: Epidemiology and Physiology', *Annals of New York Academy of Sciences,* 1990, Vol. 592.

Kronenberg, F., and J.A. Downey, 'Thermoregulatory physiology of menopauseal hot flashes: A review', *Canadian Journal of Physiology and Pharmacology,* 1987, 65:1312–1324.

Lark, Susan, M., *The Menopause Self Help Book,* Celestial Arts, California, 1990.

Linde, R., G.C. Doelle, N. Alexander, R. Kirchner, W. Vale, J. Rivier, and D. Rabin, 'Reversible inhibition of testicular steroidogenesis and spermatogenesis by a potent gonadotropin-releasing hormone agonist in normal men', *New England Journal of Medicine,* 1981, 305:663–667.

Lock, M., 'Ambiguities of aging: Japanese experience and perceptions of menopause', *Cult. Med. Psychiatry,* 1986, 10:23–46.

Montreal Health Press, *Menopause, A Well Woman Book,* Second Story Press, Canada, 1990.

Reitz, Rosetta, *Menopause A Positive Approach,* Unwin Paperbacks, London, 1985.

Sherman, B.M., R.B. Wallace, J.A. Bean, Y. Chang, and L. Schlabaugh, 'The relationship of menopausal hot flashes to medical and reproductive experience', *J. Gerontol,* 1981, 36:306–309.

Steinfeld, A.D., and C. Reinhardt, 'Male climacteric after orchiectomy in patient with prostatic cancer', *Urology,* 1980, 16:620–622.

Steingold, K.A., M. Cedars, J.K.H. Lu, D. Randle, H.L. Judd, and D.R. Meldrum, 'Treatment of endometriosis with a long-acting gonadotropin-releasing hormone agonist', *Obstet. Gynecol.*, 1987, 69:403–411.

Studd, John, and Rob Barber, 'Mastering the Menopause', Leaflet presented with the compliments of Organon Laboratories Ltd, Cambridge, UK, 1994.

Utian, W.H., 'The true clinical features of postmenopause and oophorectomy, and their responses to estrogen therapy,' *South African Medical Journal*, 1972, 46:732–737.

Walker, Barbara, G., *The Woman's Encyclopedia of Myths and Secrets*, Harper & Row, San Francisco, 1983.

Chapter Ten: Double Indemnity (and Chapter Twenty-five: Field and Forest)

American Journal of Clinical Nutrition, 1994, 60, 333–340.

Bavalve, R., et al., 'Vegetables inhibit in vivo the mutagenicity of nitrite combined with nitrosable compounds', *Mutation Research*, 1983, vol. 120, 145.

Business Week, 'Breast cancer and PCB's: A Possible Link', 1992, April 6, 36.

Cramer, D.W., et al., 'Dietary animal fat and relationship to ovarian cancer risk', *Obstetrics and Gynecology*, 1984, vol. 63, 6, 833–838.

Dickinson, L.E., et al., 'Estrogen profiles of oriental and caucasian women in Hawaii', *New England Journal of Medicine*, 1974, 291, 1211–1213.

Frenkel, K., K. Chrzan, C.A. Ryan, R. Wiesner, W. Troll, 'Chymotrypsin-specific protease inhibitors decrease H_2O_2 formation by activated human polymorphonuclear leukocytes', *Carcinogenesis*, 1987, 8, 1207–1212.

Goldin, B., et al., 'Estrogen excretion patterns and plasma levels in vegetarian and omnivorous women', *New England Journal of Medicine*, 1982, 307, 1542–1547.

Hayhow, S., and M. Messina, 'The Soy Solution', *Vegetarian Times*, 1994, March, 77-84.

Hudson, Tori, et al., 'A Pilot Study using Botanical Medicines in the Treatment of Menopause Symptoms', *Townsend Letter for Doctors*, 1994, December, 1372.

Khaw, K.T., (ed.), *Hormone Replacement Therapy*, Churchill Livingstein, London, 1992.

McDougall, J., 'Balancing the estrogen issue', *Vegetarian Times*, 1986, August, 44.

McIntyre, Anne, *The Complete Woman's Herbal*, Gaia Books Limited, London, 1994.

Mckenna, T., 'Pathogenesis and treatment of polycystic ovary syndrome', *New England Journal of Medicine*, 1988, vol. 318, 558.

MacMahan, B., et al., 'Urine estrogen profiles in Asian and North American women', *International Journal of Cancer*, 1974, 14, 161–167.

Messina, M., V. Messina, K. Setchell, *The Simple Soybean and Your Health*, Avery Publishing Group, New York, 1994.

Nakashima, H., et al., 'Inhibitory effect of glycosides like saponin from soybean on the infectivity of HIV in vitro', *AIDS*, 1989, 3, 655–658.

Pizzorno, Joseph E., and Michael T. Murray, *A Textbook of Natural Medicine*, John Bastyr College Publications, Seattle, Washington, 1985.

Ridout, C.L., et al., 'UK mean daily intakes of saponins – intestine permeabilizing factors in legumes', *Food Science & Nutrition*, 1988, 42, 111–116.

Schneider, J., et al., 'Effects of obesity on estradiol metabolism: Decreased formation of nonuterotropic metabolites', *Obstetrical and Gynecological Survey*, 1980, 38 (10), 616.

Shaffer, Willa, *Midwifery and Herbs*, Woodland Books, Utah, USA, 1986.

Shaffer, Willa, *Wild Yam, Birth Control Without Fear*, Woodland Books, Utah, USA, 1986.

Shutt, D.A. and R.I. Cox, 'Steroid and phytoestrogen binding to sheep uterine receptors in vitro', *Journal of Endocrinology*, 1972, 52, 299–310.

Snowden, D.A., letter to the editor, *Journal of the American Medical Association*, 1985, vol. 3, no 254, 356–357.

Theroux, Paul, 'Under the Spell of the Trobriand Islands', *National Geographic*, 1992, July.

U.S. Academy of Sciences, *Diet Nutrition and Cancer*, National Academy Press, Washington DC, USA, 1982.

Vines, Gail, 'Twilight Zone's New Dawn', *The Guardian*, 23 Sept. 1993.

Vines, Gail, 'The Challenge to HRT', *New Scientist*, 23 October 1993.

Walker, Morton, 'Soybean Isoflavones Lower Risks of Degenerative Diseases', *Townsend Letter for Doctors*, 1994, August/September, 874.

Weed, H.G., et al, 'Protection against dimethylhydrazine-induced adenomatous tumours of the mouse colon by the dietary addition of an extract of soybeans containing the Bowman-Birk protease inhibitor', *Carcinogenesis*, 1985, 6, 1239–1241.

Weed, Susun, S., *Menopausal Years, The Wise Woman Way*, Ash Tree Publishing, New York, 1992.

Wilcox, G., et al., 'Oestrogenic effects of plant foods in post-menopausal women', *British Medical Journal*, 1990, 301 (6757), 905–906.

Williams, D., 'The forgotten hormone', *Alternatives for the Health Conscious Individual*, 1991, Vol. 4 (6) 41–46.

Witschi, H., and A.R. Kennedy, 'Modulation of lung tumour development in mice with the soybean-derived Bowman-Birk protease inhibitor', *Carcinogenesis*, 1989, 10, 2275–2277.

Chapter Eleven: Order out of Chaos
(and Chapter Twenty-seven: Seeds of Change)

Abraham, G., 'Nutritional factors in the etiology of premenstrual tension syndromes', *Journal of Reproductive Medicine*, 1983, 28, 446–464.

Belleme, John, and Jan Belleme, *Culinary Treasures of Japan*, Avery Publishing Group, New York, USA, 1992.

Burkitt, Denis, *Refined Carbohydrate Foods and Disease*, Academic Press, New York, 1975.

Burkitt, D., and H. Trowell, *Western Diseases: Their Emergence and Prevention*, Harvard University Press, Cambridge, Mass, 1981.

Cohen, A.M., and A. Teitelbaum, 'Effect of Dietary Sucrose on Oral Glucose Tolerance and Insulin-like Activity', *American Journal of Physiology*, 1964.

Colgan, Michael, 'Pollutants and Food Degradation', *Colgan Institute Lecture Series #3*, Encinitas, CA, 1992.

Craig, Winston J., *Nutrition for the Nineties*, Golden Harvest Books, Michigan, 1992.

Crane, Milton, G., and Gerald Shavlik, 'Newstart Lifestyle

Programme. A Survey of the Results', monograph, Weimar Institute, Weimar, California, USA, 1993.

Crawford, Michael, and Sheila Crawford, *What We Eat Today*, Neville Spearman, 1972.

Facchinetti, F., et al., 'Oral Magnesium successfully relieves premenstrual mood changes', *Obstetrics and Gynecology*, 1991, 78, 177–181.

Fontana-Klaiber, H., et al., 'Therapeutic effects of magnesium in sysmenorrhoea', *Schweiz Runhdsch Med Prax*, 1990, 79, 491–494.

Foster, Vernon W., *Newstart!*, Woodbridge Press, CA, 1990.

Heaton, K.W., 'Food Intake Regulation and Fiber', in: *Medical Aspects of Dietary Fiber*, G. Spiller and R.M. Kay (eds), Plenum Press, New York, 1980.

Hur, Robin, *Food Reform: Our Desperate Need*, Heidelberg Publishers, Austin, 1975.

Jenkins, D.J.A., T.M.S. Wolever, and A.L. Jenkins, et al., 'Starchy Foods and Glycemic Index', *Diabetes Care*, 1988.

Jenkins, D.J.A., A.L. Jenkins, and T.M. Wolever, et al., 'Simple and Complex Carbohydrates', *Nutrition Review*, 1984.

Kamen, Betty, *Hormone Replacement Therapy Yes or No?* Nutrition Encounter Inc., Novato, CA, USA, 1993.

Kenton, Leslie, *Lean Revolution*, Ebury Press, London, 1994.

Kenton, Leslie, *The New Biogenic Diet*, Vermilion, London, 1995.

Kenton, Leslie, and Susannah Kenton, *The New Raw Energy*, Vermilion, London, 1995.

Lee, John R., *Optimal Health Guidelines*, BLL Publishing, Sebastapol, CA, USA, 1993.

Linder, P.G., '"Junk Foods" and medical education', *Obes Bar Med*, 1982.

McCarrison, Sir Robert, *Nutrition and Health*, The McCarrison Society, London, 1953.

National Academy Press, *Recommended Dietary Allowances 10th Edition*, Washington DC, 1989.

Ornish, Dean, *Reversing Heart Disease*, Random Century, London, 1991.

Pritiken, N., *The Pritiken Program for Diet and Exercise*, Grosset and Dunlap, New York, USA, 1979.

Recker, R.R., 'The Effect of Milk Supplements on Calcium Metabolism, Bine Metabolism, and Calcium Balance', *American Journal of Clinical Nutrition*, 1968, 41, 254.

Sanders, Hofeldt, Kirk and Levin, 'Refined carbohydrate as a contributing factor in reactive hypoglycemia', *Southern Medical Journal*, 1982.

Shurtleff, William, and Akiko Aoyagi, *The Book of Miso*, Ballantine Books, New York, 1991.

Steinman, David, *Diet for a Poisoned Planet*, Ballantine Books, New York, 1990.

Wolever, T.M.S., 'The Glycemic Index', *World Review of Nutrition and Diet*, 1990.

Wolf, G., 'Is Dietary Beta-Carotene an Anti-Cancer Agent?' *Nutritional Reviews*, 1982.

Worthington-Roberts, B., *Contemporary Developments in Nutrition*, C.V. Mosby, St Louis, Mo, 1981.

Wynne-Tyson, Jon, *Food for a Future*, Abacus, 1975.

Chapter Twelve: Body Heat
(and Chapter Twenty-nine: Second Coming)

Aloia, J.F., et al., 'Prevention of Involutional Bone Mass by Exercise', *Annals of Internal Medicine*. 1978, vol. 89, no. 3, 351–358.

American College of Sports Medicine Position Statement, 'The Recommended Quantity and Quality of Exercise for Developing and Maintaining Fitness in Healthy Adults', *Med Sci Sports*, 1979.

Ardawi, M.S., and E.A. Newsholm, *Essays in Biochemistry*, 1985, 21, 1–43.

Bahrke, M.S., 'Exercise, Meditation and Anxiety Reduction', *American Corr, Therapy Journal*, 1979, vol. 33, no. 2, 41–44.

Ballor, D.L., and E.T. Poehlman, *American Journal of Clinical Nutrition*, 1992, 56, 968.

Barry, A., et al., 'The Effects of Physical Conditioning on Older Individuals', *Journal of Gerontology*, 1966.

Belloc and Breslow, 'Relationship of Physical Fitness and Health Status', *Preventative Medicine*, 1972, vol. 1, no. 3, 109–121.

Blair, S.N., et al., *Journal of the American Medical Association*, 1989, 262, 2395–2401.

Bortz, W.J., *Journal of the American Medical Association*, 1982, 248, 1203–1208.

Brink, W.D., *The Advisor*, 1994, Winter 2.

Colgan, Michael and Ben Weider, *Bodybuilding for a Healthy Heart*, Published by International Federation of Bodybuilders.

Colgan, M., *Optimum Sports Nutrition*, Advanced Research Press, New York, USA, 1993.

Colgan, M., *Sexual Potency*, C.I. Publishers, San Diego, CA, USA, 1994.

Colgan, M., *The New Nutrition – Medicine for the Millennium*, C.I. Publications, Encinitas, CA, USA, 1994.

Eliot, D., et al., *Physician Sportsmedicine*, 1987, 15, 169.

'Exercise and Longevity: A Little Goes A Long Way', *New York Times*, 1989.

Fiatarone, M.A., et al., *New England Journal of Medicine*, 1994, 330, 1769–1775.

Fleck, Steven, J., and William J. Creamer, *Designing Resistance Training Programs*, Human Kinetics Books, Champaign, Illinois, 1987.

Franklin, B.A., E.R. Buskirk, and P.C. Mackeen, 'Eighteen Month Follow-Up of Participants in a Physical Conditioning Program for Middle-Aged Women', *Med Sci Sports*, 1978.

Griffin, S.J., and J. Trinder, 'Physical Fitness, Exercise, and Human Sleep', *Psychophysiology*, 1978, vol. 15, no. 5, 447–50.

Griffiths, M., and D. Keast, *Cell Biology*, 1990, 68, 405–408.

Gutin, B., 'Effect of Increase in Physical Fitness on Mental Ability Following Physical and Mental Stress', *Research Quarterly*, 1966, vol. 37, no. 2, 211–220.

Gwinup, G., R. Chelvam, and T. Steinbert, 'Thickness of Subcutaneous Fat and Activity of Underlying Muscles', *American International Medicine*, 1971.

Jones, H.H. et al., 'Humeral Hypertrophy in Response to Exercise', *Journal of Bone and Joint Surgery*, 1977, vol. 59, no. 2, 204–208.

Lane, Nancy, 'Exercise and Bone Status', *Complementary Medicine*, 1986, May/June.

Laragh, J.H., et al. (eds), *Frontiers in Hypertension Research*, Springer-Verlag, New York, USA, 1981.

Larson, L., *Acta Physiol Scand*, 1978, 36, Suppl. 457.

McCarthy, D.A., and M.M. Dale, *Sports Med*, 1988, 6, 333–363.

McCartney, N.A., et al., 'Usefulness of Weightlifting Training in Improving Strength and Maximal Power Output in Coronary Heart Disease', *American Journal of Cardiology*, 1991, 67, 939.

Morgan, J., et al., 'Psychological Effects of Chronic Physical Activity', *Medical Science Sports*, 1970, vol. 2, no. 4, 213–217.

Nieman, David C., *The Sports Medicine Fitness Course*, Bull Publishing, CA, USA, 1986.

Oscai, L.B., 'The Role of Exercise in Weight Control', in *Exercise and Sport Sciences Reviews*, ed. J.H. Wilmore, Academic Press, New York, 1973.

Pearl, W., *Keys to the Inner Universe. The Encyclopedia on Weight Training*, Bill Pearl Enterprises, Phoenix, Oregon, 1982.

Pollick, M.L., J. Whilmore and S.M. Fox, *Health and Fitness Through Physical Activity*, John Wiley and Sons, New York, USA, 1978.

Prior, J., 'Conditioning Exercise Decreases Premenstrual Symptoms: A Prospective, Controlled, 6 Month Trial', *Fertility and Sterility*, 1987, vol. 47, 402.

Putai, Jin, 'Changes in Heart Rate, Noradrenaline, Cortisol, and Mood During Tai Chi', *Journal of Psychosomatic Research*, 1989, vol. 33, no. 2, 197–206.

Quas, Dr Vince, *The Lean Body Promise*, Synesis Press, Oregon, USA, 1989.

Ries, L.A.G., et al., (eds), *Cancer Statistics Review*, 1973–1987, National Institute of Health Publications, Bethesda, MD, USA, 1990.

Selvey, N., and P.L. White, (eds), *Nutrition in the 1980s*, Alan R. Liss, New York, USA, 1981.

Shea, S.E., T.J. Benstead, *New England Journal of Medicine*, 1991, 324, 1517–1518.

Stamler, J., et al., *Journal of the American Medical Association*, 1986, 256, 2823–2828.

Swimme, Brian, *The Universe is a Green Dragon*, Bear & Comany, Sante Fe, MN, USA, 1983.

Young, R.J., 'Effect of Regular Exercise on Cognitive Functioning and Personality', *British Journal of Sports Medicine*, 1979, vol. 13, 3, 110–117.

Chapter Thirteen: Alchemy of Energy

Bellhouse, Elizabeth, 'Life's Flowering', unpublished manuscript, 1994.

Bellhouse, Elizabeth, personal correspondence with the author. 1994.

Borho, B., 'Therapy of the menopausal syndrome with Mulimen – Results of a multicentre post-marketing survey' *Biological Therapy*, 1972, 10, 226–229.

Borysenko, Dr Joan, *Fire in the Soul*, Warner Books, 1993.

Burton Goldberg Group, *Alternative Medicine, The Definitive Guide,* Future Medicine Publishing Inc., Puyallup, Washington, USA, 1993 (includes Dr Robert Jacobs and Ludwig).

Gorman, Teresa, and Malcolm Whitehead, *The Amarant Book of Hormone Replacement Therapy,* Pan Books, London, 1989.

Schrödinger, Erwin, *What is Life? and Mind and Matter,* Cambridge University Press, Cambridge, 1967.

Szent-Györgyi, A., *Bioenergetics,* Academic Press, New York, 1957.

Szent-Györgyi, A., *The Living State,* Academic Press, New York, 1972.

Vines, Gail, *Raging Hormones,* Virago, London, 1993.

Vines, Gail, 'Twilight Zone's New Dawn', *The Guardian,* 23 September 1993.

Vines, Gail, 'The Challenge to HRT', *New Scientist,* 23 October 1993.

Chapter Fourteen: Distant Thunder

Brown, Ellan, and Walker, *Breezing Through The Change,* Frog Ltd, Berkeley, CA, USA, 1994.

Grant, Dr Ellen, 'Long-Term Dangers of Hormonal Treatment', *The Lancet,* 9 April 1994.

Grant, Dr Ellen, 'Hormonal Mayhem', *What Doctors Don't Tell You,* 1994, vol. 5, no. 5.

Grant, Dr Ellen, 'Oral Contraceptives and the Risk of Breast Cancer', *The Lancet,* 12 November 1994.

Menopause News 2(6): *Progesterone: Irrelevant Ingredient,* Nov/Dec 1992.

Poel, W.E., 'Progesterone and Tumour Metastasis', *The Lancet,* 9 November 1963.

Poel, W.E., 'Progesterone and Mammary Carcinogenesis', *Potential Carcinogenic Hazards from Drugs,* Monograph series vol. 17, 1967, Springer-Verlag, Berlin.

Rock, John A., et al., 'Fetal Malformations Following Progesterone Therapy During Pregnancy: A Preliminary Report', *Fertility and Sterility,* 1985, 44, 1.

Sheehy, Gail, *Silent Passage,* HarperCollins, London, 1993.

Sthoeger, Z.M., et al., 'Regulation of the Immune Response by Sex Hormones', *Journal of Immunology,* 1988, 141, 91–98.

Stites, D.P., and P.K. Shteri, 'Steroids as Immunosuppressants in Pregnancy', *Immunological Review,* 1983, vol. 75.

Vessey, M.P., 'Female Hormones and Vascular Disease – An Epidemiological Overview', *British Journal of Family Planning*, 1980, October, 6, 1–12.

Chapter Twenty-three: Bad Blood

Abraham, G.E., 'Primary Dysmenorrhea', *Clinical Obstetrical Gynecology*, 1978, vol. 21, 1, 139–145.

Abraham, G.E., 'Nutritional Factors in the Etiology of the Premenstrual Tension Syndromes', *Journal of Reproductive Medicine*, 1983, 28, 446.

Abraham, G.E., and J.T. Hargrove, 'Effect of Vitamin B on Premenstrual Tension Syndrome: A Double Blind Crossover Study', *Infertility*, 1980, 3, 155.

Biskind, M.S., 'Nutritional Deficiency in the Etiology of Menorrhagia, Cystic Mastitis, Premenstrual Syndrome, and Treatment with Vitamin B Complex', *Journal of Clinical Endocrinology and Metabolism*, 1943, 3, 227–334.

Brown, Ellen, and Lynne Walker, *Breezing Through The Change*, Frog Ltd, Berkeley, California, USA, 1994.

Brown, Ellen, and Lynne Walker, *The Informed Consumer's Pharmacy*, Carol & Graf, New York, USA, 1990.

Butler, E.B., and E. McKnight, 'Vitamin E in the Treatment of Primary Dysmenorrhoea', *The Lancet*, 1955, vol. 1,844–847.

Cohen, J.D., and H.W. Rubin, 'Functional Menorrhagia: Treatment with Bioflavonoids and Vitamin C', *Current Therapeutic Research*, 1960, vol. 2, p. 539.

Coney, Sandra, *The Menopause Industry*, Penguin Books, London, 1991.

Durrant-Peatfield, Barry, 'The Premenstrual Syndrome', Monograph. Received December 1994.

Elstein, M., 'Minimal/Mild Endometriosis and Infertility: A Review', *British Journal of Obstetrics and Gynaecology*, vol. 96, no. 4, 454–450.

Endometriosis Association, Milwaukee, 'Facts and figures on endometriosis', *U.S. Pharmacist*, 1993, February, 42.

Engel, R.W., 'The Relation of B Complex Vitamins and Dietary Fat to the Lipotropic Action of Chline', *Journal of Biological Chemistry*, 1941, 37, 140.

Facchinetti, F., et al., 'Magnesium Prophylaxis of Menstrual Migraine', *Headache*, 1991, vol. 31, 298–304.

Facchinetti, F., et al., 'Oral Magnesium Successfully Relieves Premenstrual Mood Changes', *Obstetrics and Gynecology*, 1991, 78, 2, 177–181.

Feinstein, A.D., 'Conflict over Childbearing and Tumors of the Female Reproductive System: Symbolism in Disease', *Somatics*, 1983, Fall/Winter.

Friedman, A.J., et al., 'A Randomised Double-Blind Trial of Gonadotropin . . . in the Treatment of Leiomyomata Uteki', *Fertility and Sterility*, 1987, vol. 49, 404.

George, Demetra, *Mysteries of the Dark Moon*, HarperSanFrancisco, HarperCollins, New York, 1992.

Gleicher, Norbert, 'Is Endometriosis an Autoimmune Disease?' *Obstetrics and Gynecology*, 1987, July, vol. 70, no. 1.

Goci, G.S., and G.E. Abraham, 'Effect of Nutritional Supplement . . . on Symptoms of Premenstrual Tension', *Journal of Reproductive Medicine*, 1982, 83, 527–531.

Goldin, B.R., et al., 'Effect of Diet on Excretion of Estrogene in Pre- and Post-Menopausal Women', *Cancer Research*, 1981, 41, 3771–3773.

Goldin, B.R., et al., 'Estrogen Excretion Patterns and Plasma Levels in Vegetarian and Omnivorous Women', *New England Journal of Medicine*, 1982, 307, 1542–1547.

Goodale, I., A. Domar, and H. Benson, 'Alleviation of Premenstrual Syndrome Symptoms with the Relaxation Response', *Obstetrics and Gynecology*, 1990, 75, 4, 649–689.

Halme, J., S. Becker, and S. Haskill, 'Altered Maturation and Function of Peritoneal Macrophages: Possible Role in Pathogenesis of Endometriosis', *American Journal of Obstetrics and Gynecology*, 1987, vol 156, 783.

Halme, J., M.G. Hammond, J.F. Hulka, et al., 'Retrograde Menstruation in Healthy Women and in Patients with Endometriosis', *Obstetrics and Gynecology*, 1984, vol 64, 13–18.

Hargrove, J.T., W.S. Maxson, A.C. Wentz, and L.S. Burnett, 'Menopausal Hormone Replacement Therapy with Continuous Daily Oral Micronized Estradiol and Progesterone', *Obstetrics and Gynecology*, 1989, 73, 4.

Hudson, Tori, *Gynecology and Naturopathic Medicine*, TK Publications, Oregon, 1992.

Hufnagel, V., *No More Hysterectomies*, Penguin Books, New York, 1989.

Hutchins, Francis Jnr., 'Uterine Fibroids: Current Concepts in Management', *Female Patient*, 1990, October, vol. 15, 29.

Jacobs, Robert H., 'Care For Your Self', Seminar given for The Society for Complementary Medicine, 1994.

Kalma, S., et al., 'Production of Fibronectin by Peritoneal Macrophages and Concentration of Fibronectin in Peritoneal Fluid from Patients With or Without Endometriosis', *Obstetrics and Gynecology*, 1988, July, vol. 72, 13–19.

Kappas, A., et al., 'Nutrition-endocrine interactions', *Proceedings of the National Academy of Sciences*, 1983, USA, 80, 7646–7649.

Kenton, Leslie, and Susannah Kenton, *The New Raw Energy*, Ebury Press, London, 1995.

Kime, Z., *Sunlight Could Save Your Life*, World Health Publications, Penryn, CA, USA, 1980.

Landau, R.S., et al., 'The Effect of Alpha Tocopherol in Premenstrual Symptomatology: A Double Blind Trial', *Journal of the American College of Nutrition*, 1983, 2, 115–123.

Lark, Susan M., *The Menopause Self Help Book*, Celestial Arts, California, 1990.

Lee, J.R., MD, 'Clinical Uses of Natural Progesterone', Seminar given at St Thomas's Hospital, London, 4 June 1994.

Lee, J.R., MD, *Optimal Health Guidelines*, Second Edition, BLL Publishing, California, USA, 1993.

Lee, J.R., MD, 'Slowing the ageing process with natural progesterone,' Sebastopol, BLL Publishing, USA, 1992.

Lee, J.R. MD, 'The Multiple Effects of Progesterone', Seminar given at St Thomas's Hospital, London, 4 June 1994.

Lee, J.R., MD, *Natural Progesterone*, BLL Publishing, California, USA, 1993.

Lee, J.R., MD, Personal communication with the author. 1994.

Lee, J.R., MD, 'The Theory of Estrogen Dominance', Seminar given at St Thomas's Hospital, London, 4 June 1994.

Lee, J.R., MD, 'Progesterone and Estrogen', Endocrinology Notes, February 1993.

Lubran, M., and G. Abraham, 'Serum and Red Cell Magnesium Levels in Patients with Premenstrual Tension', *American Journal of Clinical Nutrition*, 1982, 34, 2364.

Montreal Health Press, *Menopause, A Well Woman Book*, Second Story Press, Canada, 1990.

Nachtigall, L., et al., *Estrogen*, HarperCollins Publishers, New York, 1991.

Norris, Ronald, 'Progesterone for Premenstrual Tension', *Journal of Reproductive Medicine*, 1983, 28, 8, 509-515.

Northrup, Christiane, *Women's Bodies, Women's Wisdom*, Bantam Books, New York, USA, 1994.

Ott, J., *Health and Light*, Pocket Books, New York, USA, 1978.

Parry, B.L., et al., 'Morning vs Evening Bright Light Treatment of Late Luteal Phase Dysphoric Disorder', *American Journal of Psychiatry*, 1991, 146, 9.

Peat, R., 'Progesterone Safe Antidote for P.M.S.', *McCall's*, 1990, October, 152–156.

Peat, R., 'The Progesterone Deception', *Ray Peat's Newsletter*, 1986, May 4, 44.

Peat, R., 'Blocking Tissue Destruction', Unpublished Paper.

Peat, R., 'Progesterone in Orthomolecular Medicine', Booklet.

Peat, R., 'Progesterone Can Be Taken Orally', Letter to the Editor, *Townsend Letter for Doctors*, 1994, November.

Peat, R., *Nutrition for Women*, Kenogen, Eugene, Oregon, USA, 1981.

Petersen, Nancy, and B. Hasselbring, 'Endometriosis Reconsidered', *Medical Self Care*, 1987, May/June.

Pizzorno, Joseph E., and Michael T. Murray, 'Premenstrual Syndrome', from *A Textbook of Natural Medicine*, John Bastyr College Publications, Seattle, Washington, USA, 1985.

Pizzorno, Joseph E., and Michael T. Murray, 'Fibrocystic Breast Disease', from *A Textbook of Natural Medicine*, John Bastyr College Publications, Seattle, Washington, USA, 1985.

Redwine, David B., 'The Distribution of Endometriosis in the Pelvis by Age Groups and Fertility', *Fertility and Sterility*, 1987, vol. 47, 173.

Reid, R.L., and S.S. Yen, 'Premenstrual Syndrome', *American Journal of Obstetrics and Gynecology*, 1981, 139, 86.

Reiter, R.C., P.L. Wagner, and J.C. Gambone, 'Routine Hysterectomy for Large Asymptomatic Leiomyomata: A Reappraisal', *Obstetrics and Gynecology*, 1992, April, vol. 79, no. 4, 481–484.

Rossignol, A.M., 'Caffeine-Containing Beverages and Premenstrual Syndrome in Young Women', *American Journal of Public Health*, 1985, 75, 11, 1335–1337.

Sampson, John, 'Peritoneal Endometriosis Due to the Menstrual Dissemination of Endometrial Tissue into the Peritoneal Cavity', *American Journal of Obstetrics and Gynecology*, 1984.

Snider, B.L., and D.F. Dietman, 'Pyridoxine Therapy for Premenstrual Acne Flare', *Archives of Dermatology*, 1974, 110.

Weed, Susun S., *Menopausal Years, The Wise Woman Way*, Ash Tree Publishing, New York, USA, 1992.

Werbach, M.R., *Nutritional Influences on Illness*, Third Line Press, Tarzana, CA, 1988.

Williams, D.G., 'The Forgotten Hormone', *Alternatives for the Health Conscious Individual*, 1991, 4(6), 41–46.

Winenman, E.W., 'Autonomic Balance Changes During the Human Menstrual Cycle', *Psychophysiology*, 1971, 8, 1, 1–6.

Chapter Twenty-four: Never Come Morning

Artz, E., S. Fernandez-Castelo, et al., 'Immunomodulation by indoleamines: Serotonin and melatonin action on DNA and interferon-y synthesis by human peripheral blood mononuclear cells', *J Clinical Immunology*, 1968, 8(6), 513–520.

Haensel, R., R. Wohlfart, and H. Cooper, 'Narcotic action of 2-methyl-3-butene-2-ol contained in hops', *Zhurnal der Natuerforschungen*, 1980, 35c, 1096–1097.

Lutomski, J., E. Signet, K. Szpunar, and K. Grisse, 'The meaning of passion flower in the healing arts', *Pharmazie in Unserer Zeit*, 1981, 10(2), 45–49.

Osol, A., and G.E. Farrar, *The Dispensatory of the United States of America*, J.B. Lippincott Co., Philadelphia, USA, 1950.

Peat, Ray, 'Insomnia and Hyperactivity', *Townsend Letter for Doctors*, April 1994, 385–386.

Seligmann, Jean, with Carl Robinson, 'No More Sag from Jet Lag', *Newsweek*, 8 May 1989, 67.

Shaffer, M., 'Melatonin could help elderly sleep better', *Medical Tribune*, 22 July 1993, 15.

Straube, C., 'The meaning of Valerian root in therapy', *Therapie der Gegenwart*, 1968, 107, 555–562.

Thrash, Agatha, M., *Health Emphasis*, Revere Publishing, London.

Weed, Susun S., *Menopausal Years the Wise Woman Way*, Ash Tree Publishing, Woodstock, New York, USA, 1992.

Wohlfart, R., R. Haensel, and H. Schmidt, 'An investigation into the sedative-hypnotic principle of hops (3)', *Planta Medica*, 1982, 45, 224.

Wohlfart, R., R. Haensel, and H. Schmidt, 'The sedative-hypnotic principle of hops (4)', *Planta Medica*, 1983, 48, 120–123.

Wren, R.W., *Potters New Cyclopedia of Botanical Drugs and Preparations*, The C.W. Daniel Company Ltd, Saffron Walden, 1975.

Chapter Twenty-five (see Chapter Ten)

Chapter Twenty-six: Resurrection

Allen, H.E., M.A. Halley-Henderson, and C.N. Hass, 'Chemical Composition of Bottled Mineral Water', *Arch Environ Health*, 1989.

Boston Collaborative Drug Surveillance Program Report, 'Coffee Drinking and Acute Myocardial Infarction', *The Lancet*, 1972.

Boughman, J., 'The Pure Truth, *Health*, 1991.

Brooks, S.M., *The Sea Inside Us: Water in the Life Processes*, Meredith Press, New York, 1968.

'Caffeine Withdrawal Headaches', *Journal of Lab & Clin Medicin*, 1942–1943.

Campion, Kitty, 'Water, not a drop to drink', *WDDTY*, Vol 3, #12.

Cantor, K.P., R. Hoover, P. Hartge, et al., 'Bladder Cancer, Drinking Water Source, and Tap Water Consumption: A Case-Control Study', *Journal of the National Cancer Inst*, 1987.

Carpenter, B., S.J. Hedges, C. Crabb, M. Reilly, and M.C. Bounds, 'Is Your Water Safe?' *US News & World Report*, 1991.

Colgan, Michael, *Prevent Cancer Now*, CI Publications, San Diego, 1992.

Colgan, Michael, 'The Importance of Pure Water', *Colgan Institute Seminar Series*, no. 21, 1991.

Craig, Winston J., *Nutrition for the Nineties*, Golden Harvest Books, Michigan, 1992.

deVries, Herbert A., *Physiology of Exercise*, William C. Brown, Dubuque, Iowa, 1966.

Dews, P.B. (ed.), *Caffeine*, Springer-Verlag, Berlin, 1984.

Disler, P.B., S.R. Lynch, et al., 'The Effect of Tea on Iron Absorption', *Gut*, 1975.

Fagliano, J., M. Berry, et al., 'Drinking Water Contamination and the Incidence of Leukemia: An Ecological Study', *American Journal of Public Health 80*, 1990.

Foster, Vernon W., *Newstart!* Woodbridge Press, CA, 1990.

Gershoff, S.N., 'Water, Water Everywhere, But is it Fit to Drink?' *Tufts Univ Diet & Nutr Letter 9*, 1991.

'Getting the Lead Out', FDA Consumer 23. 1989.

Gilber, R.J., *Caffeine. The Most Popular Stimulant,* Chelsea House Publishers, New York, 1986.

Government Printing Office, *Technologies and Management Strategies for Hazardous Waste Control,* Washington DC, 1983.

Graham, D.M., 'Caffeine – Its Identity, Dietary Sources, Intake and Biological Effects', *Nutr Rev,* 1978.

Grossman, M.I., 'Physiologic Approach to Medical Management of Duodenal Ulcer', *Am J Dig Dis. New Series,* 1961.

Hager, M., 'How Safe is Your Drinking Water?' *Consumers Digest,* 1984.

'How Safe is Your Water?' *Newsweek,* 1982.

Hunt, J., *The Conquest of Everest,* E.P. Dutton, New York, 1954.

Jankelson, O.M., et al., 'Effect of Coffee on Glucose Tolerance and Circulating Insulin in Men with Maturity Onset Diabetes', *The Lancet,* 1967.

Lechat, M.F., I. Borlee, et al., 'Caffeine Study', *Science,* 207, 1980.

Lefferts, L., 'Water: Treat it Right', *Nutrition Action Health Letter,* 1990.

Lymann, G.H., C.G., Lyman, and W. Johnson, 'Association of Leukemia with Radium Groundwater Contamination', *JAMA,* 1985.

MacNeal, Herbert P., 'Valuable Notes on a Hot Subject', *Resident and Staff Physician,* April 1981.

Morck, T.A., S.R. Lynch, and J.D. Cook, 'Inhibition of Food Iron Absorption by Coffee', *American Journal of Clinical Nutrition,* 1983.

Myers, *Medical Pharmacology,* Lange Medical Publication, Los Altos, CA, 1970.

Oglesby, P., 'Stimulants and Coronaries', *Postgraduate Medicine,* 1968.

Ostertag, W., E. Duisberg, and M. Sturman, 'The Mutagenic Actuary of Caffeine in Man', *Mutation Research,* 1965.

Pearce, Richard, 'Body Fluids', *Runners World,* 1982.

Pitts, G.C., et al., 'Factors Affecting Work Output in Hot Environments', *American Journal Physiology,* 1944.

Register, U.D., et al., 'Influence of Nutrients on Intake of Alcohol', *Journal of the American Dietary Association,* 1972.

Roth, J.L.A., A.C. Ivy, and A.J. Atkinson, 'Caffeine & Peptic Ulcer', *JAMA,* 1944.

Sabotka, T.J., 'Neurobehaviorial Effects of Prenatal Caffeine', *Ann NY Acad Sci*, 1989.

Saketkhoo, K., et al., 'Effects of Drinking Hot Water, Cold Water and Chicken Soup on Nasal Mucus Velocity and Nasal Airflow Resistance', *Chest*, 1978.

Sargent, F., and K. Weinman, In *Physiological Measurements of Metabolic Functions in Man*, (eds) C.F. Consolazio et al., McGraw-Hill, New York, 1963.

Slater, D., 'Bottled Waters. The Beverage of the Future', *Dairy and Food Sanitation*, 1991.

Smyly, D.S., B.B. Woodward, and E.C. Conrad, 'Determination of Saccharin, Sodium Benzoate and Caffeine in Beverages by Reverse Phase HPLC', *J Assoc Off Anal Chem*. 1976.

Special Report, Second International Caffeine Workshop, *Nutrition Review*, 1980.

Stollman, T., *A Manual of Pharmacology*, W.B. Saunders, Philadelphia, 1957.

Taylor, Mary, *Water Pollution: Finding The Facts*, Friends of the Earth, London, 1993.

Thrash, A.M., and C.L. Thrash, *Nutrition for Vegetarians*, Thrash Publications, Scale, AL. 1962.

Travis, C.C., and C.B. Doty, *Environmental Science and Technology*, 1990.

University of California, 'In The Heat, Drink Up', *Wellness Letter*, Vol. 1, Berkeley, CA, 1985.

University of California, 'Wrap Up: Drink Water', *Wellness Letter*, Vol. 2, 1985.

US Dept of HHES Publ., #2(FDA) 81-1081, Caffeine & Pregnancy, 1981.

US Food and Nutrition Board, 'Water Deprivation and Performance of Athletes', *American Journal of Clinical Nutrition*, 1974.

White, B.C., C.A. Lincoln, et al., 'Anxiety and Muscle Tension as Consequences of Caffeine Withdrawal', *Science*, 209, 1980.

Chapter Twenty-seven (see Chapter Eleven)

Chapter Twenty-eight: The Professionals

Balch, James, F., and Phyllis A. Balch, *Prescription for Nutritional Healing*, Avery Publishing Group Inc., Garden City Park, New York, USA, 1990.

Braverman, Eric R., with Carl, C. Pfeiffer, *The Healing Nutrients Within*, Keats Publishing Inc., New Canaan, Connecticut, USA, 1987.

Davies, Dr Stephen, and Dr Alan Stewart, *Nutritional Medicine*, Pan Books, London, 1987.

Dean, Ward, John Morgenthaler, and Steven W. Fowkes, *Smart Drugs II, The Next Generation*, Health Freedom Publications, Menlo Park, California, USA, 1993.

Garrison, Robert H., and Elizabeth Somer, *The Nutrition Desk Reference*, Second Edition, Keats Publishing Inc., New Canaan, Connecticut, USA, 1985.

Jacobs, Robert H., 'Care For Yourself', Booklet published by The Society for Complementary Medicine, London, 1994.

Kirschmann, John D., with Lavon J. Dunne, *Nutrition Almanac*, Second Edition, McGraw-Hill, New York, USA, 1984.

Lee, J.R., MD, *Natural Progesterone*, BLL Publishing, Sebastapol, California, USA, 1993.

Pearl, Bill, *Keys to the Inner Universe*, Bill Pearl Enterprises, Phoenix, Oregon, USA, 1982.

Werbach, Melvyn, R., *Nutritional Influences on Illness*, Second Edition, Third Line Press, Tarzana, California, USA, 1993.

Chapter Twenty-nine (see Chapter Twelve)

Chapter Thirty: Magnum Force

Alvarado, Donna, 'Hormone Use Cuts Risk of Heart Disease', *Press Democrat*, 1994, 18 November.

Cowan, L.D., and L. Gordis, et al., 'Breast Cancer Incidence in Women with a History of Progesterone Deficiency', *American Journal of Epidemiology*, 1981, 114, 209-217.

Dalton, Dr K., 'The Premenstrual Syndrome' *British Medical Journal*, 1953, 1, 1007.

Durrant-Peatfield, Barry J., 'Hypothyroidism and You', Monograph. Received December 1994.

Durrant-Peatfield, Barry, 'The Menopause', Monograph. Received December 1994.

Durrant-Peatfield, Barry, 'The Menopause and Natural Progesterone', Monograph. Received December 1994.

Gaby, Alan R., 'Progesterone: Oral versus Transdermal', *Townsend Letter for Doctors*, 1994, August/September, 850.

Hargrove, Joel T. 'Progesterone: Safe Antidote for PMS', *McCalls*, 1990, October.

Hargrove, Joel T., Wayne S. Maxon, and Anne Colston Wentz, 'Absorption of Oral Progesterone is Influenced by Vehicle and Particle Size', *American Journal of Obstetrics and Gynecology*, 1989, October.

Hargrove, Joel T., Wayne S. Maxon, and Anne Colston Wentz, and Lonnie Burnett, 'Menopausal Hormone Replacement Therapy with Continuous Daily Oral Micronized Estradiol and Progesterone', *Obstetrics and Gynecology*, 1989, April, 606–612.

Kradjian, Robert M., *Save Yourself from Breast Cancer*, The Berkeley Publishing Groups, 200 Madison Avenue, New York, NY 10016, 1994.

Lee, J.R., MD, *Natural Progesterone*, BLL Publishing, California, USA, 1993.

Lee, J.R., MD, 'Dr John Lee speaking at the Chelsea Hotel, London, 5 June 1994', Video.

Lee, J.R., MD, 'The Theory of Estrogen Dominance', Seminar given at St Thomas's Hospital, London, 4 June 1994.

Lee, J.R., MD, 'Clinical Uses of Natural Progesterone', Seminar given at St Thomas's Hospital, London, 4 June 1994.

Lee, J.R., MD, 'Endocrinology Notes: Progesterone and Estrogen', Monograph, 6 February 1993

Peat, Raymond F., 'Progesterone in Orthomolecular Medicine', Blake College Booklet, Eugene, Oregon, USA.

Peat, Raymond F., 'The Progesterone Deception', *Ray Peat's Newsletter*, 1986, May 4, 44.

Peat, Raymond F., 'Progesterone Can Be Taken Orally', Letter to the Editor, *Townsend Letter for Doctors*, 1994, November.

Prior, J.C., 'Progesterone as a Bone-Trophic Hormone', *Endocrine Review*, 1990, 11, 386–398.

Williams, David G., 'The Forgotten Hormone', *Alternatives*, 4 December 1991, 6.

Resources

MORE FROM LESLIE KENTON

Leslie's audio tapes including *10 Steps to A New You* and others, as well as her videos including *Ageless Ageing, Lean Revolution, 10 Day De-Stress Plan*, and *Cellulite Revolution*, can be ordered from QED Recording Services Ltd, Lancaster Road, New Barnet, Hertfordshire EN4 8AS. Telephone: 0181 441 7722. Fax 0181 441 0777. Email: QED@globalnet.co.uk

If you want to know about Leslie's personal appearances, forthcoming books, videos, workshops and projects please visit her website for the latest information:

http://www.qed-productions/lesliekenton.htm

You can also write to her care of QED at the above address enclosing a stamped, self-addressed A4 size envelope.

SOCIETY FOR COMPLEMENTARY MEDICINE

31 Weymouth Street, London W1N 3FJ.
Telephone 0171 436 0821
Fax 0171 436 1877

This charitable trust was founded in 1989. It has as its patron Lord Yehudi Menuhin and is dedicated to the development of preventative medicine, immune enhancement and holistic clinical treatment. At the society, practitioners see people by appointment. They offer leading-edge treatment using advanced energy medicine including soft laser therapy, microcurrent therapy, magnetic field therapy and homeopathy as well as advanced nutritional guidance including brain enhancement. The society cares for people fighting common illnesses as well as those striving for optimum health. It offers special care to those challenged with critical illnesses who are unable to afford treatment. Highly recommended.

VITA FONS II

Combe Castle, Elworthy, Taunton, Somerset TA4 3PX.

This company, which is owned by a charitable trust, offers a full range of Vita Fons II energy products including the water, tablets, ointment, lotion, massage oil, talcum powder and salve as well as Vita Fons II for animals and plants.

Vita Fons II Water is primarily used in the form of doses – 5 drops: neat, on food or in any beverage. It is also used in conjunction with hydrotherapy, and ocular, vaginal and colonic irrigation. It can be ordered in a spray bottle – the best for both external and internal use.

Vita Fons II Tablets are for those who prefer tablets to liquid. A compound of gypsum, calcium phosphate, kelp, sago flour and palm oil, each tablet equals one dose and may be chewed, swallowed or allowed to dissolve on the tongue.

Vita Fons II Ointment is one of the most generally useful of the preparations for external use. It contains water, hamamelis water, almond oil, wax and Vita Fons II.

Vita Fons II Talcum Powder is the most potent Vita Fons II product for external use. It can be used all over the exterior of the body. Dust on top of any other Vita Fons II product to obtain increased effect.

For Animals Use the same products and application systems as for people. For all mammals, regardless of size, the dose is 3 drops. For birds, reptiles, fish and insects the dose is 1 drop.

For Plants Vita Fons II Foliar Spray (or Dusting Powder) may be used on leaves, branches and trunks with a view to increasing crop weight, disease/parasite-resistance, helping transplanted plants and reviving wilted plants. A Seed Dressing and a Root Powder are also available.

Personal Growth

CENTRE FOR TRANSPERSONAL PERSPECTIVES
c/o Barbara Sommers, 7-11 Kensington High Street, London W8 5NP. Telephone 0171 937 9190

This organization offers excellent workshops and lectures as well as training in transpersonal psychology and personal growth. Many can be helpful for a woman in the midst of profound personal life changes. Write to them for a list of their activities and dates. Their workshops include

Initiation Initiation as the keynote of the conscious growth process. Initiation into new states of awareness, phases of life and levels of energy. Rites of Passage. Myth and Symbolism.

The Other Self The quest of the soul for wholeness through an exploration of the four functions of sensation, intuition, thinking and feeling. Discovering the polarities and splits within our nature.

Living Alchemy Its relevance to modern living, its presence in therapeutic practice, its power to link western and eastern wisdom and psychology.

Oxherding and Rainmaking Eastern approaches to life, wit and wisdom. Meditation on our personal histories will provide the fabric of this unusual and Zen-ish workshop.

The Raincloud of Knowable Things Patanjali's phrase expresses the need for individual meditation to become part of the creative world process. This is the true magical work of the soul, to make manifest the patterns, archetypes and symbols of the future.

Intuition, Inspiration and the Will Three threads of the self, linking spirit, soul and personality. This workshop is intended to help you 'map your own territory', discover the necessary conditions for your intuition, inspiration and will to work, to recognize their many and different manifestations, and to evoke and employ them in your life.

Shamanic Training and Healing in the UK Leslie Kenton now teaches shamanic workshops. For information on these or for information on where to get soul retrievals in the UK, contact Simon Buxton, The Sacred Trust, PO Box 603, Bath BA1 2ZU. Telephone 01225 852615. Fax 01225 858961.

THE FOUNDATION FOR SHAMANIC STUDIES
PO Box 1939, Mill Valley, California 94942, USA.
Telephone 415 380 8282
Fax 415 380 8416

This organization provides worldwide training in shamanic practices offering more than 180 courses to over 4,500 individuals annually. For a list of shamanic practitioners who do soul retrieval in your particular country write to Sandra Ingerman, author of *Soul Retrieval*, at the above address.

Face, Body and Beauty

THE GAGNON SYSTEM
Beth Jacobs, 31 Weymouth Street, London W1N 3FJ.
Telephone 0171 436 0821
Fax 0171 436 1877

Beth Jacobs is the originator of the Gagnon System of total body care – a unique and highly effective approach to holistic beauty which acts on the whole person to bring regeneration and rejuvenation to skin and body as a whole. The Gagnon System is built around the use of an integrated combination of specialized energy equipment such as the lightbeam generator, microcurrent, soft light laser and magnetic field tables combined with specific hands-on techniques for realigning muscles and skeleton, energizing skin and body and helping to restore homeostasis where it has been disturbed.

Natural Hormone Products and Information

For information about natural treatments for women contact:

WELL WOMAN'S INTERNATIONAL NETWORK
La Brecque, Alderney, Channel Islands GY9 3TJ, Great Britain
Residing outside UK – Telephone +44(0) 7000 437225; Fax +44(0) 7000 3299946
Residing in UK – Telephone 07000 437225; Fax 07000 3299946

The Well Woman's International Network (WWIN) is an organization for women to use as a network resource to make contact and stay in touch with natural health developments that can make a vital difference to enjoying life to the full – regardless of age. They offer information on natural supplements and Progesterone products. Patron Dr John Lee. WWIN effects a personal import service. Full range of natural hormone products (inc. Vegan) at discounted prices for its members, postal/email consultation with specialist doctors, quarterly forum/newsletter. Membership to this worldwide Well Woman's International Network is £30 (sterling) per annum.

Progesterone Body Creams & Oils (in alphabetical order)
Dr John Lee states clearly that natural progesterone oils and creams which contain less than 800 milligrams per 2 ounce jar will not supply sufficient progesterone if you are truly deficient. The following list of American products meet this criteria:

PROGEST – E Complex	Kenogen	Eugene, OR

Creams/Oils containing 400–500 mg Progesterone per Ounce

Angel Care	Angel Care, USA	Atlanta, GA
Bio Balance	Elan Care, USA	Scottsdale, AZ
Edenn Cream	SNM	Norcross, GA
E'Pro & Estrol Balance	Sarati International	Pasadena, TX
Equillibrium	Equillibrium Lab	Boca Raton, FL

Fair Lady	Village Market	Fond du Lac, WI
Femarone – 17	Wise Essentials	Minneapolis, MN
Feminique	Country Life	Hauppage, NY
Happy PMS	HM Enterprises, Inc.	Norcross, GA
Kokoro Balance Cream	Kokoro, LLC	Laguna Niguel, CA
Marpe's Wild Yam	Green Pastures	Flat Rock, NC
NatraGest	Broadmore Labs, Inc.	Ventura, CA
Natural Balance	South Market Service	Atlanta, GA
Natural Woman	Products of Nature	Ridgefield, CN
OstaDerm	Bezwecken	Beaverton, OR
PhytoGest	Karuna Corp	Novato, CR
Pro-Alo	Health Watchers Sys.	Scottsdale, AZ
ProBalance	Springboard	Monterey, CA
Pro-G	TriMedica	Scottsdale, AZ
Progessence	Young Living	Payson, UT
Pro-Gest	Prof.Tech Serv, Inc	Portland, OR
Progonol	Bezwecken	Beaverton, OR
Renewed Balance	America Image Marketing	Nampa, ID
Serenity	Health & Science Nutrition	N.Lauderdale, FL

You can purchase Pro-Gest by post from:
Woman's International Pharmacy
5708 Monova Drive
Madison WI, USA
Telephone 001 608 221 7800
Fax 001 608 221 7819

THE NATURAL PROGESTERONE INFORMATION SERVICE
NPIS
Box 131
Etchingham TN19 7ZN

For information on the multiple uses of this natural hormone for women's health from puberty to menopause, and also a list of books, tapes and videos available, write to the above address.

HIGHER NATURE LIMITED
The Nutrition Centre, Burwash Common, East Sussex TN19 7LX.
Telephone 01435 882 880
Fax 01435 883 720

This is the company which courageously introduced natural progesterone products to the British market only to find that within a few months they were forced to restrict their sales for them to prescription only. Their progesterone and oestrogen products are recognized by the Medicines Control Agency as unlicensed medicines available by doctor's prescription under the 'named patient exemption' of the Medicines Act. They give information to medical doctors on its use.

Pro-Gest Cream 50 g (2 oz) of a 3 per cent natural progesterone cream, from Mexican yam, in a base of vitamin E and aloe vera.

Pro-Gest Oil 25 g (1 oz) of a 10 per cent natural progesterone oil in a base of vitamin E. Can be used sub-lingually or applied externally.

In addition Higher Nature do a small range of first-rate nutritional products which you can order direct. They are all completely vegetarian, hypo-allergenic, innovative in their formulations and freshly prepared. They also provide excellent nutritional and health consultation both to the medical profession and health practitioners and to the general public by telephone.

Menophase Nutritional supplement to help prevent dietary deficiency of nutrients essential to the health of the female reproductive system during menopausal and postmenopausal years. Contains vitamin C, vitamin E, vitamin B3, vitamin B6, hesperidin complex, magnesium, zinc, Mexican yam extract, Dong Quai, White Peony root, Schizandra and ginseng.

Mexican Yam Capsules of concentrated wild yam extract.

Brain Food Nutrition for the brain's neurotransmitters to enhance memory and learning. Provides phosphatidyl choline, arginine pyroglutamate, DMAE, pantothenic acid and niacinamide.

Super Anti-oxidant Contains 16 protectors including minerals and vitamins, amino acids and herbal extracts. Each tablet provides beta-carotene, vitamin A, vitamin C, vitamin E, vitamin B2, iron, zinc, manganese, selenium, copper, N-acetyl cysteine, L-cysteine, reduced glutathione, milk thistle extract, bilberry extract and pycogenol.

Folacin Provides folic acid, a B vitamin essential to the workings of the central nervous system.

Organic Linseeds Rich in fibre and essential fatty acids, linseeds provide linolenic and linoleic acid.

Omega Flaxseed Oil Organic, unrefined flaxseed oil, pressed at low temperatures and bottled in containers which protect the oil from light. Must be kept refrigerated.

Herbs

PHYTO PHARMACEUTICALS LIMITED
3 Kings Mill Way, Hermitage Lane, Mansfield, Nottinghamshire NG18 5ER.
Telephone 01623 644 334
Fax 01623 657 232
Minimum order: £20

An excellent company set up 14 years ago to supply herbalists with high-quality herbs and plant products – which at that time were very difficult to come by. Every plant and herb they sell states the source of origin. All Phyto's plants are purchased only from recognizable sources.

Phyto Pharmaceuticals do a full range of tinctures, herbal skin creams, fluid extracts, herbs and the Schoenenberger plant juices, including all of those mentioned in Field and Forest pp.346–364 plus **Calendula Cream** and **Comfrey Cream**, all at very reasonable prices. The pure, pressed plant juices can be enormously useful. Virtually all the herbs mentioned in this book are supplied by this company in both tincture form and the loose dried herb. They do not supply herbs in capsules, but they now do some herbs in tablet form.

MALCOLM SIMMONDS HERBAL SUPPLIES
3 Burton Villas, Hove, West Sussex BN3 6FN.
Telephone 01273 202 401

This company has been supplying high-quality additive-free herbal aids to health practitioners in the UK and abroad since 1982. They now do a range of good-quality products for the general public as well. They offer herbal products including both single herbs and mixtures in capsule or tincture forms. Write to them for their catalogue.

Agnus Castus Available in capsules, tablets and fluid extract. Works efficiently to balance many aspects of the female reproductive system.

Echinacea Available in capsules, tablets and fluid extract. Helps boost and support the immune system.

Wild Yam Root Available in capsules.

Valerian and Passiflora Available in fluid extract form. A soothing extract to help balance the nervous system.

Fem Rep Formula Assists the cleansing of the reproductive areas. Contains Squaw Vine, Blessed Thistle, Cayenne, Helonias, Ginger, Golden Seal, Raspberry Leaf and Uva Ursi. Also available as a tea.

Horm Formula A beneficial formula to balance the hormone system. Contains Blessed Thistle, Black Cohosh, Sarsaparilla, Ginseng, Liquorice, Helonias and Squaw Vine.

HRT Formula Supports the heart and circulation of the blood. Contains Hawthorn, Motherwort, Valerian, Lily of the Valley and Dandelion.

BIOFORCE (UK) LTD
Olympic Business Park, Dundonald, Ayrshire KA2 9BE.
Telephone 01563 851 177
Fax 01563 851 173

Suppliers of herbal extracts, tinctures, homeopathic remedies and natural self-care products and foods, Bioforce is a Swiss company started by the Swiss expert in natural health, Alfred Vogel. The company always use fresh herbs in preparing their products at the Bioforce factory in Roggwil. They do over 100 different herbal and homeopathic preparations, including **Petasan tincture** and **Mistletoe & Butterbur,** all of which are very high quality. They can be ordered by post but are also often available in good health-food stores and pharmacies carrying herbal products.

Nutrition

BIOCARE
54 Northfield Road, Kings Norton, Birmingham B30 1JH.
Telephone 0121 433 3727
Fax 0121 433 3879

A science-based manufacturer of innovative nutritional and health-care products, BioCare was founded 15 years ago by practitioners for practitioners. BioCare products are now available to the public mail order (ring for a catalogue) as well as through suppliers of sophisticated nutritional products such as the Nutri Centre, 7 Park

Crescent, London, W1N 3HE, telephone 0171 436 5122, Fax 0171 436 5171. All BioCare products are formulated so carefully that they are suitable even for allergic women intolerant to the standard substances used in manufacturing. Many are vacuum packed. Their oil-based products from **Vitamin E** to **GLA** and **Linseed Oil** are all specially formulated to protect from oxidation by flushing each capsule with nitrogen. In the case of light-sensitive products, BioCare use opaque capsules. They even do chemical-free vitamins in liquid form which have been specially emulsified or micelized to enhance the absorption to 95 per cent. These can be added to juice or water or taken sub-lingually. They are excellent for allergic people or people with digestive problems. BioCare produce the very highest quality nutritional products in Britain.

B Complex (Yeast-free) Enzyme activated and containing three forms of magnesium to aid the function of the nervous system.

Vitamin B6 (Yeast-free) In the form of pyridoxal-5-phosphate, the preferred biologically active form of this vitamin.

Vitamin C In the form of magnesium ascorbate with bioflavonoids, this vitamin C is enzyme activated, buffered, and will not cause loss of minerals when taken in large doses.

Vitamin C Powder In the form of magnesium ascorbate this is a cost-effective way of taking vitamin C – simply dissolve in water.

Vitamin E Nitrogen packed, blended in pure, cold-pressed olive oil and hypoallergenic.

Multi-Mineral Complex Organically bound EAP minerals, free from iron and calcium and highly bioavailable. This is an excellent multi-mineral complex.

Magnesium EAP2 Provides support for the healthy function of the nervous system.

Zinc Citrate Easily assimilable and highly bioavailable, this form of zinc is therefore cost-effective as high doses are not needed.

Digest Aid A combination of biologically active proteolytic, lipolytic and carbolytic enzymes, all from plant sources, to aid the digestion of proteins, fats and carbohydrates.

HcL and Pepsin Provides an ideal balance of HcL (hydrochloric acid as betaine hydrochloride) to Pepsin in capsule form, to allow for quicker release while reducing the likelihood of irritation against the gastric wall.

Mega GLA Complex Emulsified to improve absorption, stabilized by the addition of vitamins E and C and nitrogen packed.

Linseed Oil (Flaxseed Oil) A rich natural source of essential fatty acids, and the richest known source of Omega 3 fatty acids in capsules. Blended with vitamins E and C and emulsified in olive oil, this is a very stable form of linseed oil in capsules.

Emulsified Efaplex A blend of essential fatty acids emulsified to improve absorption – nitrogen packed.

Oxyplex Sprouted wheat enzyme is a source of naturally occurring Superoxide Dismutase (SOD), Catalase, Peroxidases, Reductases, trace elements and co-factors.

Carbozyme To aid the digestion of beans and pulses to prevent flatulence.

XYNERGY HEALTH PRODUCTS
Lower Elsted, Midhurst, West Sussex GU29 0JT.
Telephone 01730 813 642
Fax 01730 815 109

This company specialize in selling the finest green nutritional products you can buy. They can be ordered by post from them or are available in sophisticated health-food stores. Their **spirulina** is the best. It comes in tablets or in powder form. Xynergy also import an organic spirulina in flakes which you can sprinkle on soups, miso broth, salads and other dishes. **Green drinks** are also available from Xynergy. Here are some of their best products.

Life Stream Spirulina The richest and most complete source of organic nutrients found in any food. In tablet and powder form.

Crystal Flakes Spirulina flakes ideal for sprinkling on any food – the best!

Biogenic Aloe Vera Juice Pure, fresh, with the biostimulating efficacy of freshly cut aloe leaves.

Super Green Foods Spray-dried whole juice concentrates in a choice of: **alfalfa whole juice concentrate** with the highest trace mineral content, especially calcium; **barley juice concentrate** rich in anti-oxidants and enzymes; **alfalfa/barley/chlorella** – alfalfa and barley juice concentrates along with the high RNA and chlorophyll qualities of chlorella; **carrot/barley/spirulina** – carrot and barley juice concentrates with the added organic nutrients found in spirulina.

NUTRI CENTRE

7 Park Crescent, London W1N 3HE.
Telephone 0171 436 5122
Fax 0171 436 5171

The Nutri Centre is on the lower ground floor of the Hale Clinic and has the finest selection of nutritional products under one roof in Britain. It is also able to supply homeopathic products, herbal, Ayurvedic and biochemic products, flower remedies, essential oils, skin-care and dental products, and has an extensive selection of books, all available through a good mail-order service.

BIOLAB MEDICAL UNIT

The Stone House, 9 Weymouth Street, London W1N 3FF.
Telephone 0171 636 5905
Fax 0171 580 3910

A referral centre for Nutritional Medicine. Patients can be referred by their GP or hospital consultant. Doctors can also contact the unit for advice on laboratory investigations and the correction of nutrient deficiencies or imbalances.

Miscellaneous

Ginseng A good ginseng comes in the form of Jinlin Ginseng Tea, Jinlin *Panax ginseng* dried slices and Jinlin whole root, available from health-food stores. If you have difficulty finding it contact Alice Chiu, 4 Tring Close, Barkingside, Essex IG2 7LQ. Telephone 0181 550 9900.

Mail Order Organic Foods Organic foods such as nuts, seeds, grains, miso, soy bean curd, tahini, seaweeds, bonsoy soya milk, soba noodles, brown rice syrup, amazaki, etc. can be ordered from: Freshlands, 196 Old Street, London EC1V 9FR. Telephone 0181 490 3170. Or from Wild Oats, 210 Westbourne Grove, London W11 2RH. Telephone 0171 229 1063.

Marigold Low-salt Swiss Vegetable Bouillon Powder This instant broth powder based on vegetables and sea salt is available from health-food stores or direct from Marigold Foods, Unit 10, St Pancras Commercial Centre, 63 Pratt Street, London NW1 0BY. Telephone 0171 267 7368.

Personal Trainers A personal trainer I highly recommend is Welsh champion weightlifter Rhodri Thomas, 90 Cherry Grove, Derwen

Fawr, Swansea SA2 8AX. He is often willing to spend either a week-end or a week or two working out your own personal programme in your own home which he will then monitor and readjust regularly.

Rowing If you are going to invest in an exercise machine go for a Concept II Ergometer. It is the best. Rowing provides good aerobic exercise working all the main muscle groups in the body whilst only requiring one piece of equipment. The Concept II is simple to use and requires little maintenance and gives you feedback on your workout. It is the very best rowing machine available anywhere. For further information contact Concept II, 151-153 Nottingham Road, Old Basford, Nottingham NG6 0FU. Telephone 01602 421 925. Fax 01602 424 684.

Appendix to Resources

Methods of Measuring Levels of Progesterone and Oestrogen in the Blood.

Here is what a typical lab analysis in Britain looks like.

OESTRADIOL	<37 pmol/L
Ref. range (Follicular)	(110 – 440)
Ref. range (Mid-cycle)	(550 – 1300)
Ref. range (Luteal)	(365 – 770)
Ref. range (Postmenopause)	(35 – 175)
PROGESTERONE	2.4 nmol/L
Ref. range (Follicular)	(0.3 – 5.0)
Ref. range (Luteal)	(8.0–90) (For implantation, >30)
Ref. range (Postmenopause)	(0.1 – 2.0)
* THYROID STIMULATING HORMONE	0.2 mU/L (0.3 – 3.5)
Growth hormone	5.4 mU/l (Adult <10 : Child <20)

However, in whichever country, serum progesterone levels are expressed in terms of concentration, i.e., X amount of progesterone per Y amount of serum.

My Merck Manual lists it as ng/ml (elsewhere I have seen picograms per decilitre [s s/dl] and as nmol/L. A mol is the amount of a given chemical substance equivalent to its molecular weight in grams. One nmol = 1 nanomol = one-billionth (10^9) of a mol of some substance. For progesterone, you can convert ng/ml into nmol/L by multiplying by 3.1.

One picogram = one-trillionth (10^{-12}) of a gram. A ml = one-thousandth (10^{3}) of a litre and a dl = a decilitre, or one-tenth (10^{-1}) of a litre.

Thus, the luteal range for progesterone could be written as 7-28 ng/ml or 21-84 nmol/L, and the non-ovulating level is often as low as 0.3 ng/ml or 0.9 nmol/L.

Glossary

Amenorrhea absence of menstruation.

Amino acid organic acids which are the building blocks of protein.

Analgesic something that relieves pain.

Androgens hormones secreted by the testes which produce secondary male characteristics.

Anovulatory suspension or cessation of ovulation.

Anti-oxidant a chemical or compound that inhibits reactions caused by free radicals.

Arteriosclerosis deposits of cholesterol, lipid material and cellular debris in the inner lining of arteries.

Atrophic vaginitis thinning and inflammation of the vagina.

Auto-immune the production of reactivity by an organism to its own tissues.

Autonomic self-controlling. Refers to parasympathetic and parasympathetic nervous systems.

Bacteria single-celled organisms of the plant kingdom.

Bioflavonoids brightly coloured substances in plants that are concerned with maintaining a normal state in blood vessel walls.

Carcinogen a cancer-producing substance.

Catalyst a substance which affects the rate of a chemical reaction.

Cervix mouth of the womb.

Chelating agents soluble organic compounds that can fix certain metallic ions into their molecular structure.

Collagen the main protein of connective tissue – skin, bone, tendon and cartilage.

Compression fracture break in a weakened bone which is unable to support weight and therefore becomes crushed.

Conjugated one compound combined with another.

Corpus luteum small yellow glandular mass in the ovary formed after ovulation.

Corticosteroid hormones produced by the adrenal cortex.

Diuretic a substance that promotes the secretion of urine.

DNA the acid of which chromosomes are made.

Dysmenorrhea painful menstruation.

Endocrine system composed of organs (glands) which make and secrete substances (hormones) directly into the bloodstream.

Endogenous developing or originating within the body.

Endometriosis mysterious condition where the tissue which forms the lining of the womb (the endometrium) grows outside the uterine cavity in other areas of the pelvis, sometimes causing pain and infertility.

Endometrium the inner secretory lining of the uterus.

Endorphin polypeptide hormone of the central nervous system.

Enzyme any of numerous complex proteins which act as catalysts in specific biochemical reactions.

Essential fatty acids organic acids, including linoleic and linolenic acids, required by the body for health.

Exogenous originating outside the body.

Follicle a small excretory sac or gland – e.g. the ovarian follicle that produces the ovum.

Follicle-stimulating hormone (FSH) neuropeptide hormone secreted by the pituitary that stimulates the follicle in the ovary to grow.

Free radical a compound with unbalanced electrons, capable of causing destabilizing oxidation reactions.

Gene the biological unit of heredity, a segment of DNA.

Genetic referring to reproduction, birth or heredity.

Gonadotrophic releasing hormone (GnRH) the hormone made by the hypothalamus that stimulates the pituitary gland to produce gonadotrophins.

Gonodatrophin a hormone than can stimulate the sex glands.

Half life the time it takes for an active element or substance to lose half its potency.

Homeostasis the body's ability to maintain a stable internal environment.

Hormone a substance that usually circulates in the blood and produces a specific effect on the activity of cells.

Hypoglycaemia low blood-sugar level.

Hypothalamus neural nuclei in the limbic brain just above the pituitary.

Hysterectomy surgical removal of the uterus.

Limbic brain brain cortex below the *corpus callosum* and above the pituitary that contains neural nuclei controlling autonomic functions, homeostasis, emotional sensation and responses, and regulate immune responses.

Luteinizing refers to maturation of ovarian follicles for ovulation.

Luteinizing hormone (LH) hormone produced in the pituitary which triggers the maturation of ovarian follicles. A big surge of this hormone precedes ovulation by 2 to 24 hours each month.

Menopause cessation of menstrual cycles.

Metabolism the biochemical process of living organisms by which substances are produced and energy is made available to the organism.

Menorrhagia irregular menstruation.

Microgram one millionth of a gram.

Micron one thousandth of a millimetre.

Milligram one thousandth of a gram.

Mitochondria small organelles within the cytoplasm that are the site of converting sugar into energy.

Molecule a combination of two or more atoms which form a specific chemical substance.

Nanogram one billionth of a gram.

Oestrogen the ovarian hormones that initiate the body's preparation for possible fertilization and pregnancy.

Oocytes the cell that produces the ovum.

Oophorectomy surgical removal of an ovary or ovaries.

Osteoblast bone cell that forms new bone.

Osteoclast bone cell that resorbs old bone.

Osteocyte a bone cell which may become an osteoclast or an osteoblast.

Peptide a class of low molecular weight compounds composed of several amino acids.

Perimenopausal the period in a woman's life that precedes menopause.

Phyto relating to plants.

Polyunsaturated fatty acid a fatty acid with more than one double bond in its carbon chain.

Precursor specific nutrient or body chemical required for the manufacture of a particular substance within the body.

Premenopausal before menopause – perimenopausal.

Progestogen a synthetic compound with progesterone-like action – a progestin.

Progesterone natural ovarian hormone made by the corpus luteum to sustain the endometrium and support the fertilized ovum.

Prostaglandin hormone composed of essential fatty acids with effects on smooth muscle contraction; regulates cell behaviour and inhibits hormones.

Radical a group of atoms which enter into and go out of chemical combinations without change, and which form one of the basic constituents of a molecule.

Resorption the loss or dissolving away of a substance.

RNA ribonucleic acid.

Saturated fatty acid fatty acid with full complement of hydrogen (i.e. no double bond).

Steroid any compound based on and derived from the cholesterol molecule – includes sex hormones and corticosteroids.

Sterol compounds with single hydroxyl group, soluble in fat, for example cholesterol.

Synthesis the building of a chemical compound by the union of its elements.

Trans compounds that have been altered from their natural state as in trans-fatty acids.

Triglyceride a fat composed of glycerin and 3 fatty acids.

Unsaturated fatty acid fatty acid with at least one double bond in the carbon chain.

Xeno meaning strange, or denoting relationship to foreign material, as in xenoestrogens.

Note on Measurements & Quantities

I have given approximate measurements in the recipes as cupfuls (an ordinary cup holds about 225 ml or 8 fluid ounces), table-spoons, teaspoons, and so on. Where measuring is important, I have given the imperial measurement as well as the metric. Most of the recipes are designed to feed four people. As the quantities are approximate, the amounts can easily be adjusted to suit your own particular needs.

In the main text I have mainly used metric measurements. Here are a few metric/imperial equivalents which you may find useful.

Weight

28 grams	= 1 ounce
112 grams	= 1/4 lb
450 grams	= 1 lb
1 kilogram	= 2.2 lb

Length

2.5 cm	= 1 inch
30 cm	= 1 foot
1 metre/100 cm	= 39 inches/3.3 feet
1.6 kilometres	= 1 mile

Volume

570 ml	= 1 pint
1 litre	= 1 3/4 pints
4.5 litres	= 1 gallon

Index